# NUCLEAR MEDICINE PHYSICS

## The Basics

### Seventh Edition

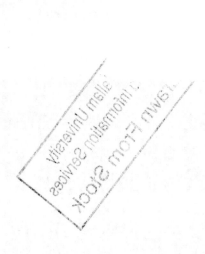

# NUCLEAR MEDICINE PHYSICS

## The Basics
## Seventh Edition

Ramesh Chandra, PhD
Emeritus Professor
Department of Radiology
New York University Langone Medical Center
New York, New York

Wolters Kluwer | Lippincott Williams & Wilkins
Health

Philadelphia · Baltimore · New York · London
Buenos Aires · Hong Kong · Sydney · Tokyo

Executive Editor: Charles W. Mitchell
Product Manager: Ryan Shaw
Vendor Manager: Bridgett Dougherty
Senior Manufacturing Manager: Benjamin Rivera

Senior Marketing Manager: Angela Panetta
Design Coordinator: Doug Smock
Production Service: Thomson Digital

Printed in China

Library of Congress Cataloging-in-Publication Data
Chandra, Ramesh, 1938-
Nuclear medicine physics : the basics / Ramesh Chandra. — 7th ed.
    p. ; cm.
    Includes bibliographical references and index.
    Summary: "This textbook will help lay the foundation on What, How and Why to document. Legal Issues, Coding, Utilization Review and utilization management are just a few of the contents areas covered"—Provided by publisher.
    ISBN 978-1-4511-0941-2 (pbk. : alk. paper)
    1. Medical physics.  2.  Nuclear medicine.  3.  Radioisotopes.  I.  Title.
    [DNLM: 1.  Health Physics.  2.  Nuclear Medicine.  3.  Radioisotopes. WN 110]
    R895.C47 2011
    616.07'575—dc22
                                                                2011013562

Care has been taken to confirm the accuracy of the information presented and to describe generally accepted practices. However, the authors, editors, and publisher are not responsible for errors or omissions or for any consequences from application of the information in this book and make no warranty, expressed or implied, with respect to the currency, completeness, or accuracy of the contents of the publication. Application of the information in a particular situation remains the professional responsibility of the practitioner.

The authors, editors, and publisher have exerted every effort to ensure that drug selection and dosage set forth in this text are in accordance with current recommendations and practice at the time of publication. However, in view of ongoing research, changes in government regulations, and the constant flow of information relating to drug therapy and drug reactions, the reader is urged to check the package insert for each drug for any change in indications and dosage and for added warnings and precautions. This is particularly important when the recommended agent is a new or infrequently employed drug.

Some drugs and medical devices presented in the publication have Food and Drug Administration (FDA) clearance for limited use in restricted research settings. It is the responsibility of the health care provider to ascertain the FDA status of each drug or device planned for use in their clinical practice.

To purchase additional copies of this book, call our customer service department at (800) 638-3030 or fax orders to (301) 223-2320. International customers should call (301) 223-2300.

Visit Lippincott Williams & Wilkins on the Internet: at LWW.com. Lippincott Williams & Wilkins customer service representatives are available from 8:30 am to 6 pm, EST.

10 9 8 7 6 5 4 3 2 1

RRS1104

*To the future,*
*my grandsons,*
*Aidan, Liam, and Alexander*

# Contents

# Preface

The purpose and the audience for this new edition of this book and the subject matter remains the same as in previous editions. I quote with a minor change,

"This book is primarily addressed to resident physicians in nuclear medicine and radiology, as well as fellows in nuclear cardiology who wish to acquire knowledge of nuclear medicine. Nuclear medicine technologists wishing to advance in their field should also find this book useful.

I have tried to write in a simple and concise manner, including not only essential details but also many examples and problems taken from the routine practice of nuclear medicine. Basic principles and underlying concepts are explained. Mathematical equations or in some cases their derivations have been included only when it was felt their inclusion will help the reader and when it was essential for the proper development of the subject matter. However, the reader is warned that this is not an introductory book of physics, and, therefore, familiarity on his or her part with the elementary concepts of physics, such as units, energy, force, electricity, and light, is assumed by the author."

However, since the publication of 6th edition, a new detector, CZT, is threatening the prime position occupied by the NaI(Tl) detector in nuclear medicine since its inception for almost 60 years ago. Therefore, some major and some minor changes have been made in Chapters 8, 10, 11, and 14 to reflect this. Five new figures have been added and all the old figures have been redrawn to show a uniform style. Chapter 15 has been rearranged and a table of effective doses in nuclear medicine has been added. There are minor changes in most of the other chapters, some in addition or deletion of content and others in arrangement of the subject matter. As there was a good response to the problems at the end of each chapter, these have been enlarged.

Again, I thank all the readers and teachers who wrote to me or e-mailed with their commendations and/or criticism, or who brought the errors to my attention. I would also like to thank Martha Helmers for all her hard work in the preparation of figures. Last, but not the least, I thank the publisher and his staff for their help and cooperation in bringing my labor to fruition.

Ramesh Chandra
New York, New York

From a physicist's point of view, nature consists mainly of matter and the forces governing the behavior of matter. This chapter reviews briefly some aspects of the atomic structure of matter that are essential for the understanding of subsequent subject matter.

## Matter, Elements, and Atoms

All matter is composed of a limited number of elements (118 so far, see Periodic Table, Table 1.1) that in turn are made of atoms. An atom is the smallest part of an element that retains all its chemical properties. In general, atoms are electrically neutral; that is, they do not show any electric charge. However, atoms are not indivisible as once was thought but are composed of three elementary particles: electrons, protons, and neutrons.

An electron is a tiny particle that possesses a negative charge of $1.6022 \times 10^{-19}$ coulomb (unit of charge) and a mass of $9.109 \times 10^{-31}$ kg. A proton is a particle with a positive charge equal in amount to that of an electron. A neutron does not have any electric charge and weighs slightly more than a proton. Protons and neutrons have masses of $1.6726 \times 10^{-27}$ and $1.6749 \times 10^{-27}$ kg, respectively; hence, they are about 2000 times heavier than an electron.

## Simplified Structure of an Atom

An atom is generally neutral because it contains the same number of electrons and protons. The number of protons in an atom is also known as the atomic number Z. It specifies the position of that element in the periodic table (Table 1.1) and therefore specifies its chemical identity. The electrons, protons, and neutrons in an atom are arranged in a planetary structure in which the protons and neutrons (the sun) are located at the center and the electrons (planets) are revolving over the surface of spherical shells (or orbits) of different radii. The center in which the protons and neutrons are located is known as the nucleus and is similar to a packed sphere. The size of atoms of different elements varies greatly but is in the range of 1 to $2 \times 10^{-10}$ m. The nucleus is really small in comparison to the atom (about $10^5$ times smaller or $10^{-15}$ m in size).

The attractive coulomb (electrical) force between the positively charged nucleus (due to the protons) and the negatively charged electrons provides stability to the electrons revolving in the spherical shells. The first shell (having the smallest radius) is known as the K shell, the second shell as L, the third shell as M, and so on. There is a limit to the number of electrons that can occupy a given shell. The K shell can be occupied by a maximum of 2 electrons, the L shell by a maximum of 8 electrons, the M shell by a maximum of 18 electrons, and the N shell by a maximum of 32 electrons. However, the outermost shell in a given atom cannot be occupied by more than eight electrons. In a simple atom such as hydrogen, there is only one electron that under normal circumstances occupies the K shell. In a complex atom such as iodine, there are 53 electrons that are arranged in the K, L, M, N, and O orbits in numbers of 2, 8, 18, 18, and 7, respectively. The arrangement of electrons in

**Table 1.1.**

## Periodic Table

| 1 | 2 | 3 | 4 | 5 | 6 | 7 | 8 | 9 | 10 | 11 | 12 | 13 | 14 | 15 | 16 | 17 | 18 |
|---|---|---|---|---|---|---|---|---|----|----|----|----|----|----|----|----|----|
| Hydrogen 1 **H** | | | | | | | | | | | | | | | | | Helium 2 **He** |
| Lithium 3 **Li** | Beryllium 4 **Be** | | | | | | | | | | | Boron 5 **B** | Carbon 6 **C** | Nitrogen 7 **N** | Oxygen 8 **O** | Fluorine 9 **F** | Neon 10 **Ne** |
| Sodium 11 **Na** | Magnesium 12 **Mg** | | | | | | | | | | | Aluminium 13 **Al** | Silicon 14 **Si** | Phosphorus 15 **P** | Sulfer 16 **S** | Chlorine 17 **Cl** | Argon 18 **Ar** |
| Potassium 19 **K** | Calcium 20 **Ca** | Scandium 21 **Sc** | Titanium 22 **Ti** | Vanadium 23 **V** | Chromium 24 **Cr** | Manganese 25 **Mn** | Iron 26 **Fe** | Cobalt 27 **Co** | Nickel 28 **Ni** | Copper 29 **Cu** | Zinc 30 **Zn** | Gallium 31 **Ga** | Germanium 32 **Ge** | Arsnic 33 **As** | Selenium 34 **Se** | Bromine 35 **Br** | Krypton 36 **Kr** |
| Rubidium 37 **Rb** | Strontium 38 **Sr** | Yttrium 39 **Y** | Zirconium 40 **Zr** | Niobium 41 **Nb** | Molybdenum 42 **Mo** | Technetium 43 **Tc** | Ruthenium 44 **Ru** | Rhodium 45 **Rh** | Palladium 46 **Pd** | Silver 47 **Ag** | Cadmium 48 **Cd** | Indium 49 **In** | Tin 50 **Sn** | Antimony 51 **Sb** | Tellurium 52 **Te** | Iodine 53 **I** | Xenon 54 **Xe** |
| Caesium 55 **Cs** | Barium 56 **Ba** | †57-70 | Lutetium 71 **Lu** | Hafnium 72 **Hf** | Tantalum 73 **Ta** | Tungsten 74 **W** | Rhenium 75 **Re** | Osmium 76 **Os** | Iridium 77 **Ir** | Platinum 78 **Pt** | Gold 79 **Au** | Mercury 80 **Hg** | Thallium 81 **Tl** | Lead 82 **Pb** | Bismuth 83 **Bi** | Polonium 84 **Po** | Astatine 85 **At** | Radon 86 **Rn** |
| Francium 87 **F** | Radium 88 **Ra** | ‡89-102 | Lawrencium 103 **Lr** | Rutherfordium 104 **Rf** | Dubnium 105 **Db** | Seaborgium 106 **Sg** | Bohrium 107 **Bh** | Hassium 108 **Hs** | Meitnerium 109 **Mt** | Darmstadtium 110 **Ds** | Roentgenium 111 **Rg** | Copernicium 112 **Cn** | 113 **Uut** | 114 **Uuq** | 115 **Uup** | 116 **Uuh** | 117 **Uus** | 118 **Uuo** |

†Lanthanide Series

| Lanthanium 57 **La** | Cerium 58 **Ce** | Praseodymium 59 **Pr** | Neodymium 60 **Nd** | Promethium 61 **Pm** | Samarium 62 **Sm** | Europium 63 **Eu** | Gadolinium 64 **Gd** | Terbium 65 **Tb** | Dysprosium 66 **Dy** | Holmium 67 **Ho** | Erbium 68 **Er** | Thulium 69 **Tm** | Ytterbium 70 **Yb** |
|---|---|---|---|---|---|---|---|---|---|---|---|---|---|

‡Actinide Series

| Actinium 89 **Ac** | Thorium 90 **Th** | Protactinium 91 **Pa** | Uranium 92 **U** | Neptunium 93 **Np** | Plutonium 94 **Pu** | Americium 95 **Am** | Curium 96 **Cm** | Berkelium 97 **Bk** | Californium 98 **Cf** | Einsteinium 99 **Es** | Fermium 100 **Fm** | Mendelevium 101 **Md** | Nobelium 102 **No** |
|---|---|---|---|---|---|---|---|---|---|---|---|---|---|

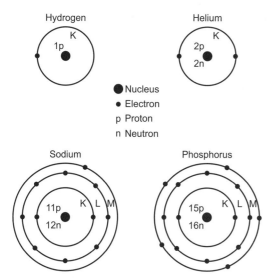

**Fig. 1.1.** Simplified atomic structure of four elements in their ground state—hydrogen atom contains only one electron and its nucleus one proton, helium atom contains two electrons and its nucleus contains two protons and two neutrons, sodium atom contains 11 electrons and its nucleus 11 protons and 12 neutrons, phosphorus atom contains 15 electrons and its nucleus contains 15 protons and 16 neutrons. Distribution of the electrons in various orbits for each atom is also depicted.

various shells for hydrogen and three other typical atoms is shown in Figure 1.1. This is a simplified description of the atomic structure that, in reality, is more complex as each shell is further divided into subshells. For our purpose, however, it is more than sufficient.

## Molecules

Molecules are formed by the combination of two or more atoms (e.g., a molecule of water, $H_2O$, is formed by the combination of two hydrogen atoms and one oxygen atom). The combination of atoms is accomplished through the interaction of electrons (also known as valent electrons) in the outermost orbits of the atom. Valent electrons participate in the formation of the molecules in several ways—for example, in ionic binding, covalent binding, and hydrogen binding. In theory, most chemical reactions and chemical properties of atoms or molecules can be explained on the basis of the interaction of the valent electrons.

## Binding Energy, Ionization, and Excitation

Each electron in a given shell is bound to the nucleus with a fixed amount of energy. Therefore, if one wishes to remove an electron from a particular shell to make it free and no longer associated with that atom, energy will have to be provided to the electron from outside the atom. The minimum amount of energy necessary to free an electron from an atom is known as the binding energy of the electron in that atom. The unit in which energy is measured on the atomic scale is known as an electron volt (eV), which is the energy acquired by an electron accelerated through 1 volt of potential difference. The electrons in the K shell are the most tightly bound electrons in an atom and therefore require the most energy to be removed from the atom. Electrons in the outermost shell, on the other hand, are the least tightly bound electrons and therefore require the least amount of energy for their removal from the atom. The binding energy of electrons in various shells increases rapidly with the atomic number Z. Table 1.2 lists the K- and L-shell average binding energies of electrons in the atoms of various elements.

Under normal conditions, electrons occupy the lowest possible shells (those closest to the nucleus) consistent with the maximum number of electrons by which a given shell can be occupied. However, electrons can be made to move into higher shells (unoccupied shells) temporarily by the absorption of energy. This absorption can take place in various ways—for example, by heating a substance, by subjecting matter to high electric fields, by passage of a charged particle through matter, or even by a high mechanical impact. When an electron absorbs sufficient energy for its removal from the atom, the process is called ionization and the remaining atom, an ion. When the electron absorbs amounts of energy that are just sufficient to move it into a higher unoccupied shell, the process is known as excitation and the atom as an excited atom. Excited atoms are, in general, unstable and acquire their normal configuration by emitting electromagnetic radiation (light, ultraviolet light, or x-rays), generally within $10^{-9}$ seconds.

| Table 1.2. | Average Binding Energies of K- and L-Shell Electrons in Various Elements | | |
|---|---|---|---|
| | | Average Binding Energy (keV) | |
| Element | Atomic Number Z | K Shell | L Shell |
| H | 1 | 0.014 | — |
| C | 6 | 0.28 | 0.007 |
| O | 8 | 0.53 | 0.024 |
| P | 15 | 2.15 | 0.19 |
| S | 16 | 2.47 | 0.23 |
| Fe | 26 | 7.11 | 0.85 |
| Zn | 30 | 9.66 | 1.19 |
| Br | 35 | 13.47 | 1.78 |
| Ag | 47 | 25.51 | 3.81 |
| I | 53 | 33.17 | 5.19 |
| Tm | 69 | 59.40 | 10.12 |
| W | 74 | 69.52 | 12.10 |
| Pb | 82 | 88.00 | 15.86 |

For example, let us consider a sodium atom, which has an atomic number of 11 and therefore 11 electrons and 11 protons. The electrons are arranged in K, L, and M shells in numbers of two, eight, and one, respectively. The energies of these electrons in the K, L, and M shells are approximately −1072, −63, and −1 eV, respectively. To remove an electron from the K shell of a sodium atom, it is necessary to provide an amount of energy equal to 1072 eV, whereas from the M shell only 1 eV of energy is necessary. An electron from the L shell can move to the M shell by absorbing 62 eV of energy, thereby producing an excited atom of sodium. When this excited atom decays (i.e., when the electron jumps back into the L shell), an electromagnetic radiation of 62 eV will be emitted.

It should be pointed out here that in the case of electrons, the zero of energy scale, by convention, is chosen to be the state when the electron is just free and not bound to the atom. As a result, when an electron is bound in the atom, its energy is represented as negative and when an electron is free and moving (i.e., possesses kinetic energy); its energy is represented

as positive. This convention is different from the one used in the case of a nucleus discussed in the next chapter (p. 14).

## Forces or Fields

Force is a general term related to the interaction of various constituents of matter. At present, four kinds of forces (or fields) are known: gravitational, weak, electromagnetic, and strong. Gravitational forces are produced as a result of the mass of matter and play a significant role in holding our solar system intact, but they are negligible between atoms and molecules and therefore not discussed here. Weak forces play a significant part in nuclear transformation, and are described in Chapter 2. Electromagnetic forces play a dominant role in our daily life because they hold the atom together and are responsible for interactions between atoms, molecules, biomolecules, and so on, and are discussed below. Strong forces are the forces that hold a nucleus together and act between proton–proton, proton–neutron, and neutron–neutron and are described in Chapter 2. The relative strengths of these forces are listed below.

| Type of Force | Strength |
|---|---|
| Strong | 1 |
| Electromagnetic | $10^{-2}$ |
| Weak | $10^{-13}$ |
| Gravitational | $10^{-39}$ |

**Electromagnetic Forces** Electromagnetic forces or fields are produced by charged particles. During interactions between charged particles, quite often energy is emitted as electromagnetic radiation. Electromagnetic radiation can propagate either as waves or as particles. When electromagnetic radiation behaves like particles, these particles are called photons. A photon does not have any rest mass or charge. It is a packet of energy that interacts with matter in a specified manner or according to the laws of electromagnetic forces. The dual nature of radiation, which is now an established fact, is true of matter (i.e., electrons) as well. Electromagnetic radiation is characterized by its energy or wavelength only. Electromagnetic radiation of varying energies is known by different names (Fig. 1.2). The energy of electromagnetic radiation is related to the wavelength by a simple relationship:

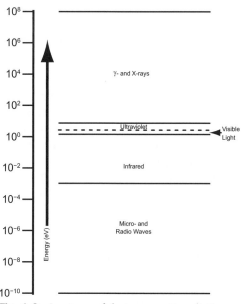

Fig. 1.2. Spectrum of electromagnetic radiations. Electromagnetic radiations of different energies are known by various names. For example, x- or $\gamma$-radiations are electromagnetic radiations with energies higher than 100 eV.

$$E = hc/\lambda$$

where h is Planck's constant, c is the velocity of light or electromagnetic radiation, and $\lambda$ is the wavelength. The above relationship is further reduced if one measures energy in keV and the wavelength in nanometers (1 nm = $10^{-9}$ m):

$$E \text{ (keV)} = 1.24/\lambda$$

# Characteristic X-Rays and Auger Electrons

As can be seen from Figure 1.2, x-rays are part of the electromagnetic radiation spectrum. Electromagnetic radiations with energies of approximately 100 eV or more are called x-rays. X-rays are primarily distinguished from other forms of electromagnetic radiation by their ability to produce ionization in matter and to penetrate substances. Characteristic x-rays are produced by the transition of electrons from outer to inner orbits of atoms (the K or L shell in most cases). The inner orbits of an atom under normal circumstances are fully occupied; therefore, to cause the transition of an electron from an outer to an inner orbit, it is necessary to create a vacancy or hole in the inner orbit. This can be accomplished in various ways. The well-known example is an x-ray tube, where high-energy electrons sometimes collide with the inner-shell electrons, knocking them out of the target atoms and thus creating a vacancy in the inner shells of the target atoms. Other examples of vacancy creation in inner shells are discussed in Chapter 2.

Once a vacancy is created in the inner shell of an atom, an electron from the outer shell falls to fill this hole. The difference between the potential energies of the two shells involved in the transition is emitted as electromagnetic radiation. This is called a characteristic x-ray of the atom if the energy emitted is approximately 100 eV or more. If the vacancy was in the K shell, the x-rays emitted are known as K x-rays; if the vacancy was in the L shell, they are known as L x-rays. Because the energy of a characteristic x-ray emitted by an atom is unique, it is possible to identify an atom (and therefore an element) by the energy of its characteristic x-rays.

Let us consider the example of a sodium atom where electrons in the K, L, and M shells have −1072, −63, and −1 eV of energies, respectively. Now if a vacancy is created in the K shell of this atom, it will be filled by one of the L- or M-shell electrons. Let us assume it is filled by the L-shell electron. The L-shell electron, which originally had −63 eV of energy, now in the K shell has only −1072 eV of energy. The difference of the two energies, $e_L − e_K = [−63 − (−1072)] = 1009$ eV, will be emitted as a characteristic K x-ray and this energy is unique for a sodium atom.

An alternate process to characteristic x-ray emission is the emission of Auger electrons (named in honor of their discoverer, P. Auger). In this process, the vacancy in the K shell is filled by an electron from the L or M shells; however, the balance of energy that would have been emitted as an x-ray is taken by another electron from the L or M shell. Thus, in Auger-electron emission, two electrons are removed from L and/or M shells: one fills the vacancy in K shell, and the other is emitted from the atom with the balance of energy. The atom is now doubly ionized. A similar process may occur if the vacancy is in the L or M shell. The Auger process occurs most frequently in elements with low atomic numbers ($Z < 24$, e.g., C, N, O, Al, Ca), whereas x-ray emission is characteristic of elements with high atomic numbers ($Z > 45$, e.g., I, Cs, W, Pb). These two processes, characteristic x-ray emission and Auger-electron emission, are graphically depicted in Figure 1.3.

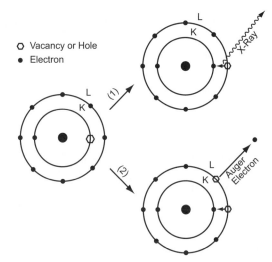

**Fig. 1.3.** X-ray emission and Auger-electron emission. When there is a vacancy (or hole) in the K shell of an atom, one of two processes may occur: either an electron from the L shell (or higher shells) fills the vacancy in the K shell and the balance of energy between the K and L shells is emitted as a characteristic x-ray, or one of the electrons from the L shell fills the vacancy in the K shell and the balance of energy is taken by another electron in the L shell (or higher shell), which is then emitted as an Auger electron.

## Interchangeability of Mass and Energy

In 1905, Einstein derived an expression on theoretical grounds that showed the interconvertibility of mass and energy. With subsequent advances in experimental atomic and nuclear physics, his assertion proved to be correct. The expression that relates mass and energy is simply

$$E = mc^2$$

where E is the energy, m is the mass, and c is the velocity of light. Mass on an atomic or nuclear scale is measured in atomic mass units (amu), defined as 1/12 of the mass of a carbon atom. From Einstein's equation for mass and energy conversion, 1 amu is equivalent to 931 MeV of energy. The masses in amu and their equivalent energy in MeV for an electron, proton, and neutron are given in Table 1.3.

| Table 1.3. | Mass and Energy Equivalence for Electrons, Protons, and Neutrons | |
|---|---|---|
| **Particle** | **Mass (amu)** | **Mass Energy (MeV)** |
| e | 0.000549 | 0.511 |
| p | 1.00728 | 938.28 |
| n | 1.00867 | 939.57 |

## Key Points

1. Matter is made of a relatively small number of elements (Table 1.1). An atom is the smallest chemical unit of an element.
2. An atom is made of elementary particles: electrons, protons, and neutrons. Electrons revolve in fixed orbits, K, L, M, and so on, around the nucleus that contains both protons and neutrons. Electrons are bound in orbits with fixed amount of energies, called binding energy. Number of electrons equals number of protons, Z (atomic number), in a neutral atom.
3. Electrons can move to higher orbits by absorption of energy in discrete amounts, thus producing excited atoms. Electrons can be completely removed from an atom by absorption of energies that exceed the binding energies of the electrons, causing the atom to be ionized.
4. Excited atoms release their energy in the form of electromagnetic radiation.
5. Elementary particles interact with each other through four types of forces of which electromagnetic force is the dominant force between electrons and the nucleus. It provides stability to electrons revolving in the orbits.
6. Electromagnetic force manifests itself as waves or particles called photons. Photons of different energies are known by different names, such as x- or $\gamma$-rays (gamma rays), ultraviolet light, visible light, infrared light, microwaves, and radio waves. The energy of a photon is related to its frequency or wavelength by the following expression: $E = hc/\lambda$.
7. Mass and energy are interchangeable and are related through Einstein's equation, $E = mc^2$.

## Questions

1. Find the energies of radiations emitted from the atoms of (a) iodine and (b) lead when there is a vacancy in the K shell of these atoms (use Table 1.2).
2. Determine the minimum energy needed to create a vacancy in (a) the K shells of P, Fe, and Tm atoms and (b) the L shells of Zn, I, and Pb atoms (use Table 1.2).
3. Using Table 1.2, find the minimum energy of radiation that can ionize a hydrogen atom, carbon atom, or iodine atom.
4. A 100-keV electron knocks out a K-shell electron from an iodine atom and is left with 50-keV energy. What is the kinetic energy of the electron emitted from the K-shell? Use Table 1.2.
5. If a 20-keV x-ray is absorbed by an atom of P, I, or Pb, what are the possible energies of the electrons emitted in each case? Use Table 1.2 for binding energy information.
6. What are the wavelengths of the 10, 100, and 1000 keV x-rays?
7. X-ray or $\gamma$-rays can convert their energies into light. If a 140-keV $\gamma$-ray converts 10% of its energy into a 5-eV light photon, how many light photons will be generated? (This process occurs in scintillator detectors discussed in Chapter 8.)
8. Can a micro or radio wave remove electrons from K or L shell electrons from any of the atoms listed in Table 1.2?
9. If a vacancy is created by the absorption of a 20-keV x-ray in the K shell of an atom of P, Fe, or Ag, and it is filled by the emission of an Auger electron from L shell, what is the energy of the Auger electron emitted by each atom in such a transition (use Table 1.2)?
10. If the rest mass of an electron is converted into electromagnetic energy, what is the energy of this radiation? What is its name?
11. If the mass difference between a neutron and a proton can be converted into electrons, what is the maximum number of electrons produced?

# Nuclides and Radioactive Processes

In the previous chapter, I discussed the structure of the atom and pointed out the importance of electrons and their interactions. In this chapter, I discuss the properties of the nucleus (the central core of an atom) and the radioactive processes that are strictly nuclear phenomena.

## Nuclides and Their Classification

As in the case of an atom, different types of atoms are called elements; in the case of a nucleus, different types of nuclei are termed nuclides. An element is characterized by its atomic number (Z) alone, whereas a nuclide is characterized by its mass number (A) and by its atomic number (Z). The mass number (A) of a nuclide is the sum of the number of its protons (Z) and neutrons (N), that is, A = Z + N.

As an example, $^{131}_{53}$I, a nuclide of iodine contains 53 protons and 78 neutrons, which add up to 131, the mass number of this nuclide. A general notation for a nuclide is $^{A}_{Z}$X, where A and Z, respectively, are the mass number and the atomic number of the nuclide and X is the element to which this nuclide belongs.

Nuclides are classified according to their mass number, neutron number, and atomic (proton) number. Nuclides having the same atomic mass are called isobars (e.g., $^{131}_{53}$I and $^{131}_{54}$Xe; both of these nuclides have the same mass number, 131). Nuclides having the same number of protons are called isotopes (e.g., $^{12}_{6}$C and $^{13}_{6}$C). Because they contain the same number of protons, and therefore have the same atomic

number, isotopes always belong to the same element. Nuclides having the same number of neutrons are called isotones (e.g., $^{13}_{7}$N and $^{14}_{8}$O both of these nuclides contain six neutrons). As an aid to memory, a pair of corresponding letters in each definition is italicized.

| | |
|---|---|
| Same number of *p*rotons | isoto*p*es |
| Same *a*tomic mass | iso*ba*rs |
| Same number of *n*eutrons | isoto*n*es |

## Nuclear Structure and Excited States of a Nuclide

How are neutrons and protons (a common name for the two combined is nucleon) arranged inside the nucleus? We have only a partial answer to this question so far. Our understanding of the structure of a nucleus as compared with the structure of an atom (i.e., arrangement of electrons in various shells and their interactions) is quite limited. It is postulated—with a wealth of supportive experimental data—that nucleons are arranged in spherical shells inside the nucleus in a manner similar to that of electrons in an atom. Not much is known, however, of the manner in which nucleons are stacked in these shells or about the transitions of nucleons between different shells. What is known and is important for the present discussion is that nucleons, just as electrons in an atom, can also be excited to higher unoccupied shells by absorption of energy from outside the nucleus. The lowest possible arrangement of nucleons in the nucleus is known as the ground state of a nuclide. The higher shells are commonly referred to as energy levels or excited states. Again, similar to electrons in an atom, nucleons in a nucleus are also bound with different binding energies. The binding energy (BE) of a nucleon (amount of energy needed to pull it out of the nucleus) varies from nuclide to nuclide. However, the average BE of nucleons for most nuclides is in the range of 5 to 8 MeV. This is about 1000 times higher (MeV rather than keV) than the average binding energies of electrons in atoms. Therefore, it is hard to remove a proton or neutron from a nucleus. It requires transfer of a large amount of energy from outside that is, in general, only possible in nuclear reactors, accelerators, or cyclotrons.

The excited states of a nuclide, in general, are of a short duration ($<10^{-11}$ seconds) and decay to the ground state or lower energy states by emission of high-energy radiation in a manner similar to that of the excited states of an atom, which decay to the ground state of an atom by emitting light or x-rays.

Excited states have the same mass number, same atomic number, and the same number of neutrons as the ground state and therefore are called isomers (i.e., an isom*e*r is an *e*xcited state of a nuclide). Note that the letter "e" has been italicized twice in the above definition, again as an aid to memory. The isomer of a nuclide is generally distinguished from its ground state by placing an asterisk after the symbol of the nuclide (e.g., $^{12}_{6}C^*$ is an excited state of $^{12}_{6}C$). In a few cases, however, the lifetime of the excited state of a nuclide can be very long (seconds, minutes, or even years). When this occurs, the excited state is called a metastable state. Well-known examples of nuclides having metastable states are $^{99m}Tc$ and $^{113m}In$. The letter "m" after the mass number in these two nuclides stands for metastable state and distinguishes them from their respective ground states of $^{99}Tc$ and $^{113}In$.

# Radionuclides and Stability of Nuclides

Even in their ground state, many nuclides are unstable. These unstable nuclides are called radionuclides. Radionuclides try to become stable by emitting electromagnetic radiation or charged particles. Electromagnetic radiation or charged particle emission is called radioactive decay. What makes a nuclide stable or radioactive? Two kinds of forces, strong and electromagnetic, determine the stability of a nuclide. The strong forces act between a pair of nucleons (e.g., proton–proton, proton–neutron, or neutron–neutron). They are attractive and act only when the distance between the two nucleons is very small. Electromagnetic forces act between protons only (because there is no charge on neutrons) and are repulsive (similar charges repel each other). The balance between these two forces—one attractive, the other repulsive—determines the stability of a nuclide. Whenever the balance between these two forces is disturbed, the nuclide becomes unstable and therefore radioactive. There are approximately 259 stable nuclides found in nature.

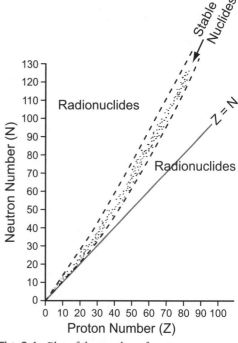

**Fig. 2.1.** Plot of the number of neutrons as a function of number of protons (atomic number) for stable nuclides. In the low–atomic number elements, the number of protons is roughly equal to the number of neutrons, but in the high–atomic number elements, more neutrons are needed than protons for stability. Radionuclides lie on either side of the stability curve.

If one plots the number of neutrons (N) contained as a function of the number of protons (Z) in a nuclide for all stable nuclides, a curve as shown in Figure 2.1 results. This curve initially starts as a straight line and then slowly bends toward the neutron number (N) for higher atomic numbers. From this curve it can be seen that for a lighter nuclide (A < 50), the number of protons in stable nuclides is equal to the number of neutrons; for example, $^{16}_{8}O$ a stable oxygen nuclide, contains eight neutrons and eight protons. For heavier nuclides (A > 100), however, the number of neutrons needed for the stability of a nuclide is much more than the number of protons; for example, $^{127}_{53}I$, a stable iodine nuclide, contains 53 protons and 74 neutrons. The region on either side of the curve in Figure 2.1 is called the domain of radionuclides. If a radionuclide lies in the upper region, it contains an excess number of neutrons that cause the "unstability" of the radionuclide. On the other hand, if the radionuclide lies in the lower region, it is the excess of protons that makes the nuclide unstable.

## Radioactive Series or Chain

A radionuclide tries to attain stability through radioactive decay. The stability may be achieved either by direct (single-step) decay to a stable nuclide or by decaying to several radionuclides in multiple steps and, finally, to a stable nuclide. For example, $^{131}_{53}I$ directly decays to a stable nuclide $^{131}_{54}Xe$. On the other hand, $^{226}_{88}Ra$ first decays to $^{222}_{86}Rn$, which decays to $^{218}_{84}Po$ and so on and finally to $^{210}_{82}Pb$, a stable nuclide. The complete series for this is given below (the arrows denote the sequence of decay).

$$^{226}_{88}Ra \rightarrow {}^{222}_{86}Rn \rightarrow {}^{218}_{84}Po \rightarrow {}^{214}_{82}Pb \rightarrow {}^{214}_{83}Bi \rightarrow {}^{214}_{84}Po \rightarrow {}^{210}_{82}Pb \text{ (stable nuclide)}$$

This sequence is often referred to as a radioactive series or chain. Well-known examples of a radioactive series in nuclear medicine are the decay of $^{99}Mo$ and $^{113}Sn$, which go through the following sequences:

$$^{99}Mo \rightarrow {}^{99m}Tc \rightarrow {}^{99}Tc \rightarrow {}^{99}Ru \text{ (stable)}$$

$$^{113}Sn \rightarrow {}^{113m}In \rightarrow {}^{113}In \text{ (stable)}$$

## Radioactive Processes and Conservation Laws

The three processes through which a radionuclide tries to attain stability are called alpha, beta, and gamma decay. These names were given because at the time of the discovery of these processes their exact nature was not known. Three important conservation laws are pertinent here because they always hold true in radioactive processes or nuclear transformations. These are the law of conservation of energy, the law of conservation of mass number, and the law of conservation of electric charge.

The law of conservation of energy states that the total energy (mass energy + kinetic energy + energy in any other form, e.g., a photon) remains unchanged during a radioactive process or nuclear transformation. The law of conservation of mass number states that the sum of mass numbers remains unchanged in radioactive or nuclear processes. The mass number of a neutron or proton is assumed to be one and that of an electron zero. Similarly, the law of conservation of electric charge states that the total charge during a radioactive process or nuclear transformation remains unchanged.

**Alpha Decay** In alpha decay, a radionuclide emits a heavy, charged particle called $\alpha$ particle. An $\alpha$ particle is four times heavier than a proton or neutron and carries an electric charge that is twice that of a proton. In fact, $\alpha$ particle is a stable nuclide with atomic mass number A = 4 and atomic number Z = 2. This happens to be the nucleus of a helium atom.

From the conservation laws of the mass number and electric charge, it follows that during alpha decay the mass number and the atomic number of the resulting nuclide (also known as the daughter nuclide) will be reduced by 4 and 2, respectively. Alpha decay can be expressed by the following equation:

$$^{A}_{Z}X = {}^{(A-4)}_{(Z-2)}Y + {}^{4}_{2}He \text{ ($\alpha$ particle)}$$

Notice that the mass number and the electric charge (in this case the sum of atomic numbers) on both sides of the equation are the same. An example of alpha decay is the decay of radium 226 to radon 222:

$$^{226}_{88}Ra = {}^{226}_{86}Rn + \alpha$$

**Example.** $^{222}_{86}$Rn is a radionuclide that decays through alpha decay. Determine the nature of its daughter nuclide. Because $^{222}_{86}$Rn decays through the alpha decay process, the mass number of the daughter nuclide will be 4 less than that of the parent, that is, $222 - 4 = 218$. Similarly, the atomic number will be reduced by 2, that is, $86 - 2 = 84$. Therefore, the daughter nuclide has a mass number 218 and its atomic number is 84. According to the periodic table, the atomic number 84 belongs to the element Po. Therefore, the daughter nuclide is $^{218}_{84}$Po.

Radon 222 is a radioactive gas that escapes into the environment from the rocks or soil containing radium 226. A small amount of radium, and therefore radon, is present everywhere. Such amounts increase the background radiation and constitute a major part of background radiation exposure to humans. In rare cases, a combination of relatively large concentrations of radium in the soil and rocks and poor circulation in a house can sometimes produce hazardous concentrations of radon in the house. This should be dealt with effectively for the safety of the occupants.

Two salient facts concerning alpha decay to remember are that it occurs mostly with radionuclides whose atomic mass number A is greater than 150 and the kinetic energy of the emitted $\alpha$ particle is fixed and discrete for a given decay. In the above example of $^{226}_{88}$Ra alpha decay, the kinetic energy of $\alpha$ particle emitted is 4.780 MeV.

**Beta Decay**  During this transformation, a neutron or a proton inside the nucleus of a radionuclide is converted into a proton or a neutron, respectively. When a proton is converted into a neutron, the positive charge inside the nucleus is decreased by one, thus reducing the repulsive forces between protons. On the other hand, when a neutron is converted into a proton, the positive charge inside the nucleus is increased by one, and therefore the repulsive forces between protons are increased. The result of the decrease or increase in the repulsive force within the nucleus is to balance the two forces (electromagnetic and strong) in an attempt to stabilize the nuclide (see Radionuclides and Stability of Nuclides, p. 10).

The conversion of a neutron into a proton or of a proton into a neutron is controlled by weak (as opposed to strong, electromagnetic, and gravitational) forces (see Chapter 1). The exact nature of weak forces is not known and is not pertinent to our discussion of beta decay. Beta decay occurs through one of the following processes: $\beta^-$ emission or electron emission, $\beta^+$ emission or positron emission, or electron capture.

**$\beta^-$ Emission.**  In this process, a neutron inside the radionuclide is converted into a proton and the excess energy is released as a pair of particles, an electron and an antineutrino ($\bar{\nu}$). As such, there are no electrons or antineutrinos inside the nucleus. These are created from excess energy at the instant of radioactive decay. An antineutrino is a particle that has no rest mass and no electric charge ($Z = 0$). It rarely interacts with matter and therefore is of no biological significance. Its existence was postulated so that the law of energy conservation would not be violated. However, its existence has now been confirmed experimentally. $\beta^-$ decay can be expressed as

$$^A_Z X = {}^A_{Z+1} Y + e^- + \bar{\nu}$$

Note that both the mass number and the electric charge are conserved. Some well-known examples of $\beta^-$ decay are $^3_1$H, $^{14}_6$C, and $^{32}_{15}$P, which can be expressed as follows:

$$^3_1 H = {}^3_2 He + e^- + \bar{\nu}$$
$$^{14}_6 C = {}^{14}_7 N + e^- + \bar{\nu}$$
$$^{32}_{15} P = {}^{32}_{16} S + e^- + \bar{\nu}$$

As can be seen, during $\beta^-$ decay the mass number (A) remains unchanged and the atomic number (Z) is increased by one. The kinetic energy of the emitted electron is not fixed because the total available energy in the decay (difference between the mass energy of the parent radionuclide and the daughter nuclide) has to be shared between the electron and the antineutrino.

In the above example, the difference between the mass energies of $^3_1$H and $^3_2$He, $^{14}_6$C and $^{14}_7$N, and $^{32}_{15}$P and $^{32}_{16}$S during decay is shared by the electron and the antineutrino. The sharing of the available energy is random; therefore, the electrons are emitted with varying amounts of kinetic energy (known as the $\beta^-$ spectrum) ranging from 0 to a maximum of $E_{\beta\,max}$. $E_{\beta\,max}$

is the total available energy in the case of a particular $\beta^-$ decay. In the above examples $E_{\beta\,max}$ for ³H decay is 0.018 MeV, for ¹⁴C decay 0.156 MeV, and for ³²P decay 1.71 MeV. The probability of an electron emission with a given kinetic energy $E_\beta$, $P(E_\beta)$, varies greatly with the kinetic energy $E_\beta$. The variation of $P(E_\beta)$ with $E_\beta$ (i.e., $\beta^-$ spectrum) is shown in Figure 2.2 for a typical $\beta^-$ decay.

In calculations of radiation dose to a patient with $\beta^-$emitting radionuclides, one is interested in the average energy, $\bar{E}_\beta$, of the electrons. The computation of $\bar{E}_\beta$ depends on knowledge of the exact shape of the $\beta$ spectrum. However, as a rule of thumb, in cases where high accuracy is not desired, $\bar{E}_\beta$ can be obtained by dividing $E_{\beta\,max}$ by 3 (i.e., $\bar{E}_\beta = E_{\beta\,max}/3$). Generally, $E_{\beta\,max}$, and sometimes $\bar{E}_\beta$, is listed in the table of nuclides.

### $\beta^+$ or Positron Emission

In this process, a proton inside the nucleus is converted into a neutron and the excess energy is emitted as a pair of particles, in this case a positron and a neutrino. (Neutrinos and antineutrinos can be considered identical for our purposes.) A positron is an electron with a unit-positive instead of a unit-negative charge. It has the same mass as an electron and interacts with matter in a manner similar to that of an electron. Positron decay can be expressed as

$$_Z^A X = \, _{Z-1}^A Y + e^+ + \nu$$

This equation is consistent with the laws of conservation of mass number and electric charge. However, for the total energy to be conserved, the mass of the nuclide X should be greater than the mass of the Y nuclide by at least 1.02 MeV (2x mass of an electron). This is because the mass of a nuclide includes in it the mass of the nucleus and the electrons associated with it. Therefore, the mass of the X nuclide contains the mass of Z electrons, whereas the mass of the Y nuclide contains the mass of only $(Z-1)$ electrons. Also an $e^+$ is created from the nuclear energy of X nuclide. Hence, the mass of the X nuclide has to be greater than two times the mass of an electron plus the mass of the Y nuclide. Some examples of positron emission are

$$_6^{11}C = \, _5^{11}B + e^+ + \nu$$
$$_8^{15}O = \, _7^{15}N + e^+ + \nu$$
$$_9^{18}F = \, _8^{18}O + e^+ + \nu$$

Note that during $\beta^+$ emission, the mass number does not change, but the atomic number is decreased by one. In $\beta^+$ emission, too, the energy of the emitted positron varies from 0 to maximum $E_{\beta\,max}$, which is known as the $\beta^+$ spectrum. The exact computation of the average $\beta^+$ energy, $\bar{E}_{\beta+}$, in this case, too, is quite involved. As an approximation one can determine $\bar{E}_{\beta+}$ again by dividing the $E_{\beta+\,max}$ by three.

### Electron Capture

In this process, a proton inside the nucleus is converted into a neutron by capturing an electron from one of the atomic shells (e.g., K, L, or M). No electron or positron but only a neutrino is emitted. The capture of an electron from the K shell of the atom is known as K capture; capture of an electron from the L shell is known as L capture, and so on. Electron capture is one of the few instances (another will be encountered in the case of gamma decay) in which a nucleus interacts directly with the orbital (K, L shells, etc.) electrons of an atom. Once an electron is captured from the K, L, or M shell, a vacancy is created in the inner shell of an atom. This vacancy is subsequently filled by electrons from higher

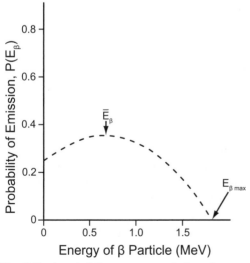

**Fig. 2.2.** A typical $\beta$-ray spectrum. In beta decay, electrons (or positrons) are emitted with varying energies up to a maximum $E_{\beta\,max}$. A $\beta$ spectrum gives the probability of emission of an electron with a given energy $E_\beta$.

shells with simultaneous emission of a characteristic x-ray or Auger electron (see Chapter 1). The probability of a capture from the K shell is generally much higher than that from the L or M shell. Electron capture is expressed as

$$_Z^A X + e^- \text{ (orbital)} = {_{Z\text{-}1}^A} Y + \nu$$

This is also consistent with the laws of conservation of mass number and electric charge. Common examples of electron capture are

$$_{24}^{51}\text{Cr} + e^- \text{ (orbital)} = {_{23}^{51}}\text{V} + \nu$$
$$_{55}^{131}\text{Cs} + e^- \text{ (orbital)} = {_{54}^{131}}\text{Xe} + \nu$$

Note that during electron capture, as in positron emission, the mass number does not change but the atomic number is reduced by one.

During all three processes of beta decay, the mass number A remains unchanged. For this reason, beta decay is quite often referred to as an isobaric transition.

**Gamma Decay or Isomeric Transition** It has already been explained that a nucleus can be excited by the absorption of energy to an excited state (isomer). Isomers in general are of very short duration except in cases of metastable states. The decay of an excited state to a lower energy or ground state is known as isomeric transition (as opposed to isobaric transition in the case of beta decay) and proceeds through either of two processes: an emission of a high-energy photon or internal conversion. These are graphically shown in Figure 2.3.

**High-energy Photon Emission** In this process, the excess energy of an isomer is released in the form of a high-energy photon known as a $\gamma$-ray. A $\gamma$-ray is an electromagnetic radiation with high energy (>100 eV; see Chapter 1). A $\gamma$-ray and an x-ray of the same energy cannot be distinguished from each other because both interact with matter in exactly the same manner. The only difference between the two is that of origin. Energy emitted from the nucleus as a high-energy photon is known as a $\gamma$-ray; energy emitted by an atom (i.e., transition of electrons in atomic shells) as a high-energy photon is called an x-ray. This difference in nomenclature of a high-energy photon is of no practical significance in nuclear medicine.

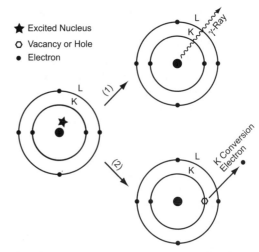

★ Excited Nucleus
○ Vacancy or Hole
● Electron

**Fig. 2.3.** Isomeric transition. An excited nucleus in isomeric transition can release its energy in two ways: by the emission of a $\gamma$-ray (photon) or by the transfer of its energy directly to an orbital electron, generally in the K shell. The electron acquiring the energy is ejected from the atom and is known as the conversion electron. The vacancy thus created in the inner shell of the atom is subsequently filled in the manner discussed in Chapter 1.

**Internal Conversion** Sometimes a nuclide in an excited state, instead of emitting a $\gamma$-ray, transfers its excess energy directly to an orbital electron (in the K, L, or M shell). This process is called internal conversion and is another example of the direct interaction of a nucleus with the orbital electrons revolving around it. The first example is electron capture in beta decay and is described on p. 13.

Internal conversion is an alternate process to $\gamma$-ray emission. A single nucleus will emit either a $\gamma$-ray or an electron. However, in a collection of nuclei, some will emit $\gamma$-rays and some conversion electrons. The ratio of the number of electrons to the number of $\gamma$-rays emitted by a collection of excited nuclei is called the coefficient of internal conversion (ic) for that excited state:

$$\text{ic} = \frac{\text{total number of electrons emitted}}{\text{total number } \gamma\text{ - rays emitted}}$$

When considering only the electrons knocked from the K shell, the above ratio is known as the coefficient of K conversion, $\text{ic}_K$. When considering only the electrons knocked out of the L shell, the above ratio is known as the coefficient of L conversion, $ic_L$. The total conversion coefficient, then, is the sum of the individual K, L, M conversion coefficients (i.e., $ic = ic_K + ic_L + ic_M$).

As an example, if $ic = 1/5$, the emission of a $\gamma$-ray is five times more likely than the emission of an electron by internal conversion; or, out of six decays, five will be through $\gamma$-ray or photon emission, and only one will be through the conversion process. Therefore, if there are 100 decays of excited nuclei, then in $(5/6)100 \simeq 83$ decays a $\gamma$-ray will be emitted, and in the remaining 17 decays a conversion electron will be emitted. If the internal conversion coefficient, $ic$, is 2, then the emission of an electron is twice as likely as the emission of a $\gamma$-ray, or out of three decays, one will be through $\gamma$-ray emission and two will be through conversion electron emission. Therefore, if there are 100 decays of the excited nuclei, then the number of $\gamma$-rays emitted will be $(1/3)100 \simeq 33$, whereas the number of conversion electrons emitted will be 67. When I discuss later the ideal properties of a radionuclide for nuclear medicine (Chapter 5), it will be seen that radionuclides that do not emit particulate radiation are desirable. Since even in gamma decay, because of internal conversion, electrons can be emitted, it follows that the coefficient of internal conversion should be as small as possible.

The probability of K conversion is generally quite high compared with L and M conversion because of the closeness of the K-shell electrons to the nucleus compared with the L- and M-shell electrons. Also, the probability of internal conversion is higher if the excited state is long-lived (metastable state) and the energy of the excited state is low ($<100$ keV).

Because in internal conversion an electron is emitted from the inner shell of an atom (K, L, or M), a vacancy is created in that shell. This vacancy is subsequently filled by electrons from higher shells, leading to the emission of an x-ray or Auger electron. The process of vacancy filling in atomic shells is the same as that following K capture in beta decay. As the electrons in each shell (K, L, ...) of the atom are bound with a certain amount of energy known as BE, the conversion electron carries a kinetic energy that is the difference of the energy of the excited state (nucleus) and the BE of the electron in a given shell. For example, $^{113m}$In, a metastable state with an energy of 393 keV, emits a $\gamma$-ray of 393 keV but emits a K conversion electron with a kinetic energy of $393 - 29.7$ (BE of K electrons in In atom) $= 363.3$ keV.

# Decay Schemes

In this discussion of alpha, beta, and gamma decay, various examples of radioactive processes have been presented. How does one know that a given radionuclide will decay by the emission of $\alpha$ particle, $\beta$-ray, or $\gamma$-ray or by a combination of two or more? Actually, there are no theoretical laws to supply this information. Such data are experimentally determined for each radionuclide and then tabulated in a pictorial form known as a decay scheme. A decay scheme is a collection of experimental information regarding the modes and frequency of decay, process of decay, energy of different radiation emitted, half-life, and other information of interest for a given radionuclide.

In one commonly used approach, decay schemes of isobars (or $\beta$ transitions) are graphically represented on one page, with radionuclides arranged in order of increasing atomic number from left to right. In this representation, all $\beta^-$ decaying radionuclides decay to the nuclide on their right (↘) and all the K-capture or $e^+$-decaying radionuclides to their left (↙ or ↵). A broken arrow is the indication for positron decay. It signifies that the mass of the parent nuclide has to be greater than the mass of the daughter nuclide by at least 1.02 MeV. The excited states of the nuclides are shown as horizontal bars above the ground state. The energy of these states increases from the bottom to the top of the page. Isomeric transitions between two states are shown by vertical lines connecting the two states.

In this instance, as opposed to the energy of electrons in an atom (p. 3), the zero of the energy scale is, by convention, chosen to be the ground state of a nuclide. It is as if the K shell of an atom has been arbitrarily chosen to have zero energy. According to this convention, all other shells of the atom (L, M, etc.) will have positive energy. In nuclear convention, then, the energy of the electrons in the K, L, and M shells of a sodium atom will, instead of $-1072$, $-63$, and $-1$ eV, be 0, 1009, and 1071 eV, respectively.

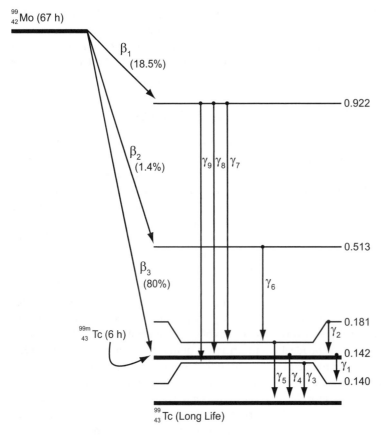

**Fig. 2.4.** Decay scheme of $^{99}$Mo. $^{99}$Mo decays via $\beta$ emission to the 0.142, 0.513, and 0.922 MeV excited states of $^{99}$Tc. These excited states then decay to the ground state by the emission of a number of $\gamma$-rays shown in the figure. Less likely transitions have been omitted from the decay scheme. Except for the 0.142 MeV excited state, which has a half-life of 6 hours, other excited states are short-lived.

A decay scheme is shown in Figure 2.4 for $^{99}$Mo, the parent of $^{99m}$Tc that has revolutionized the field of nuclear medicine. Briefly, the decay scheme of $^{99}$Mo shows that $^{99}$Mo decays 80% of the time to an excited state of $^{99}$Tc, which has an energy of 0.142 MeV (a metastable state because of its relatively long life), by emission of a $\beta^-$ particle with $E_{\beta\,max} = 1.23$ MeV. For 18.5% of the time, the decay proceeds to another excited state (isomer) of $^{99}$Tc, which has an energy of 0.922 MeV, by emission of a particle with $E_{\beta\,max} = 0.45$ MeV. For the remaining 1.4% of the time, the decay takes place to other excited states of $^{99}$Tc. The excited state of $^{99}$Tc at 0.922 MeV is short-lived and quickly ($<10^{-9}$ seconds) decays to the ground state or to lower energy excited states by emission of $\gamma$-rays or conversion electrons. Two radionuclides, $^{99}$Mo and $^{99m}$Tc, form a radionuclidic generator that is created whenever the parent's ($^{99}$Mo) half-life is greater than daughter's ($^{99m}$Tc). This is discussed in detail in Chapter 4.

Table 2.1 lists the number of radiations eventually emitted in the decay of $^{99}$Mo ($\beta$-rays, $\gamma$-rays, characteristic x-rays, conversion electrons, and Auger electrons) with their respective energies, $\bar{E}_i$, and the frequency of emission $n_i$ ($n_i$ is defined as the probability of emission of radiation i with energy $E_i$ per decay of a radionuclide). The information given in Table 2.1, however, cannot be obtained from Figure 2.4 alone because additional data and complex computations are required. The Society of Nuclear Medicine (New York, NY) has published such information for a large number of radionuclides (*MIRD: Radionuclide Data and Decay Schemes*; Weber, Eckerman, Dillman, and Ryman, 1989). An important thing to notice in Table 2.1 is that the number of radiations emitted in *the decay of one $^{99}$Mo nucleus(atom)* is more than one (add all the $n_i$ in Table 2.1). For different radionuclides this number will vary. Sometimes it can be less than one but quite often it is more than one.

| Table 2.1. | Radiations Emitted in the Decay of $^{99}$Mo | | |
|:---|:---|:---|:---|
| **Number** | **Radiation (i)** | **Frequency of Emission ($n_i$)** | **Mean Energy (MeV) ($\bar{E}_i$)** |
| 1 | $\beta 1$ | 0.185 | 0.140 |
| 2 | $\beta 2$ | 0.014 | 0.298 |
| 3 | $\beta 3$ | 0.797 | 0.452 |
| 4 | $\gamma 1$ | — | — |
| 5 | M conversion electron | 0.851 | 0.002 |
| 6 | $\gamma 2$ | 0.130 | 0.041 |
| 7 | K conversion electron | 0.043 | 0.019 |
| 8 | $\gamma 3$ | 0.815 | 0.140 |
| 9 | K conversion electron | 0.085 | 0.120 |
| 10 | L conversion electron | 0.011 | 0.138 |
| 11 | $\gamma 4$ | — | — |
| 12 | $\gamma 5$ | 0.066 | 0.181 |
| 13 | $\gamma 6$ | 0.014 | 0.366 |
| 14 | $\gamma 7$ | 0.137 | 0.740 |
| 15 | $\gamma 8$ | 0.048 | 0.778 |
| 16 | X-rays—K($\alpha$) | 0.094 | 0.018 |
| 17 | X-rays—K($\beta$) | 0.017 | 0.021 |
| 18 | KLL Auger electron | 0.022 | 0.015 |
| 19 | KLX Auger electron | 0.01 | 0.018 |
| 20 | LMM Auger electron | 1.53 | 0.002 |
| 21 | MXY Auger electron | 1.20 | 0.001 |

Two more examples of decay schemes, $^{99m}$Tc and $^{125}$I, are also given here. Appendix A gives in tabular form radiations emitted by a number of other radionuclides commonly used in nuclear medicine. Only those radiations emitted more than 1.0% of the time in the decay are included in these tabulations, which are primarily derived from the above source. For radionuclides not given here or in Appendix A, the reader should consult the above reference. Although information regarding the decay of $^{99m}$Tc can be derived from the decay scheme of $^{99}$Mo, the decay scheme of $^{99m}$Tc is shown separately in Figure 2.5 because of its great importance in nuclear medicine. Table 2.2 lists the relevant data for $^{99m}$Tc.

Decay scheme for $^{125}$I, a radionuclide widely used in radio–immunoassays, is shown in Figure 2.6. The number of $\gamma$-rays, x-rays, conversion electrons, and so on and their respective energies and frequency of emission in the decay of $^{125}$I are given in Table 2.3.

It is important to remember that in the decay of $^{99}$Mo and $^{125}$I, the $\gamma$-rays and x-rays emitted are not from $^{99}$Mo and $^{125}$I nuclides but from $^{99}$Tc and $^{125}$Te nuclides, respectively, even though in laboratory jargon these are referred to as iodine 125 $\gamma$-rays or molybdenum 99 $\gamma$-rays. This is a misnomer. The decay actually takes place in the following series:

$$^{99}\text{Mo} \xrightarrow{\beta^-} {}^{99}\text{Tc}^* \xrightarrow{\gamma} {}^{99}\text{Tc}$$

$$^{125}\text{I} \xrightarrow{\text{K Capture}} {}^{125}\text{Te}^* \xrightarrow{\gamma} {}^{125}\text{Te}$$

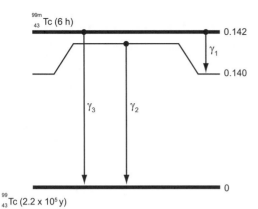

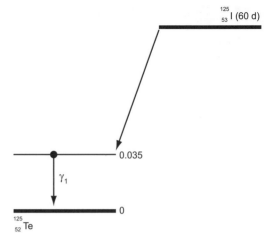

**Fig. 2.5.** Decay scheme of $^{99m}$Tc: the 6-hour half-life isomeric state of $^{99}$Tc at 0.142 MeV primarily (99% probability) decays to another isomeric state at 0.140 MeV. It has a very short half-life ($10^{-9}$ seconds) and therefore decays almost instantaneously to the ground state by the emission of a 0.140-MeV γ-ray or a corresponding conversion electron. The ground state or the nuclide $^{99}$Tc itself is a radionuclide. However, its half-life is so long that for all practical purposes it may be considered stable.

**Fig. 2.6.** Decay scheme of $^{125}$I. $^{125}$I decays through electron capture to an isomeric state of $^{125}$Te at 0.035 MeV, which subsequently decays to the ground state by the emission of a γ-ray (7% probability) or a conversion electron (93% probability). Because in electron capture (E.C.) and internal conversion a vacancy is created in the K shell, K x-rays of $^{125}$Te (29.8 keV) are also emitted in the decay of $^{125}$I.

Another decay scheme of interest to us, and shown in Figure 2.7, is that of $^{18}$F that emits positrons. Positrons are used in PET (positron emission tomography), an imaging modality that is acquiring an increasingly important role in nuclear medicine. Positrons as such cannot be used for external imaging of a radionuclidic distribution. However, due to their annihilation (Chapter 6), resulting gamma rays can be used for imaging. Table 2.4 lists the radiations emitted in the decay of $^{18}$F.

**Table 2.2.** Radiations Emitted in the Decay of $^{99m}$Tc

| Number | Radiation (i) | Frequency of Emission ($n_i$) | Mean Energy (MeV) ($\bar{E}_i$) |
|---|---|---|---|
| 1 | γ1 (conversion electron) | 0.986 | 0.002 |
| 2 | γ2 (photon) | 0.883 | 0.140 |
| 3 | K conversion electron | 0.088 | 0.119 |
| 4 | L conversion electron | 0.011 | 0.138 |
| 5 | M conversion electron | 0.004 | 0.140 |
| 6 | γ3 (conversion electron) | 0.01 | 0.122 |
| 7 | K (α) x-ray | 0.064 | 0.018 |
| 8 | K (β) x-ray | 0.012 | 0.021 |
| 9 | KLL Auger electron | 0.015 | 0.015 |
| 10 | LMM Auger electron | 0.106 | 0.002 |
| 11 | MXY Auger electron | 1.23 | 0.0004 |

**Table 2.3.** Radiations Emitted in the Decay of $^{125}$I

| Number | Radiation (i) | Frequency of Emission ($n_i$) | Mean Energy (MeV) ($\bar{E}_i$) |
|---|---|---|---|
| 1 | $\gamma 1$ | 0.068 | 0.035 |
| 2 | K conversion electron | 0.746 | 0.004 |
| 3 | L conversion electron | 0.107 | 0.031 |
| 4 | M conversion electron | 0.080 | 0.035 |
| 5 | X-ray—K($\alpha$) | 1.176 | 0.027 |
| 6 | X-ray—K($\beta$) | 0.240 | 0.031 |
| 7 | X-ray—L | 0.215 | 0.004 |
| 8 | KLL Auger electron | 0.137 | 0.023 |
| 9 | KLX Auger electron | 0.058 | 0.026 |
| 10 | KXY Auger electron | 0.01 | 0.030 |
| 11 | LMM Auger electron | 1.49 | 0.003 |
| 12 | MXY Auger electron | 3.59 | 0.001 |

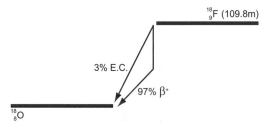

**Fig. 2.7.** Decay scheme of $^{18}$F, a positron emitting radionuclide commonly used in PET imaging. It only emits a positron that then annihilates to give two $\gamma$ rays of 0.511 MeV.

**Table 2.4.** Radiations Emitted in the Decay of $^{18}$F

| Radiation (i) | Frequency of Emission ($n_i$) | Mean Energy, $\bar{E}_i$ (MeV) |
|---|---|---|
| Electron capture | 0.03 | 0 |
| $\beta^+$ | 0.97 | 0.25 |
| Annihilation $\gamma$ rays | 1.97 | 0.511 |
| KLL Auger electron | 0.027 | 0.0005 |

## Key Points

1. In a nucleus or a nuclide, the number of neutrons (N) plus the number of protons (Z) equal its mass number (A). A nuclide is represented as $^A_Z X$, where X is the chemical symbol of the element to which this nucleus belongs. Quite often, Z is omitted from the symbol, for example, $^{131}$I, which represents a radionuclide of iodine with mass number of 131 (53 protons and 78 neutrons).

2. A nuclide is stable only for certain combinations of Z and N given by the curve of stability (Fig. 2.1). In lighter nuclides, Z = N, and in heavier nuclides, N > Z. Nuclides can also exist temporarily in excited states called isomers. Whenever an isomer has a half-life of 1 $\mu$s or longer, it is called a metastable state and is denoted with letter "m" next to the mass number as in $^{99m}$Tc.

3. Any other combination of Z and N, away from the stability curve, results in an unstable nuclide (radionuclide).

4. Radionuclides decay through alpha, beta, and gamma processes. In each of these

decays, energy, electric charge (Z), and mass number (A) are conserved.

5. In alpha decay, a helium nucleus is given off. The daughter nuclide's mass and atomic numbers are A − 4 and Z − 2, respectively, where A and Z are the parent radionuclide's mass and atomic numbers, respectively.

6. In beta decay, an electron or positron is emitted from a nucleus, or an electron is captured from an orbit. In each case, a neutrino is also emitted. Mass number remains unchanged, but atomic number of the daughter nuclide can increase (electron emission) or decrease (positron emission or electron capture) by one unit.

7. In electron capture, a vacancy is created in an orbit. It results in the emission of a characteristic x-ray.

8. In gamma decay, a photon or a conversion electron is emitted. Mass and atomic numbers are not affected. In conversion electron emission, too, a vacancy is formed in the orbit, resulting in emission of a characteristic x-ray.

9. Decay schemes summarize the various decay processes and radiations emitted in the decay of a particular radionuclide.

## Questions

1. Separate the following nuclides into pairs of isotopes, isobars, isotones, or isomers:

   $^{3}_{1}H$, $^{4}_{2}He$, $^{3}_{2}He$, $^{12}_{6}C$, $^{12}_{7}N$, $^{14}_{6}C$, $^{99}_{43}Tc$, $^{99}_{42}Mo$, $^{99m}_{43}Tc$, $^{100}_{44}Ru$.

2. Identify the following decay processes in which (a) the mass number is unchanged, (b) the atomic number decreases by one, (c) the atomic number increases by one, (d) the mass number decreases by four, and (e) the mass and atomic numbers remain constant.

3. The $E_{\beta\,max}$ for $^{3}H$ and $^{32}P$ are 0.0186 and 1.710 MeV, respectively. What are the average energies of $\beta$ emission in these decays?

4. In electron capture, an electron is removed from the K or L shell of an atom. Is the daughter atom in the ground state or excited state? Is it ionized?

5. Can a radionuclide decay with all three (alpha, beta, and gamma) processes?

6. What makes two isomers or an isomer and a metastable state different from each other?

7. Find the following radiations in the decay tables given in this chapter or in Appendix A: (a) x-ray with the highest energy in the decay of $^{99m}Tc$; (b) $\gamma$-rays in the energy range of 100 to 300 keV in the decay of $^{111}In$; (c) $\beta$-ray with the least frequency of emission, $\beta$-ray with the most energy of emission, and $\gamma$-rays in the energy range of 700 to 800 keV in the decay of $^{99}Mo$; and (d) % emission and the energies of x-rays in the decay of $^{201}Tl$.

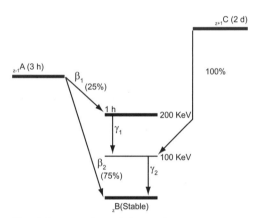

**Fig. 2.8.** Hypothetical decay scheme.

In the hypothetical decay scheme shown in Figure 2.8 (questions 8–10 only):

8. How many $\gamma_1$ and $\gamma_2$ will be emitted for 100 disintegrations of radionuclide A and C, respectively? What is the energy of $\gamma_1$ and $\gamma_2$?

9. Which radionuclide, A or C, can be used as a radionuclidic generator? Identify the metastable state of nuclide B.

10. How many positrons will be emitted in 100 disintegrations of radionuclide C?

11. The average energy of a $\beta$ particle emitted in the decay of $^{18}F$ is 0.25 MeV.
    What is the approximate $E_{\beta max}$ for this transition?

12. Determine approximately the mass difference in MeV between an $^{18}F$ and $^{18}O$ atom (use the result of question 11).

# Radioactivity: Law of Decay, Half-Life, and Statistics

Radionuclides are unstable and decay to other nuclides by the processes discussed previously. At what rates do radionuclides decay? Do all radionuclides decay at the same rate? How many radioatoms (i.e., an atom whose nucleus is radioactive) remain after a given period of time? The answers to these and related questions constitute the primary subject matter of this chapter.

## Radioactivity: Definition, Units, and Dosage

The number of disintegrations of a sample of nuclei (atoms) per unit of time (decay rate) is called the radioactivity or simply the activity of a sample of a radionuclide. For example, if we have a collection of 1,000 atoms of a radionuclide at a given time and 50 of these disintegrate in the next 5 seconds, the activity of the sample is 50/5 = 10 disintegrations per second (dis/s). In algebraic terms, if out of a number $N_t$ of radioatoms at a time t, a number of radioatoms $dN_t$ decays in a small time interval dt, the radioactivity $R_t$ of the sample is calculated by dividing the number of radioatoms decayed ($dN_t$) by the interval (dt) during which the decay took place. In other words,

$$R_t = \frac{-dN_t}{dt} \qquad (1)$$

In this equation, the minus sign denotes that the radioatoms are decreasing in number.

A caveat: radioactivity is defined in terms of disintegrations or decays of parent nuclei and not in terms of particular type of radiations or total number of radiations emitted. As we saw in chapter 2, p 16, the number of radiation emitted per decay of parent nucleus varies from radionuclide to radionuclide. Therefore number of radiations being emitted per unit time from a radioactive sample will be different from the actual disintegration per unit time of nuclei in the sample.

The unit of radioactivity is the becquerel (Bq) in the current system of units système international (SI) and the curie (Ci) in the older system of units (centimeter-gram-seconds CGS). SI units have now replaced the older system of units in scientific work. Unfortunately, in clinical nuclear medicine, old units are still sometimes used. I use the new units here. However, to accommodate the users of the old units, these are included in parentheses for the important data, results, or problems. The major differences between the two systems of units are given in Appendix B.

A becquerel is defined as the radioactivity of a sample that is disintegrating at a rate of 1 disintegration/s, whereas a curie is defined as the radioactivity of a sample that is disintegrating at a rate of $3.7 \times 10^{10}$ disintegrations/s. Because the becquerel is a small unit, larger units derived from it are used. On the other hand, the curie is a large unit; therefore smaller units derived from it are often used. Some of these derived units for the curie and the becquerel and their interrelationships are given below:

$Bq = 1 \, dis/s = 27.03 \times 10^{-12} \, Ci = 27.03 \, pCi$

Kilobecquerel (KBq) $= 10^3 \, Bq = 27.03 \, nCi$

Megabecquerel (MBq) $= 10^6 \, Bq = 27.03 \, \mu Ci$

Gigabecquerel (GBq) $= 10^9 \, Bq = 27.03 \, mCi$

and

Curie (Ci) = $3.7 \times 10^{10}$ dis/s = 37 GBq
Millicurie (mCi) = $10^{-3} \times$ Ci = $3.7 \times 10^7$ dis/s
= 37 MBq
Microcurie ($\mu$Ci)= $10^{-6} \times$ Ci = $3.7 \times 10^4$ dis/s
= 37 KBq
Nanocurie (nCi) = $10^{-9} \times$ Ci = $3.7 \times 10$ dis/s
= 37 Bq
Picocurie (pCi) = $10^{-12} \times$ Ci = 3.7
$\times 10^{-2}$ dis/s or 0.037 Bq.

In nuclear medicine, the amount of radioactivity (MBq or mCi) administered to a patient is called dosage and not dose (to avoid confusion with another term, radiation dose, discussed in Chapter 7).

## Law of Decay

When a sample of a radionuclide is observed for a long period of time, it is found that the radioactivity R of a sample at a given time t depends on the number of the radioatoms $N_t$ present at that time and a constant $\lambda$ that is characteristic of a given radionuclide and is different for various radionuclides.

The constant $\lambda$, also known as the decay constant, is defined as the probability of decay per unit time for a single radioatom. Therefore, if there are $N_t$ radioatoms present at time t, then the number of nuclei disintegrating per unit time $R_t$, at time t, will be simply the product of $\lambda$ and $N_t$ or

$$R_t = \lambda \cdot N_t \qquad (2)$$

From this equation it can be seen that for the different radionuclides (i.e., different $\lambda$), number of radioatoms $N_t$ that must be present to produce the same amount of radioactivity $R_t$ varies. For example, the number of radioatoms present in a sample of $^{99m}$Tc, which has a radioactivity of 37 MBq (1 mCi), is not the same as the number of radioatoms present in a sample of $^{131}$I, which has a radioactivity of 37 MBq (1 mCi). This is true because the decay constant for $^{99m}$Tc ($\lambda$ = $3.2 \times 10^{-5}$/sec) is different from the decay constant for $^{131}$I ($\lambda = 10^{-6}$/sec). The number of radioatoms of $^{99m}$Tc or of $^{131}$I that must be

present in a sample to produce a radioactivity of 37 MBq can easily be determined from equation (2). For $^{99m}$Tc,

$$R_t = 37 \text{ MBq (1 mCi)} = 37 \times 10^6 \text{ dis/s and}$$
$$\lambda \ (^{99m}\text{Tc}) = 3.2 \times 10^{-5}/\text{s}$$

Therefore, from equation (2),

$$N_t \ (^{99m}\text{Tc}) = \frac{R_t}{\lambda} = \frac{37 \times 10^6}{3.2 \times 10^{-5}}$$
$$= 1.15 \times 10^{12} \text{ radioatoms}$$

For $^{131}$I,

$$R_t = 37 \text{ MBq (1 mCi) and } \lambda \ (^{131}\text{I}) = 10^{-6}/\text{sec}$$

Therefore, from equation (2),

$$N_t(^{131}\text{I}) = \frac{37 \times 10^6}{10^{-6}} = 3.7 \times 10^{13} =$$
$$32 \times N_t \ (^{99m}\text{Tc}) \text{ radioatoms}$$

(i.e., for the same amount of radioactivity, there are approximately 32 times more radioatoms present in a sample of $^{131}$I than in a sample of $^{99m}$Tc).

**Calculation of the Mass of a Radioactive Sample** Once we know the number of radioatoms $N_t$ present in a 1-mCi sample of a radionuclide of mass number A, it is simple to calculate the mass of the radionuclide present in that sample. Here we assume that the radioactive sample contains only the radionuclide under consideration and none of its isotopes.

From equation (2), for a 1-MBq sample,

$$N_t = \frac{1 \times 10^6}{\lambda}$$

From Avogadro's hypothesis, A grams of this radionuclide contain $6 \times 10^{23}$ radioatoms.

Therefore, mass of 1 radioatom = $\dfrac{A}{6 \times 10^{23}}$ g

or, mass, M, of $N_t$ radioatoms = $\dfrac{N_t \cdot A}{6 \times 10^{23}}$ g

or, substituting value of $N_t$,

$$\text{mass M} = \frac{1 \times 10^6 \times A}{6 \times 10^{23} \times \lambda} \text{ g/MBq}$$
$$= 1.67 \times 10^{-18} \cdot \text{A}/\lambda \text{ g/MBq}$$
$$[6 \times 10^{-17} \cdot \text{A}/\lambda \text{ g/mCi}]$$

Example:

**What is the mass of a 1 MBq sample of $^{99m}$Tc? The mass number for this radionuclide is 99 and the decay constant is $3.2 \times 10^{-5}$/s. Therefore,**

$$M = 1.67 \times 10^{-18} \times \frac{99}{3.2 \times 10^{-5}} = 5.17 \times 10^{-12}\,g$$

**Specific Activity** In the above calculations the mass of a 1-MBq sample was determined. In many instances, however, one is interested in the reciprocal of the above (i.e., the amount of radioactivity per unit mass of the radionuclide of interest). This, the radioactivity per unit mass of a radionuclide, is known as the specific activity of a radioactive sample. It is generally expressed in units such as MBq/mg (mCi/mg) or disintegration/min/mg. In the above example, the specific activity of the $^{99m}$Tc sample is simply the inverse of M or equal to $1/(5.17 \times 10^{-12})$ MBq/g or equal to $1.93 \times 10^{11}$ MBq/g or $1.93 \times 10^{8}$ MBq/mg.

In this example, it was assumed that all atoms of technetium were radioactive and no stable or longer-lived technetium atoms were present in the sample. Such a sample that contains only the radionuclide of interest and no other isotope or long-lived radioisotope of that radionuclide is generally called a "carrier-free" sample. Therefore, the above calculation of the specific activity applies only to a carrier-free sample. The specific activity of a sample with carrier (which contains stable or longer-lived isotopes of the radionuclide of interest) will always be less than that of a carrier-free sample and will depend on the amount of the carrier in the sample.

When a radionuclide is not present in its elemental form but is a part of a molecule, the concept of specific activity can be generalized to the mass of the molecule rather than the element. For instance in the above sample, if the technetium radioactivity is present as pertechnetate ($^{99m}$TcO$_4^-$) rather, than as $^{99m}$Tc, the specific radioactivity of the sample can also be expressed as radioactivity per unit mass of pertechnetate. Again, if the sample is carrier free (i.e., no molecules of pertechnetate exist in the sample that does not contain $^{99m}$Tc as its part or $^{99}$TcO$_4^-$ molecules are absent), the specific activity of a pertechnetate sample can be calculated as above by simply taking the inverse of M and

substituting the molecular weight of TcO$_4^-$ for A in the above formula. Because the molecular weight of TcO$_4^-$ is about 163, the specific activity of a 1-MBq sample of $^{99m}$TcO$_4^-$

$$= \frac{1}{M} = \frac{\lambda}{A \times 1.67 \times 10^{-18}} = \frac{3.2 \times 10^{-5}}{163 \times 1.67 \times 10^{-18}}$$

$= 1.18 \times 10^{11}$ MBq/g ($3.4 \times 10^{9}$ mCi/g). Of course, when the sample is not carrier free, the specific activity of the sample will be lower than that of a carrier-free sample and will depend on the amount of carrier present. In nuclear medicine, the knowledge of the specific activity of a sample is important for several reasons. First, the toxicity of a chemical or drug is always dependent on the amount of the chemical or drug administered to the patient. Therefore, it is important to know the amount of a particular chemical or drug in the radioactive sample. Second, the distribution of a radiochemical in a biological system many times depends on the amount of carrier present in the sample. Third, the labeling efficiency of a radionuclide to a chemical is also sometimes dependent on the specific activity of the radionuclide.

**The Exponential Law of Decay** If we combine equations (1) and (2), then

$$-\frac{dN_t}{d_t} = \lambda\,N_t$$

This is a differential equation whose solution is given by the following expression:

$$N_t = N_0 e^{-(\lambda \cdot t)} \qquad (3)$$

This equation relates the number of radioatoms $N_t$ remaining at time t when we initially started (at t = 0) with a number $N_0$ and is known as the exponential law of decay. When we plot this expression as a linear graph, curves similar to those shown in Figure 3.1 result for different radionuclides (different $\lambda$). When we plot the same expression on semi-log graph paper, as in Figure 3.2, we obtain straight lines of different slopes (steepness) for different radionuclides.

The exponential law of decay is also true for the radioactivity $R_t$; that is, $R_t$ is also related to the original radioactivity $R_0$ by an expression similar to equation (3). This can be seen easily

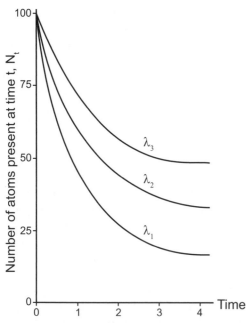

**Fig 3.1.** Linear plot of the number of radioatoms remaining at a time t as a function of time for three radionuclides with different decay constants: $\lambda_1$, $\lambda_2, \lambda_3$.

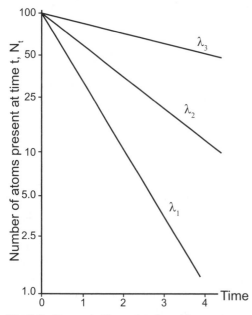

**Fig 3.2.** Data as in Figure 3.1 plotted here on a semi-logarithmic graph. Plot of an exponential function, on semi-log graph paper, results in a straight line. The slope of the straight line is determined by the decay constant or the half-life of the radionuclide.

by substituting equation (3) on the right side of equation (2):

$$\begin{aligned}
R_t &= \lambda\, N_t \\
&= \lambda \cdot N_0 \cdot e^{-(\lambda \cdot t)} \qquad (4) \\
\text{or} \quad R_t &= R_0 \cdot e^{-(\lambda \cdot t)}
\end{aligned}$$

where $R_0 = \lambda \cdot N_0$ is the radioactivity at time 0. If one plots activity $R_t$ as a function of time, curves similar to those shown in Figs. 3.1 and 3.2 result except that y axis will now represent the radioactivity.

## Half-Life

How does one determine the decay constant $\lambda$? Experimentally, it is more convenient to measure another parameter $T_{\frac{1}{2}}$, known as the half-life. This is defined as the time interval for a given number of nuclei (or their radioactivity) to decay to one-half of the original value. For example, if initially there are 10,000 nuclei in a radionuclide and 5000 of them decay in 5 days, then the half-life of this radionuclide is 5 days. Therefore, by definition of the half-life, when

$$N_t = \frac{N_0}{2}, \quad \text{then } t = T_{\frac{1}{2}}$$

If we substitute these values in equation (3), we obtain

$$\frac{N_0}{2} = N_0 e^{-(\lambda \cdot T_{\frac{1}{2}})}$$

Or

$$\frac{1}{2} = e^{-(\lambda \cdot T_{\frac{1}{2}})}$$

Because $e^{-0.693}$ is equal to 1/2 (see Appendix C), it follows that

$$\lambda \cdot T_{\frac{1}{2}} = 0.693 \qquad (5)$$

Equation (5) relates the decay constant to the half-life of a radionuclide. From this, if one knows the half-life of the radionuclide, one can calculate the decay constant or vice versa.

**Example:**
**Half-life of $^{131}$I = 8 days. Determine the decay constant for $^{131}$I**

$$T_{\frac{1}{2}} = 8 \text{ days} = 8 \times 24 \times 60 \times 60 \text{ seconds}$$

$$= 0.631 \times 10^6 \, s$$

**From equation (5),**

$$0.691 \times 10^6 \times \lambda = 0.693 \text{ or } \lambda = 10^{-6}/s$$

**Problems on Radioactive Decay** Equations (1) to (5) are the basic equations necessary for solving routine problems in nuclear medicine. In general, to solve such problems, use of exponential tables is necessary (Appendix C). However, in special cases, where multiples of half-life are involved, equation (3) can be written in a simpler form by substituting the value of $\lambda$ from equation (5).

$$N_t = N_0 e^{\frac{-(0.693t)}{T_{\frac{1}{2}}}}$$
$$= N_0(e^{-0.693})^{\frac{t}{T_{\frac{1}{2}}}} \tag{6a}$$
$$= N_0\left(\frac{1}{2}\right)^{\frac{t}{T_{\frac{1}{2}}}}$$

When t is a multiple of $T_{\frac{1}{2}}$, it is easier to make calculations using the above expression than to use exponential tables. For example, if one is interested in finding the number of radioatoms remaining after an interval t = 3 $\times$ the half-life of a radionuclide, the above expression becomes

$$N_t = N_0 \cdot \left(\frac{1}{2}\right)^{\frac{3 \times T_{\frac{1}{2}}}{T_{\frac{1}{2}}}} = N_0\left(\frac{1}{2}\right)^3$$
$$= N_0/8$$

or one-eighth of the original number. A similar simplification occurs for the activity:

$$R_t = R_0\left(\frac{1}{2}\right)^{\frac{t}{T_{\frac{1}{2}}}} \tag{6b}$$

Example 1:
A radioactive sample of $^{99m}$Tc contains 370 MBq (10 mCi) radioactivity at 9:00 a.m. What will be the radioactivity of this sample at 3:00 p.m. on the same day? (The half-life of $^{99m}$Tc is 6 hours.) In this example,

$R_0 = 370$ MBq (10 mCi)
$T_{\frac{1}{2}} = 6$ hours
$\quad$ t = 3:00 p.m. $-$ 9:00 a.m. = 6 hours

Now, using equation (6b)

$$R_t = 10 \cdot \left(\frac{1}{2}\right)^{6/6} = 10/2 = 185 \text{ MBq (5 mCi)}$$

Example 2:
A preparation of $^{99m}$Tc was calibrated at 7 a.m. and contained 555 MBq/mL (15 mCi/mL) of radioactivity at that time. If the prescribed dosage to the patient is 555 MBq (15 mCi), determine the volume of the preparation that will have to be injected at 10 a.m.

$R_0 = 555$ MBq/mL
$T_{\frac{1}{2}} = 6$ hours or $\lambda = \dfrac{0.693}{6}$/h
$\quad$ t = 10 a.m. $-$ 7 a.m. = 3 hours

Using equations (4) and (5)

$$R_t \text{ (at 10 a.m.)} = 555 \cdot e^{\frac{-0.693 \times 3}{6}}$$
$$= 555e \cdot {}^{-0.346}$$
$$= 555 \times 0.70 \text{ (from Appendix C)}$$
$$= 388.5 \text{ MBq/mL (10.5 mCi/mL)}$$
$$\text{Amount desired} = 555 \text{ MBq (15 mCi)}$$

$$\therefore \text{ Volume needed} = \frac{555 \text{ MBq}}{388.5 \text{ MBq/ml}} = 1.43 \text{ mL}$$

Example 3:
An iodine-123 capsule is calibrated to contain 100 $\mu$Ci (3.7 MBq) at noon. However, the capsule is given to a patient early in the morning at 9 a.m. Find the dosage of $^{123}$I administered to the patient. (Half-life of $^{123}$I = 13 hours.)

Let us assume that the radioactivity at 9 a.m. is $R_0$. Then, the radioactivity at noon (i.e., 3 hours later) is $R_t = 100$ $\mu$Ci. Using equations (4) and (5), we get

$$100 = R_0 \cdot e^{\frac{-0.693 \times 3}{13}} = R_0 \cdot e^{-0.16}$$
$$= R_0 \times 0.85 \text{ (from Appendix C)}$$
$$R_0 = \frac{100}{0.85} = 117.6 \text{ } \mu\text{Ci (4.3MBq)}$$

Quite often, the term $e^{-\lambda \cdot t}$ is tabulated for various intervals of time for a given radionuclide. These are known as decay factors. In example 3, the decay factor for $^{123}$I for 3-hour decay is 0.85. If the table of decay factors is available, then the relationship of $R_t$ and $R_0$ becomes simplified as $R_t = R_0 \times$ decay factor, where decay factor = $e^{-\lambda \cdot t}$. Table 3.1 lists some decay factors for $^{99m}$Tc.

For practical considerations, a simple fact to remember is that the radioactivity remaining after 10 half-lives of a radionuclide is about one-thousandth of the original radioactivity (i.e., MBq amounts are reduced to kBq amounts or millicurie amounts are reduced to microcurie amounts). This is so because $(1/2)^{10} \sim 1/1000$.

**Average Life ($T_{av}$)** Occasionally, we encounter the use of another term known as average life of a radionuclide. It is related to the half-life of the radionuclide or the decay constant $\lambda$ as follows:

$$T_{av} = 1.44 \times T_{\frac{1}{2}} = \frac{1}{\lambda}$$

Because in radioactive decay not all radioatoms decay at the same time, each individual radioatom exists for a different period of time. Average life is therefore the mean of all these intervals for which individual radioatoms remain in existence.

| **Table 3.1.** | Decay Factors for $^{99m}$Tc | | |
|---|---|---|---|
| **Elapsed Time (hr)** | **Decay Factor** | **Elapsed Time (hr)** | **Decay Factor** |
| 0.5 | 0.94 | 3.5 | 0.67 |
| 1.0 | 0.89 | 4.0 | 0.63 |
| 1.5 | 0.84 | 4.5 | 0.59 |
| 2.0 | 0.79 | 5.0 | 0.56 |
| 2.5 | 0.74 | 5.5 | 0.53 |
| 3.0 | 0.71 | 6.0 | 0.50 |

**Biological Half-Life**  Under many circumstances, the disappearance with time of a biochemical or drug in a biological system (e.g., thyroid, liver, lungs, bone, blood, plasma, or reticuloendothelial cells) can be described by an exponential law similar to that which holds true for radionuclidic decay. In this case, the disappearance of the biochemical or drug is accomplished through metabolism, excretion, simple diffusion, or some other ill-defined biomechanism. The amount $M_t$ of the biochemical or drug present in the biological system at time t can be determined by an equation similar to that used to determine radioactivity $R_t$ [equation (4)], provided the original amount $M_0$ of the biochemical or drug and the probability of its disappearance $\lambda_{Bio}$ in the biological system under consideration is known. In that case,

$$M_t = M_0 e^{-(\lambda_{Bio} \cdot t)} \qquad (7)$$

The disappearance probability $\lambda_{Bio}$ is related to the biological half-life $T_{\frac{1}{2}}(Bio)$, by an equation similar to equation (5):

$$\lambda_{Bio} \cdot T_{\frac{1}{2}}(Bio) = 0.693 \qquad (8a)$$

The biological half-life is defined as the interval during which a given amount of a biochemical or drug in a biological system is reduced to one-half its original value.

Often the disappearance of a biochemical or drug in the biological system cannot be described by equation (7). In these cases, the disappearance of the biochemical or the drug can be described by a sum of several exponential terms as follows:

$$M_t = M_0 \{A_1 e^{-\lambda 1 Bio \cdot t} + A_2 e^{-\lambda 2 Bio \cdot t} + ....\} \quad (8b)$$

where $A_1$, $A_2$... and $\lambda 1_{Bio}$, $\lambda 2_{Bio}$... are constants and are determined experimentally for a given drug in a given biological system.

**Effective Half-Life**  In nuclear medicine, one is interested in the distribution and the disappearance with time of radioactive substances or drugs from biological systems as a result of both physical decay and biological elimination (metabolism, diffusion, or excretion). Such information is crucial in radiation dose calculations to a patient and to determine the optimum time for imaging after the administration of the radiopharmaceutical.

In the simple case of mono-exponential biological distribution and disappearance [equation (7)], the probability of disappearance of a radiopharmaceutical from a biological system is the sum of both the physical and biological disappearance probabilities, i.e.:

$$\lambda + \lambda_{Bio} = \lambda_{eff} \qquad (9)$$

where $\lambda_{eff}$ is the effective disappearance probability for a radioactive substance or drug. If one converts the various disappearance constants in equation (9) to their respective half-lives, equation (9) becomes

$$\frac{0.693}{T_{\frac{1}{2}}} + \frac{0.693}{T_{\frac{1}{2}}(Bio)} = \frac{0.693}{T_{\frac{1}{2}}(eff)}$$

or

$$\frac{1}{T_{\frac{1}{2}}} + \frac{1}{T_{\frac{1}{2}}(Bio)} = \frac{1}{T_{\frac{1}{2}}(eff)} \qquad (10)$$

From this relationship [equation (10)], one can determine the effective half-life of a radiopharmaceutical if the physical half-life of the radionuclide and the biological half-life of the drug (or chemical) are known. As a rule, however,

$T_{\frac{1}{2}}$(eff) will always be less than or equal to the shorter of the two, $T_{\frac{1}{2}}$ and $T_{\frac{1}{2}}$(Bio).

In the complex case of biological distribution and disappearance [equation (8a)], it becomes difficult to define a single effective half-life unless each exponential represents a separate biological compartment or organ. Then, each compartment or organ has an effective half-life determined by the physical half-life and the biological half-life for that organ or compartment.

Example:

(1) The biological half-life of iodine in human thyroid is about 64 days, and the physical half-life of $^{131}$I is 8 days. Determine the effective half-life of $^{131}$I in the thyroid.

Given:

$$T_{\frac{1}{2}} = 8 \text{ days}, T_{\frac{1}{2}} \text{ (Bio)} = 64 \text{ days}$$

Therefore, from equation (10),

$$\frac{1}{T_{\frac{1}{2}} \text{ (eff)}} = \frac{1}{8} + \frac{1}{64} = \frac{9}{64}$$

or

$$T_{\frac{1}{2}} \text{ (eff)} = \frac{64}{9} = 7.1 \text{ days}$$

(2) Xenon-133, a radioactive inert gas, is used for lung-function studies. Its physical half-life is 5.3 days and its biological half-life in the lungs is about 0.35 minutes. Determine the effective half-life of $^{133}$Xe in the lungs. Given:

$$T_{\frac{1}{2}} = 5.3 \text{ days} = 5.3 \times 24 \times 60 \text{ minutes}$$
$$= 7632 \text{ minutes}$$
$$T_{\frac{1}{2}} \text{ (Bio)} = 0.35 \text{ minutes}$$

Therefore, from equation (10),

$$\frac{1}{T_{\frac{1}{2}} \text{ (eff)}} = \frac{1}{7632} + \frac{1}{0.35}$$

or

$$T_{\frac{1}{2}} \text{ (eff)} = 0.35 \text{ minutes}$$

In this example, $T_{\frac{1}{2}}$ (eff) = $T_{\frac{1}{2}}$ (Bio). Actually, whenever one of the half-lives, $T_{\frac{1}{2}}$ or $T_{\frac{1}{2}}$ (Bio), is very large (10 times or more) in comparison with the other, then $T_{\frac{1}{2}}$ (eff) is equal to the other half-life ($T_{\frac{1}{2}}$ (Bio) or $T_{\frac{1}{2}}$). In mathematical terms,

when $T_{\frac{1}{2}} \gg T_{\frac{1}{2}}$ (Bio), then $T_{\frac{1}{2}}$ (eff) $\approx T_{\frac{1}{2}}$ (Bio)

or

when $T_{\frac{1}{2}}$ (Bio) $\gg T_{\frac{1}{2}}$, then $T_{\frac{1}{2}}$ (eff) $\approx T_{\frac{1}{2}}$

# Statistics of Radioactive Decay

Although $\lambda$ is defined here as the probability of decay per unit time per atom, in earlier discussions it has been tacitly assumed that the number of radioatoms that decay in time t can be accurately determined. This is not so, nor is there any way to predict exactly which particular atom will decay at a given moment. In practice, the number of radioatoms that decay in a given time t fluctuate around an average value, and for this reason the equations described in the preceding sections express only the relationships of the average values of $N_t$ and $R_t$.

Because of these statistical variations in nuclear measurements, it is essential to know what contribution these fluctuations make to the total error of a measurement. Barring blunders, error in any measurement has two causes, systematic and random. Systematic errors are caused by the use of improperly calibrated instruments and will always either underestimate a measurement or overestimate it, depending on which way the error has been made in calibration. Random errors are caused by some uncontrollable factors. Therefore, when a number of repeat measurements are made, these tend to be randomly distributed. The term "accuracy" is used to describe systematic errors, whereas "precision" is used to describe random errors. In radioactivity measurements, random errors that are the result of the natural decay process dominate over the systematic errors and therefore are taken into account only. I should point out here that this discussion of errors is not limited only to counting but is of importance in imaging as well.

## Poisson Distribution, Standard Deviation, and Percent Standard Deviation

The probability that a given number of disintegrations N will actually occur in a radioactive sample in time t, when the mean number of disintegrations for that sample is $\overline{N}$ is determined by the Poisson distribution. The mathematical or graphic description of Poisson distribution is complicated. Therefore, it is generally approximated with a Gaussian or standard distribution, shown in Figure 3.3. A Gaussian distribution,

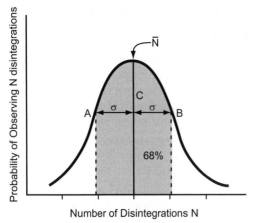

Probability of Observing N disintegrations

Number of Disintegrations N

**Fig 3.3.** Poisson distribution (for large values of N, it is similar to a Gaussian distribution) showing the random nature of radioactivity. The width $\sigma$ (AC or BC) is known as standard deviation SD. A range of N + $\sigma$ to N − $\sigma$ (A to B) covers about 68% of the total area of the distribution curve.

which is completely determined by two parameters, mean $\overline{N}$ and standard deviation $\sigma$, is given by the following expression

$$P(N) = \frac{1}{\sigma\sqrt{2\pi}} \cdot e^{-\frac{1}{2}\left(\frac{N-\overline{N}}{\sigma}\right)^2}$$

where P(N) is the probability for observing N disintegrations, $\overline{N}$ is the average number of disintegrations, and $\sigma$ is the standard deviation SD. SD determines the spread or width of a Gaussian (or Poisson) distribution and is commonly used as a measure of random error, or precision, of a radioactive measurement.

A range of N − $\sigma$ to N + $\sigma$ (1 SD) implies that the probability of a given measurement lying within this range is about 68%. When the range is extended to include 2 SDs (N − $2\sigma$ to N + $2\sigma$), the probability increases to 95%. Further extension of the range to include 3 SDs (N − $3\sigma$ N + $3\sigma$) increases the probability to 99%.

An important characteristic of Poisson distribution is the relation of its SD to the mean number of disintegrations $\overline{N}$ as follows:

$$\sigma = \sqrt{\overline{N}} \qquad (11)$$

For large values of $\overline{N}$, this equation allows a rapid determination of the SD of a given measurement if we replace $\overline{N}$ by N.

A more useful index of statistical error or precision of a measurement than SD is percent

standard deviation % SD. The % SD of a measurement is determined as follows:

$$\%SD = \frac{\sigma}{N} \times 100 = \frac{\sqrt{N}}{N} \times 100 = \frac{100}{\sqrt{N}} \quad (12)$$

This equation states that the precision of a given radioactive measurement can be increased by increasing the observed number of disintegration. In practical terms, this means that if we measure a radioactive sample for 1 minute and obtain 100 disintegrations during this time, then its % SD, as determined from the above relationship, will be equal to

$$\frac{100}{\sqrt{100}}$$

or 10%. However, if we measure the sample long enough (approximately 100 times longer) so that there are 10,000 disintegrations during this interval, the % SD in this case will be equal to

$$\frac{100}{\sqrt{10000}}$$

or 1%. In other words, by increasing the time of counting (approximately 100 times), we have decreased the percent error in our results (only by a factor of 10). When the time of counting is limited, a compromise has to be made between the length of counting time and precision.

**Propagation of Statistical Errors** In many nuclear applications, we have to add, subtract, multiply, or divide two or more measurements. How does one determine the precision of the final result? To answer this question, let us assume that N1 and N2 are two measurements from which the final result N is obtained by adding, subtracting, dividing, or multiplying N1 and N2. Without going into detail, then, the SD of N is given by the following expressions:

$$SD\,(N1 \pm N2) = \sqrt{SD\,(N1)^2 + SD\,(N2)^2}$$

$$SD\,(N1 \times N2) = (N1 \times N2)$$
$$\times \sqrt{\left\{\frac{SD(N1)}{N1}\right\}^2 + \left\{\frac{SD(N2)}{N2}\right\}^2}$$

$$SD\,(N1/N2) = (N1/N2)$$
$$\times \sqrt{\left\{\frac{SD(N1)}{N1}\right\}^2 + \left\{\frac{SD(N2)}{N2}\right\}^2}$$

The % SD of N is given by the following expressions:

When adding:

$$\%SD = \frac{100}{\sqrt{N1 + N2}} \qquad (13)$$

When subtracting:

$$\%SD = \frac{100 \cdot \sqrt{N1 + N2}}{N1 - N2} \quad (14)$$

When multiplying or dividing:

$$\%SD = \sqrt{(\%SD \text{ of } N1)^2 + (\%SD \text{ of } N2)^2} \quad (15)$$

**Error in Count Rate** Count rate R of a sample is determined by dividing the number of counts N observed in a time interval t by the time interval t or

$$R = \frac{N}{t} \quad \text{or} \quad N = R \cdot t \quad (16)$$

Because the error in the measurement of time t is generally very small, the error in R mainly results from the error in N. Therefore,

$$\sigma_R = \frac{\sigma_N}{t} = \frac{\sqrt{N}}{t} \quad (17)$$

Substituting $N = R \cdot t$ from equation (16), we get

$$\sigma_R = \frac{\sqrt{R \cdot t}}{t} = \sqrt{\frac{R}{t}} \quad (18)$$

To reduce the error of a count rate R, one has to increase the averaging time t. The % $\sigma_R$ of a count rate is given by the following expression:

$$\%\sigma_R = \frac{\sigma_R \times 100}{R} = \sqrt{\frac{R}{t}} \cdot \frac{100}{R}$$
$$= \frac{100}{\sqrt{R \cdot t}} = \frac{100}{\sqrt{N}} \quad (19)$$

**Room Background** Even when there is no radioactive sample near a radiation detector, it will still record a certain number of disintegrations known as room background. This is due to the presence of minute amounts of radioactivity in the surrounding earth and/or building material. Part of the room background is also contributed by the high-energy radiations of cosmic rays. Room background can be reduced to a low level by shielding the radiation detector. However, it cannot be reduced to zero because of the presence of trace amounts of radioactive substances in the detector and shielding materials themselves and because of the inability to completely shield against high-energy background radiation. In situations where the sample count rate is very low (less than ten times of background), it is important to take into consideration the room background and its effect on the precision of the final result.

Examples

(1) In the thyroid uptake measurement of a patient, it is found that the neck activity gives 900 counts per minute, whereas the standard is 2500 counts per minute. Calculate the % uptake by the thyroid and its precision.

$$\%uptake = \frac{counts \text{ in neck}}{counts \text{ in standard}} \times 100$$
$$= \frac{900}{2500} \times 100 = 36\%$$

Using equation (12),

$$\%SD \text{ in neck counts} = \frac{100}{\sqrt{900}} = 3.3\%$$

and

$$\%SD \text{ in standard counts} = \frac{100}{\sqrt{2500}} = 2\%$$

Using equation (15),

$$\%SD \text{ of thyriod uptake} = \sqrt{3.3^2 + 2^2}$$
$$= \sqrt{11 + 4} = 4\%$$

Therefore,

Thyroid uptake = (36 ± 4%) %

Because 4% of 36 is 1.4,

Thyroid uptake = (36 ± 1.4) %

(2) A radioactive sample registers a total (sample + background) of 3200 counts in 1 minute. The room background is 1000 counts per minute. Calculate the net counts of the sample and the % SD of the total counts, background, and the net counts, respectively.

Net counts in the sample

$$= total \text{ counts} - background \text{ counts}$$
$$= 3200 - 1000$$
$$= 2200 \text{ counts}$$

Using equation (12),

$$\%SD \text{ of the total counts} = \frac{100}{\sqrt{3200}} = 1.7\%$$

and

$$\%SD \text{ of the background counts} = \frac{100}{\sqrt{1000}} = 3.1\%$$

Using equation (14),

$$\%SD \text{ of the net counts} = \frac{100\sqrt{3200 + 1000}}{3200 - 1000}$$
$$= \frac{100\sqrt{4200}}{2200} = 2.9\%$$

This clearly demonstrates the manner in which the room background degrades the precision of a radioactive measurement.

## Key Points

1. Radioactivity of a sample is defined as the rate of decay. Its unit is Bq (1 disintegration/s) in SI units and curie ($3.7 \times 10^{10}$ disintegration/s) in old units.
2. Radioactivity of a sample at time t, $R_t$ depends on the radioatoms $N_t$ present at that instant and a characteristic decay constant of the radionuclide, $\lambda$ and $R_t = \lambda N_t$.
3. $N_t$ and $R_t$ decay with time through law of exponential (i.e., $N_t$ or $R_t = N_0$ or $R_0 e^{-\lambda t}$).
4. Half-life of a radionuclide is related to the decay constant, $\lambda$ as $\lambda T_{\frac{1}{2}} = 0.693$.
5. Biological half-life and effective half-life are defined in a similar fashion to physical half-life of a radionuclide for a biochemical and a biochemical labeled with a radionuclide, respectively.

6. Radioactive decay is random and follows Poisson statistics. It is impossible to predict how many decays will occur exactly in a given second or minute.
7. Standard deviation SD is used to measure the range in which such decay may lie. This is used to quantify error of a radioactive measurement.
8. For Poisson distribution, SD is related to the average count of a measurement as

$$SD = (\text{average count})^{1/2}.$$

9. One SD range has a 68%, two SD range a 95%, and three SD range a 99% confidence level.
10. When two measurements of radioactivity are added, subtracted, multiplied, or divided, special rules for propagation of errors apply.

## Questions

1. Determine the radioactivity of a sample disintegrating at a rate of 10,000 disintegrations per second in (a) millicuries and (b) megabecquerels.
2. What is a 10-mCi dosage of $^{99m}$Tc radiopharmaceutical equivalent to in SI units?
3. If the decay constant $\lambda$ of the radionuclide in problem 1 is (a) 0.1 per second and (b) 0.1 per hour, how many radioatoms are present in this sample?
4. Determine the radioactivity of a $^{99m}$Tc sample (370 MBq at 0 time) after (a) 9 hours, (b) 12 hours, and (c) 60 hours of decay.
5. A $^{99m}$Tc radiopharmaceutical at 8 a.m. contained 850 MBq/ml of radioactivity. Determine the volume to be injected to a patient at 9 a.m., 11:30 a.m., 2:15 p.m. and 3 p.m. if the dosage to be injected in the patient is 1,000 MBq.
6. How long will it take for the radioactivity of a sample to decay to its 25% value if the radionuclide is (a) $^{201}$Tl, (b) $^{99}$Mo, or (c) $^{67}$Ga?
7. The biological half-life of $^{99m}$Tc macroaggregated albumin in the lungs is 6 hours. What is the effective half-life of this agent in the lungs?
8. How many counts are needed to make the standard deviation equal to 1%?

9. A series of 100 1-minute measurements were made, giving an average count rate of 1600 counts per minute. Of these, how many are in the range of $1600 \pm 80$?
10. A 99% confidence level of counts taken at the rate of 1,200 counts per minute for 3 minutes is _____ counts.
11. If one obtains 10,000 counts in 5 minutes, what is the standard deviation of the count rate?
12. Sample A yields 900 counts per minute and sample B 500 counts per minute. What is the % SD of quantity C if it relates to A and B as (a) C = count rate of sample A/count rate of sample B and (b) C = count rate of sample A − count rate of sample B.
13. How many gamma rays of 140 keV are emitted by one mCi of $^{99m}$Tc sample (use Table 2.2)?
14. How many gamma rays of 172 keV are emitted by 1 Mbq of $^{111}$In sample (use Appendix A)?
15. How many gamma rays of 364 keV are emitted by 10 microcurie of $^{131}$I sample (use appendix A)?
16. What is the SD and % SD of the light photons produced in question 7, Chapter 1?

# 4

# Production of Radionuclides

In 1896, Henry Becquerel discovered that uranium was radioactive. Soon after, other naturally occurring radionuclides such as radium and polonium were discovered. Most naturally occurring radionuclides have long half-lives (greater than 1000 years) and are not used in nuclear medicine. The radionuclides most commonly used in nuclear medicine (see Appendix D) are artificial and produced by three basic methods:

1. Irradiation of stable nuclides in a reactor (reactor produced)
2. Irradiation of stable nuclides in an accelerator or cyclotron (accelerator or cyclotron produced)
3. Fission of heavier nuclides (fission produced).

## Methods of Radionuclide Production

**Reactor-Produced Radionuclides** A nuclear reactor (for a description of a nuclear reactor, see Fission-Produced Radionuclides) is a source of a large number of thermal neutrons. Thermal neutrons are those neutrons whose kinetic energy is very small ($\sim 0.025$ eV, which is the kinetic energy of atoms or molecules at room temperature). At these energies, neutrons can be easily captured by stable nuclides because neutrons that are neutral particles do not experience the repulsive coulomb forces of the positively charged nucleus. The capture reaction of neutrons with a given nuclide $_{Z}^{A}X$ is represented by either of the following notations:

(i) $_{Z}^{A}X + _{0}^{1}n \rightarrow {}_{Z}^{A+1}X + \gamma\text{-rays}$

(ii) $_{Z}^{A}X \, (n, \gamma) \, _{Z}^{A+1}X$

In (i), the reactants are to the left of the arrow, and the products of the reaction are to the right. The first equation is written as a chemical reaction; the second equation is a short notation for the same. It can be seen that in the above nuclear reaction, the atomic number (and therefore the chemical nature or element) of the resulting nuclide ($_{Z}^{A+1}X$) does not change; only the mass number A increases by one. Because in this reaction a neutron is being added, the resulting nuclide (if radioactive) quite often decays through $\beta^-$ emission. I say "if radioactive" because for many neutron capture reactions, the resulting nuclide is stable [e.g., $_{6}^{12}C \, (n, \gamma) \, _{6}^{13}C$]. In this example, the $_{6}^{13}C$ nuclide is a stable nuclide. Another feature of reactor-produced nuclides is that these, in general, are not carrier free. In a carrier-free sample, only the desired radionuclide is present without contamination from its other isotopes. A sample of $_{53}^{131}I$ can be called carrier free only if no other stable isotope or radioisotope of iodine is present in the sample.

Some of the reactor-produced radionuclides used in nuclear medicine and the nuclear reactions producing them, are given below:

(i) $_{24}^{50}Cr + _{0}^{1}n \rightarrow {}_{24}^{51}Cr + \gamma$

$^{51}Cr$ is used for labeling red blood cells and spleen scanning.

(ii) $_{42}^{98}Mo + _{0}^{1}n \rightarrow {}_{42}^{99}Mo + \gamma$

$^{99}Mo$ is the source of $^{99m}Tc$, which is so commonly used in nuclear medicine. Presently this is the only method of commercial production of this radionuclide. In North America, there is only one reactor that is the source of all $^{99}$Mo and periodic shutdown of this reactor causes shortage of this important radionuclide. Other methods for its production are being explored as described in next section.

$$\text{(iii)} \quad ^{132}_{54}\text{Xe} + {}^{1}_{0}\text{n} \rightarrow {}^{133}_{54}\text{Xe} + \gamma$$

$^{133}$Xe is used for lung ventilation studies.

### Accelerator- or Cyclotron-Produced Radionuclides

An accelerator or cyclotron is the source of a large number of high-energy (MeV range) charged particles such as p (protons), $^{2}_{1}$D (deuterons), $^{3}_{2}$He (helium 3), and $^{4}_{2}$He $\alpha$) particles. The classification of an accelerator or a cyclotron depends on the way in which these charged particles are accelerated and is not relevant here. The probability of a nuclear reaction occurring with charged particles is highly dependent on the energy of the bombarding particles. For each charged particle and target, there is a threshold energy below which the nuclear reaction does not occur at all. This is due to the repulsive coulomb forces between the positively charged particle and the positively charged target nuclide. Generally, the threshold energy is in the MeV range. The most common reactions for protons are

$$\text{(i)} \quad ^{A}_{Z}\text{X} + {}^{1}_{1}\text{p} \rightarrow {}^{A}_{Z+1}\text{Y} + \text{n}$$

or

$$^{A}_{Z}\text{X} \ (\text{p,n}) \ ^{A}_{Z+1}\text{Y}$$

$$\text{(ii)} \quad ^{A}_{Z}\text{X} + {}^{1}_{1}\text{p} \rightarrow {}^{A-1}_{Z+1}\text{Y} + 2\text{n}$$

or

$$^{A}_{Z}\text{X} + (\text{p, 2n}) \ ^{A+1}_{Z+1}\text{Y}$$

The most common reactions for deuterons, $^{2}_{1}$D (also known as heavy hydrogen), are (in short notations)

$$\text{(iii)} \quad ^{A}_{Z}\text{X}({}^{2}_{1}\text{D, n}) \ ^{A+1}_{Z+1}\text{Y}$$
$$\text{(iv)} \quad ^{A}_{Z}\text{X} \ ({}^{2}_{1}\text{D, p}) \ ^{A+1}_{Z}\text{Y}$$
$$\text{(v)} \quad ^{A}_{Z}\text{X} \ ({}^{2}_{1}\text{D, 2n}) \ ^{A}_{Z+1}\text{Y}$$

Common nuclear reactions for $^{3}_{2}$He particles are

$$\text{(vi)} \quad ^{A}_{Z}\text{X} \ ({}^{3}_{2}\text{He, n}) \ ^{A+2}_{Z+2}\text{Y}$$

$$\text{(vii)} \quad ^{A}_{Z}\text{X}({}^{3}_{2}\text{He, p}) \ ^{A+2}_{Z+1}\text{Y}$$

Common reactions for $\alpha$ ($^{4}_{2}$He) particles are

$$\text{(viii)} \quad ^{A}_{Z}\text{X} \ ({}^{4}_{2}\text{He, n}) \ ^{A+3}_{Z+2}\text{Y}$$
$$\text{(ix)} \quad ^{A}_{Z}\text{X} \ ({}^{4}_{2}\text{He, 2n}) \ ^{A+2}_{Z+2}\text{Y}$$

Most of the above reactions occur in the range of 5 to 30 MeV. As the energy of the bombarding particles further increases, other nuclear reactions occur. Sometimes these additional reactions may also be useful for producing radionuclides. Some radionuclides used routinely in nuclear medicine and produced in an accelerator or cyclotron, are given below:

$$\text{(i)} \quad ^{16}_{8}\text{O} + {}^{3}_{2}\text{He} \rightarrow {}^{18}_{9}\text{F} + \text{p}$$

$^{18}$F is used for labeling radiopharmaceuticals for positron emission tomography.

$$\text{(ii)} \quad ^{68}_{30}\text{Zn} + \text{p} \rightarrow {}^{67}_{31}\text{Ga} + 2\text{n}$$

$^{67}$Ga is widely used for soft tumor and occult abscess detection.

$$\text{(iii)} \quad ^{98}_{42}Mo + D \rightarrow {}^{99}_{42}Mo + \text{p}$$

This is currently being explored as an alternative to reactor produced $^{99}$Mo.

In the above examples, the radionuclide of interest is formed directly as a result of a particular nuclear reaction. Sometimes, the radionuclide of interest may be formed indirectly by the decay of another radionuclide that is formed first with a nuclear reaction. Two examples of these indirect methods are the production of radionuclides $^{123}$I and $^{201}$Tl:

(1) Production of $^{123}$I

  (i) Nuclear reaction, $^{122}_{52}\text{Te} + {}^{4}_{2}\text{He} \rightarrow {}^{123}_{54}\text{Xe}$ + 3n (2 hours, half-life)

  (ii) Decay, $^{123}_{54}\text{Xe} \xrightarrow{\text{E.C.}\beta}$ (13 hours, half-life)

(2) Production of $^{201}$Tl

  (i) Nuclear reaction, $^{203}_{81}\text{Tl} + \text{p} \rightarrow {}^{201}_{82}\text{Pb}$ + 3n (9.4 hours, half-life)

  (ii) Decay, $^{201}_{82}\text{Pb} \xrightarrow{\text{E.C.}} {}^{201}_{83}\text{Tl}$ (73 hours, half-life)

Because in charged-particle nuclear reactions the resultant radionuclide generally has an atomic number different from that of the target nuclide, one can chemically separate the two. Therefore, the radionuclides produced by charged particle reactions are generally carrier free. Also, because in these reactions protons are added to a nuclide, these are generally $\beta^+$- or electron-capturing radionuclides.

**Fission-Produced Radionuclides** Soon after the discovery of radioactivity, naturally occurring radioactive nuclides such as $^{226}_{88}\text{Ra}$, $^{232}_{90}\text{Th}$, or $^{210}_{84}\text{Po}$ were found to be good sources of $\alpha$ particles. The reactions of these $\alpha$ particles produced neutrons by $^A_Z\text{X} \, (\alpha, \, n)$, $^{A+3}_{Z+2}\text{Y}$. When the reactions of the neutrons thus generated were systematically studied, a surprising discovery was made. For many heavier nuclei (A $\sim$ 200), it was found that capture of a neutron, instead of producing a heavier radionuclide, resulted in the production of several radionuclides whose mass numbers were about one-half that of the target nuclide. For example, in the case of $^{235}\text{U}$, $^{235}_{92}\text{U} + ^1_0\text{n} \rightarrow ^{236}_{92}\text{U} + \gamma$ seldom occurs. Instead, $^{235}_{92}U + ^1_0n \rightarrow ^{141}_{56}Ba + ^{91}_{36}Kr + 4\,^1_0n$ is a much more frequent reaction.

This process of splitting a heavier nucleus into two small nuclei is called fission. Barium and krypton are not the only elements formed in fission. Actually, every element from zinc (Z = 30) to dysprosium (Z = 66) has been identified in fission reaction. Besides the production of radionuclides of intermediate elements (Z = 30 to 66) during fission, another important result is the production of a large number of neutrons (in the above example, four). A neutron initiates the fission by being captured, yet more than one neutron is produced during fission. These extra neutrons can then cause further fission, thereby producing an even larger number of neutrons. This process is a chain reaction and will theoretically continue until the supply of fissionable material is exhausted. An uncontrolled chain reaction of fissionable material is called an atomic bomb. A controlled chain reaction, however, that is a very good source of a large number of neutrons and of energy (for producing electricity) is known as a nuclear reactor. Iodine-131, so commonly used in nuclear medicine, is produced by fission. Another example of a fission-produced radionuclide is $^{99}\text{Mo}$, the parent radionuclide of

$^{99m}\text{Tc}$. Like cyclotron- or accelerator-produced radionuclides, fission-produced radionuclides are also generally carrier free.

## General Considerations in the Production of Radionuclides

The amount of radioactivity $R_t$ produced in time t in a nuclear reaction depends on the following factors:

1. The number of bombarding particles/s/$cm^2$ known as Flux, I;
2. The total number of the target nuclei irradiated, n × V, when n is the number of the target nuclides in 1 $cm^3$ and V is the volume of the target material being irradiated;
3. The time of irradiation t;
4. The half-life or the decay constant of the radionuclide produced (i.e., $T_{\frac{1}{2}}$ or $\lambda$);
5. The probability of the given nuclear reaction, called the cross section $\sigma$. The unit for cross section is a barn, which is equal to $10^{-24}$ $cm^2$.

In the case of neutron capture reactions (reactor-produced radionuclides), the formula relating the above factors to the activity produced after time t is

$$R_t = \sigma \cdot I \cdot n \cdot V \cdot (1 - e^{-\lambda t}) \qquad (1)$$

Because of the factor $(1 - e^{-\lambda t})$, it does not pay to irradiate a target for more than one half-life of the desired radionuclide. In cases where the half-life of the desired radionuclide is sufficiently long (in days), the above equation can be reduced to a simpler form:

$$R_t = \sigma \cdot I \cdot n \cdot V \cdot \lambda \cdot t \qquad (2)$$

A similar equation can be written for charged particle nuclear reactions. In practice, however, the flux of charged particles is measured as $\mu$amp (a unit of electric current) instead of the number per s/$cm^2$. In this case, too, the amount of activity produced will depend on the five factors given above. In general, the values quoted for the activity produced by charged-particle reactions are in units of MBq/$\mu$amp/h and are known as the yield of a particular reaction. The higher the yield for a particular nuclear reaction, the easier it is to produce large quantities of the given radionuclide. In selecting the best method of radionuclide production, one has to take into account yield, which is an economical consideration, and purity and the specific activity of the radionuclide, which are biological or scientific considerations and therefore depend on the particular use of the radionuclide.

## Production of Short-Lived Radionuclides Using a Generator

Because of the reduction in radiation dose to the patient, short-lived radionuclides are often the agents of choice in nuclear medicine. In general, however, the use of short-lived radionuclides entails many problems due to their fast decay. For example, the short half-life of a radionuclide limits the available time for such purposes as processing, transportation, storage, and quality control. For this reason, $^{18}$F, with a half-life of 100 minutes, does not have widespread use as a bone-scanning agent. Similar limitations apply to the widespread use of other short-lived radionuclides such as $^{11}$C (20.3 minutes), $^{13}$N (10 minutes), and $^{15}$O (2 minutes), which are quite attractive from other considerations. A radionuclide generator described below (also referred to as a "cow") solves some of the above problems and allows the use of short-lived radionuclides at long distances from the site of production (e.g., a cyclotron or reactor).

**Principles of a Generator** A radionuclidic generator is a two- or three-step radioactive series in which a long-lived radionuclide (also called "parent") decays into a short-lived radionuclide (also known as "daughter") of interest.

The following are some examples of radionuclide generators. The first generator system is the most common in use today with scintillation camera imaging. The second generator produces $^{81m}$Kr is used in lung ventilation studies. The third and fourth generators are receiving attention because of their special advantages for positron tomography. The fifth and sixth gen-

erators are used in radiotherapy for variety of diseases because the daughter radionuclides mainly emit β particles.

(i)     $^{99}$Mo → $^{99m}$Tc → $^{99}$Tc → $^{99}$Ru

Half-life:   67 hours   6 hours   long   stable

(ii)     $^{81}$Rb → $^{81m}$Kr → $^{81}$Kr

Half-life:   4.7 hours   13 seconds   stable

(iii)     $^{68}$Ge → $^{68}$Ga → $^{68}$Zn

Half-life:   275 days   1.1 hours   stable

(iv)     $^{82}$Sr → $^{82}$Rb → $^{82}$Kr

Half-life:   25 days   75 seconds   stable

(v)     $^{90}$Sr → $^{90}$Y → $^{90}$Zr

Half-life:   28 years   64 hours   stable

(vi)     $^{188}$W → $^{188}$Re → $^{188}$Os

Half-life:   69 days   16.7 hours   stable

In a radioactive series, the daughter radionuclide is being continuously produced by the decay of the parent radionuclide and is being continuously destroyed by its own decay. If the half-life of the parent radionuclide is longer than the half-life of the daughter radionuclide, an important phenomenon occurs that is the basis of the generators presently used in nuclear medicine. Under this condition (i.e., $T_{\frac{1}{2}}$ parent greater than $T_{\frac{1}{2}}$ daughter) and in due course, equilibrium is established between the parent and daughter radionuclides. In the state of equilibrium, the ratio of the amounts (number of radionuclei present) of the two radionuclides becomes constant. The two radioactivities also maintain a constant ratio (this ratio is in general very close to unity) with time even though the half-lives of the two radionuclides are quite different. In effect, the daughter radioactivity decays with an apparent half-life of the parent radionuclide rather than its own. For example, in a $^{99}$Mo–$^{99m}$Tc generator, the $^{99m}$Tc radioactivity in equilibrium with $^{99}$Mo decays with a half-life of 67 rather than 6 hours. The growth and decay of the daughter activity in a generator can be exactly predicted using the decay laws given in Chapter 3. Rather than going through complicated mathematics, we show this relationship graphically in Figures 4.1

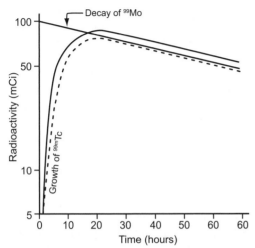

**Fig. 4.1.** Growth and decay of $^{99m}$Tc radioactivity in the decay of $^{99}$Mo. It takes about 24 hours for equilibrium to establish. For the solid curve, it is assumed that all disintegrations of $^{99}$Mo produce technetium, $^{99m}$Tc. The broken curve represents the actual radioactivity of $^{99m}$Tc because only 92% of disintegrations of $^{99}$Mo produce $^{99m}$Tc. The remaining 8% of $^{99}$Mo disintegrations produce the ground state, $^{99}$Tc, via short-lived isomers.

and 4.2 for the two most common generators. In both cases, it can be seen that it takes about four daughter half-lives to reach equilibrium. For a $^{99}$Mo–$^{99m}$Tc generator, it is about 24 hours, whereas for a $^{68}$Ge–$^{68}$Ga generator it is about

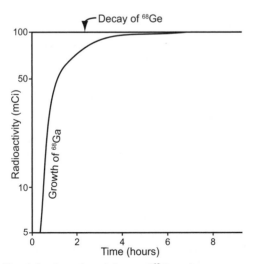

**Fig. 4.2.** Growth and decay of $^{68}$Ga radioactivity in the decay of $^{68}$Ge. It takes approximately 4.4 hours for equilibrium to be established.

4.4 hours. It is also evident from Figures 4.1 and 4.2 that the growth of the daughter radioactivity is not linear with time. Instead, it takes about one daughter half-life to reach 50%, two daughter half-lives to reach 75%, and three daughter half-lives to reach 87% of the equilibrium level. Similar considerations apply to other generator systems cited above.

Caveat: The Figures 4.1 and 4.2 are showing the radioactivities of the parent and daughter radionuclides (disintegration rate of the radionuclei of each radionuclide). These are not the actual number of radionuclei present in the sample. Actual number of parent nuclei will always be much larger than the number of daughter radionuclei (for $^{99}$Mo–$^{99m}$Tc generator there about 11 times $^{99}$Mo radionuclei present at a given time than those of $^{99m}$Tc). Simply put we cannot create more daughter radionuclei than the number of parent radionuclei present in the sample.

Once equilibrium has been achieved between the parent and daughter radioactivities, it can be disturbed only by chemical separation of the two radionuclides. Chemical separation is also referred as elution of daughter radionuclide or "milking." After chemical separation, the daughter radioactivity again grows and reestablishes equilibrium (in about four daughter half-lives) with the parent radioactivity, although at a new level. In other words, one has a fresh supply of the daughter radionuclide available for milking each four daughter half-lives after the previous milking. However, one does not necessarily have to wait four daughter half-lives before milking. Four daughter half-life intervals provide the maximum obtainable yield from a generator. If an emergency supply of the daughter radionuclide is needed, the generator can be re-milked sooner. For example, after one daughter half-life, re-milking will provide about 50% of the maximum obtainable radioactivity of the daughter radionuclide.

The state of equilibrium between the parent and daughter radionuclides is sometimes classified in two categories, transient and secular. When the half-life of a parent radionuclide is not long in comparison with the half-life of the daughter radionuclide, the equilibrium is called transient. $^{99}$Mo–$^{99m}$Tc generator is an example of transient equilibrium. On the other hand, when the half-life of the parent radionuclide is much longer than that of the daughter radionuclide, the equilibrium is termed secular. An example of secular equilibrium is $^{68}$Ge–$^{68}$Ga generator. In secular equilibrium, the activities of the parent and daughter radionuclides become nearly equal, whereas in transient equilibrium, the daughter radioactivity is slightly higher than the parent radioactivity. This distinction between secular and transient equilibrium is of academic interest only, as it carries no practical significance.

Because, in the case of a generator, a daughter radionuclide is chemically separated from the parent, the daughter radionuclide is produced almost carrier free. I say almost carrier free because the daughter radionuclide, being a metastable state, decays to the same element (e.g., $^{99m}$Tc → $^{99}$Tc). As a consequence, and particularly when the generator has not been milked for some time, sufficient amounts of the stable (or almost stable in the case of $^{99}$Tc, a long-lived radionuclide) isotope build up in the generator. At the time of milking, this stable isotope will also be milked with the desired radioisotope (e.g., $^{99m}$Tc eluate always contains small, but variable, amounts of $^{99}$Tc), and therefore such a sample cannot be strictly classified as carrier free.

**Description of a Typical Generator** A typical generator comprises a glass column filled with a suitable exchange material such as alumina ($Al_2O_3$). The bottom of the glass column is fitted with a porous glass disk to retain the alumina in the column (Fig. 4.3). The parent radionuclide in equilibrium with its daughter is firmly absorbed on the top of the alumina. The daughter radionuclide is separated (eluted or milked) from its parent radionuclide by passing a special liquid (eluting solution) through the column at a suitable flow rate. The daughter is dissolved in the eluting solution, whereas the parent is retained by the column.

In a typical $^{99}$Mo–$^{99m}$Tc generator, the column is filled with alumina, $^{99}$Mo is part of the molecule, sodium molybdate, and the eluting solution is oxidant-free physiologic saline (0.9% sodium chloride solution). The technetium radioactivity elutes in the form of sodium pertechnetate ($Na^{99m}TcO_4$). Molybdenum-99 used in these generators is produced either by irradiation of $^{98}$Mo with neutrons or by fission of $^{235}$U in a reactor. Molybdenum-99 produced in fission reactions is essentially carrier free, and therefore has very high specific activity. On the other hand, $^{99}$Mo produced by neutron irradiation of $^{98}$Mo is generally of low specific activity. The other difference between these two types of $^{99}$Mo is the presence of very minute amounts of other radionuclides (radionuclidic impurities). In the $^{99}$Mo produced by neutron irradiation, the most common radionuclidic impurities are $^{134}$Cs, $^{60}$Co, $^{86}$Rb, $^{124}$Sb, and $^{95}$Zr, whereas in the fission produced $^{99}$Mo, the most common radionuclidic impurities are $^{131}$I, $^{132}$I, $^{89}$Sr, $^{90}$Sr, and $^{103}$Ru. Because some radionuclides may be eluted with $^{99m}$Tc during the milking of the generator, their amounts in the $^{99}$Mo sample should be as small as possible.

For any generator system to be of practical use in nuclear medicine, the milking process should be convenient and rapid. The eluate, as described in the next chapter, must be sterile, apyrogenic, and its pH in physiologic range (4.5–7.5). In the selection of a suitable generator, one has to consider several other factors such as efficiency, amount of parent breakthrough, radiation shielding, and specific concentration. These factors are discussed below with special reference to the $^{99}$Mo–$^{99m}$Tc generator system.

**Efficiency**
The efficiency of a generator is defined in the following manner:

$$\text{Efficiency} = \frac{\text{Amount of activiy eluted}}{\text{Total daughter activity on the column}} \times 100$$

This is also referred to as the yield of the generator. Present day $^{99}$Mo–$^{99m}$Tc generators give a high yield of $^{99m}$Tc, generally between 70% and 90%.

**Parent Breakthrough**
This is the amount of the parent radioactivity that is eluted with the daughter radioactivity. The amount should be as small as possible because any contamination by a long-lived radionuclide (in this case, the parent) increases the radiation

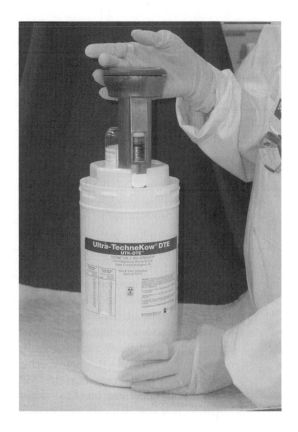

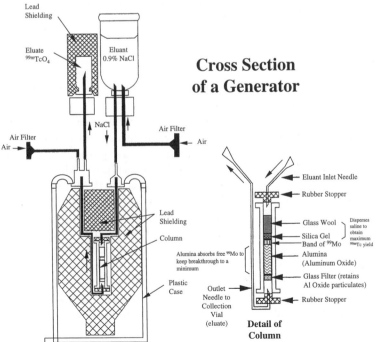

**Cross Section of a Generator**

**Fig. 4.3.** Picture and outline of a typical $^{99}$Mo/$^{99m}$Tc generator (Reproduced from Bushberg JT, Siebert JA, Leidholdt EM Jr, et al. The Essential Physics of Medical Imaging. 2nd ed. Philadelphia: Lippincott Williams & Wilkins; 2002, with permission).

dose without providing any benefit to the patient. The maximum allowable level of breakthrough depends primarily on the radiation dose delivered by this contaminant. For the $^{99}$Mo–$^{99m}$Tc generator, the maximum allowable level is 0.15 $\mu$Ci (5.6 kBq) of $^{99}$Mo for each mCi (37MBq) of $^{99m}$Tc. In general, the $^{99}$Mo breakthrough in $^{99}$Mo–$^{99m}$Tc generators is about 1/10 of the maximum allowable level. Breakthrough of $^{99}$Mo is easily measured with a dose calibrator described in Chapter 8.

### Chemical Purity

Because these generators contain large amounts of alumina, occasionally some aluminum may also be eluted with technetium pertechnetate. Aluminum, depending on its amount, may form colloid. This is an undesirable chemical impurity whose amount should be tested. Its amount should not exceed 10 $\mu$g/mL of the eluate. Commercial kits are available to measure simply and quickly the content of aluminum in the eluate.

### Radiation Shielding

Because the generators presently in use routinely contain curie amounts of radionuclides,

the generator should be properly shielded for the safety of nuclear medicine personnel. The exact amount of shielding depends on the total amount of radioactivity present and the energy of the $\gamma$-rays of the parent and daughter radionuclides. Commercial generators conform to the radiation safety rules and regulations described in Chapter 16.

### Specific Concentration

This is defined as the number of MBq/mL of the milked eluting solution. This number should be generally high for two reasons:

1. In dynamic studies, such as cardiac or brain blood flow, it is important to have a small concentrated bolus;
2. When labeling a variety of pharmaceuticals with the daughter radionuclide, various dilution steps are required. Therefore, to obtain a reasonably high specific concentration of the labeled compound, it is necessary to begin with a very high specific concentration of the radionuclide. Too high a specific concentration of the radioactivity is, however, of no practical value.

Present generators yield up to GBq/mL of specific concentration for $^{99m}$Tc.

## Key Points

1. Radionuclides used in nuclear medicine are artificial and are produced in a reactor, particle accelerator, or cyclotron.
2. A reactor is a source of neutrons. Most radionuclides produced in reactors decay through electron emission and contain large amounts of carrier (stable isotope).
3. In some nuclides, capture of a neutron leads to fission. In fission, large numbers of carrier-free radionuclides are generated.
4. Particle accelerators or cyclotrons are sources of high-energy charged particles. Radionuclides produced through charged particle reactions decay mainly through positron emission and/or electron capture and are carrier free.
5. Radioactivity produced depends on the amount of target, number of bombarding particles, reaction cross section, time of

irradiation, and half-life of the radionuclide being produced.
6. Radionuclidic generators are a source of short-lived radionuclides for hospitals that are some distance away from a reactor or cyclotron. In a generator ($^{99}$Mo–$^{99m}$Tc), a long-lived radionuclide ($^{99}$Mo) decays into a short-lived radionuclide ($^{99m}$Tc). Under these conditions, equilibrium is established in the radioactivities of the parent and daughter radionuclides after a certain interval.
7. The daughter radionuclide can be easily separated from the parent radionuclide. After the chemical separation, a new equilibrium is established.
8. Parent breakthrough should be a minimum and there are regulatory limits on it. For $^{99}$Mo, it is 0.15 $\mu$Ci/mCi of $^{99m}$Tc.

## Questions

1. What particle causes the nuclear reactions in a nuclear reactor and what is the typical energy of this particle?
2. What particles are typically used in a cyclotron and what are the typical ranges of energy of these particles?
3. Why do reactor-produced radionuclides generally decay with $\beta-$ and accelerator-produced radionuclides with $\beta+$ and/or electron capture?
4. List the factors that determine the amount of radionuclide produced in a reactor or accelerator.
5. Why are carrier-free radionuclides desirable in nuclear medicine?
6. Why is the $^{99}$Mo–$^{99m}$Tc radionuclidic generator so popular in nuclear medicine?
7. Can $^{99m}$Tc produced from a generator be strictly considered carrier free?

8. Why is the parent breakthrough in a generator undesirable and to be kept to a minimum?
9. What is the permissible amount of parent breakthrough in the $^{99}$Mo–$^{99m}$Tc generator?
10. A radionuclidic generator consisting of $^{132}$Te (half-life = 78 hours) and $^{132}$I (half-life = 3.2 hours) is in transient equilibrium. If the radioactivity of $^{132}$Te at this time is 16 GBq, how much radioactivity of $^{132}$I will be available 156 hours later if no milking took place during this interval?
11. The above generator is completely milked at 156 hours. The $^{132}$I-radioactivity thus obtained is left to decay for 16 hours. How much radioactivity of $^{132}$I remained at this time?
12. How often can the above generator be milked for optimum daughter radioactivity?

# Radiopharmaceuticals

In nuclear medicine, radionuclides are rarely used in their simplest chemical form. Instead, they are incorporated in a variety of chemical compounds that may be of interest because of their favorable biochemical, physiologic, or metabolic properties. A chemical compound tagged with a radionuclide and prepared in a form suitable for human use is known as a radiopharmaceutical. As with all pharmaceuticals, the U.S. Food and Drug Administration (FDA) also approves radiopharmaceuticals for human use.

A radiopharmaceutical is used (with a few exceptions discussed at the end of this chapter) to obtain diagnostic information rather than to produce therapeutic results. It is usually administered in tracer quantities in a single dose and produces no pharmacologic effects.

## Design Considerations for a Radiopharmaceutical

Because a radiopharmaceutical consists of a radionuclide and a biochemical, two considerations apply in designing or developing a radiopharmaceutical, one relating to the radionuclide and the other relating to the biochemical.

**Selection of a Radionuclide** The choice of a radionuclide for imaging purposes is chiefly dictated by the necessity of minimizing the radiation dose to the patient and the detection characteristics of present-day nuclear medicine instrumentation.

To minimize the radiation dose to the patient, a radionuclide should have as short a half-life as

is compatible with the biological phenomena under study. For example, a radionuclide with a 1-hour half-life, despite its smaller radiation dose, cannot be used in studies of physiologic or metabolic functions that span months. A suggested rule of thumb in this connection is that the physical half-life of the radionuclide should be about $0.693 \times T_{obs}$, where $T_{obs}$ is the time interval between the time of administration of the radionuclide and the time at which measurement or imaging is to be performed. It should not emit any corpuscular radiations (e.g., $\beta$ particles, conversion electrons), as these result in a radiation dose to a patient without providing any benefit.

A radionuclide should preferably emit a monochromatic (single-energy) $\gamma$-ray with energy between 100 and 300 keV. The upper limit of the desired energy of the $\gamma$-ray is the consequence of the detection characteristics of the scintillation camera routinely used to image diagnostic radiopharmaceuticals. As the energy of $\gamma$-rays increases, they become more and more penetrating; therefore, a smaller number of them interact within the detector. This reduces the sensitivity of the system. The concept of sensitivity and its importance in nuclear medicine is discussed in later chapters. The lower limit of the desired energy of the $\gamma$-ray is arrived at from the consideration of attenuation of $\gamma$-rays in the patient. Because $\gamma$-rays should be able to penetrate the patient's body effectively, their energy has to be high enough to be transmitted out of the patient's body; hence, the lower limit.

In addition, a radionuclide should be available easily, economically, and in an uncontaminated form. Technetium 99m, with its 6-hour half-life and 140-keV γ-ray emission, little emission of corpuscular radiation, and easy economical availability from a generator, comes very close to fulfilling the above requirements. This accounts for its wide use in nuclear medicine.

**Selection of a Chemical**  Besides being nontoxic in the desired amounts, the choice of the biochemical or pharmaceutical substance in a radiopharmaceutical is dictated by the requirement that it be distributed or localized in the desired organ or compartment and that the uptake by that organ (or part of the organ) in a normal condition differs substantially from uptake in a pathologic condition. This is generally expressed as target to nontarget ratio. The higher the ratio, the higher the contrast in the image and easier it becomes to visualize a disease (see Chapter 13).

To help in the selection of a suitable biochemical, a wealth of information has been acquired in the field of pharmacology. A number of physiochemical variants determine or affect the distribution and localization of drugs in tissues. Three important determinants in this regard are route of administration, blood flow to the organ or tissues, and extraction by the tissues. Radiopharmaceuticals, with few exceptions, are nearly always administered intravenously, primarily because this is the fastest way to introduce a drug into the circulatory system of the body. Blood flow or perfusion (which can be severely affected in diseases) essentially determines the fraction of the administered dose that will be delivered to a particular organ or tissue during the first transit (10–20 seconds). Because blood serves as a carrier for the drug, another property, binding to plasma proteins, plays an important role in the localization of a drug or a chemical in a given tissue. In general, drugs or chemicals strongly bound to plasma proteins remain in blood for a longer period (hours to days) and localize to a lesser extent in tissues than those not so tightly bound to plasma proteins.

Extraction of a drug or chemical from circulation and localization in tissue may occur in a number of ways. Simple diffusion, filtration through small pores in the membranes, active transport, receptor binding, and phagocytosis are some examples. It is evident from Table 5.1 that all of these mechanisms were used in the development of the radiopharmaceuticals.

# Development of a Radiopharmaceutical

When appropriate radionuclides and chemicals have been selected, the following steps are involved in the eventual development of a radiopharmaceutical.

**Chemical Studies**  These are aimed at establishing the best method of radiolabeling the chemical, defining the optimum condition of labeling

---

**Table 5.1.**  Mechanism of Localization of Radiopharmaceuticals

| Mechanism | Example |
|---|---|
| Active transport | Thyroid uptake and scanning with iodine |
| Compartmental localization | Blood pool scanning with human serum albumin, plasma, or red blood cell volume determinations |
| Simple exchange or diffusion | Bone scanning with $^{99m}$Tc-labeled phosphate compound |
| Phagocytosis | Liver, spleen, and bone marrow scanning with radiocolloids |
| Capillary blockade | Lung scanning with macroaggregate (size 8–75 $\mu$m organ perfusion studies with intra-arterial injection of macroaggregates |
| Cell sequestration | Spleen scanning with damaged red blood cells |
| Receptor binding/ antibody–antigen | Tumor imaging with somatosin receptor-binding $^{111}$In-pentetreotide, $^{111}$In-OncoScint for tumors |

and in vitro stability, and determining the nature and the extent of the radiochemical impurities.

### Animal Distribution and Toxicity Studies

The main purpose of these studies is to determine biodistribution of labeled material and establish safe amounts (radioactivity mainly, as the mass of the chemical used is in trace amounts) of the radiochemicals that can be administered to humans without subjecting them to undue risk. Biodistribution establishes the pattern of distribution (major organ or tissues of uptake) of the radioactivity at different times after the administration of the radiochemical in animals considered normal (control) and those in which the appropriate pathologic condition has been induced. From these, one estimates the optimum time for imaging after administration of the radiopharmaceutical and radiation dose delivered to various tissues.

### Human or Clinical Studies

Because biodistribution of a radiopharmaceutical in animals may be different from that in humans, initial studies (phase I) in only a small number of humans are performed to establish the distribution patterns, clearance time, mode of excretion, and optimum imaging time for the radiopharmaceutical. In phase II, these studies are extended to include patients with known diseases and provide further evidence of safety and initial proof of the diagnostic or therapeutic efficacy and final estimates of radiation doses to various human tissues. Finally (phase III), a large series of patients are studied that establishes the overall usefulness (i.e., safety and efficacy) of the agent.

Human or clinical studies are performed as an Investigational New Drug under a Notice of Claimed Exemption to the FDA. Once these data are collected, a New Drug Application is submitted to the FDA, which must approve it before its commercial use.

## Quality Control of a Radiopharmaceutical

Because all radiopharmaceuticals are intended eventually for human use, strict quality control is very important. To ensure optimum quality, the following properties of a radiopharmaceutical must be considered.

### Radionuclidic Purity

Ideally, the radiopharmaceutical should contain only the desired radionuclide. Often, however, it is not possible to avoid some contamination by other radionuclides, and therefore it is essential to hold this contamination to a low level. A contaminating radionuclide does not add to diagnostic information, but it does increase the radiation dose to the patient and, in many cases, may degrade the image quality. A good example is provided by the radionuclide, $^{123}$I, which is difficult to produce without $^{124}$I as radiocontaminant. Iodine-124, besides significantly increasing the radiation dose to the patient, degrades image quality because of its emission of high-energy $\gamma$-rays.

The amount of impurity is generally given as $\mu$Ci (kBq) of radiocontaminant per $\mu$Ci (kBq) or mCi (MBq) of the desired radionuclide. Sometimes the limit of the allowable contamination is set by governmental agencies, as in the case of $^{99m}$Tc, for which the amount of $^{99}$Mo must not exceed more than 0.15 $\mu$Ci for each mCi of $^{99m}$Tc. In cases where no such limits are prescribed, the rule of thumb is to keep the radiation dose to the patient from the radiocontaminants to less than 10% of that due to the radionuclide of interest.

Another important aspect of radionuclidic purity is that it does not stay constant with time. Where the half-life of the desired radionuclide is shorter than that of the radiocontaminant, radionuclidic purity degrades with time and vice versa. For example, because the half-life of $^{124}$I, a common radiocontaminant in $^{123}$I, is longer than $^{123}$I, the radionuclidic purity is best at the time of the production of this radionuclide, and as the radionuclide is stored, it becomes progressively less pure.

The most common method of determining the nature and extent of radionuclidic impurity is with $\gamma$ spectroscopy using a NaI (Tl) or Ge (Li) detector, both of which are discussed in Chapter 8.

### Radiochemical Purity

Because a radionuclide may form several compounds with a given chemical, it is important to ascertain that a given radiopharmaceutical is in the desired chemical form. Any radiochemical impurities present should be precisely stated. In this regard, it is also important to consider that although a radiochemical may be pure to begin with, it may not be stable over a period as a result of the action of radiation or the nature of the chemical itself. To avoid this deterioration, the radiochemical should be stored properly according to the instructions of the manufacturer. For example, radioiodinated human serum albumin (RIHSA) which, among other things, is used as a blood pool scanning agent, may be 99.9% pure when freshly prepared. With time, however, some of the radioiodine becomes free. The amount of free radioiodine strongly depends on storage conditions. The contamination with free radioiodine is several times higher if RIHSA is stored at room temperature than if it is refrigerated. A significant amount of free radioiodine will interfere with the intended study.

A common method for the detection of radiochemical impurities is thin-layer or paper chromatography.

**Chemical Purity** A radiopharmaceutical should contain only the desired chemical. In the final preparation of the radiopharmaceutical, there may be a number of chemicals involved besides the radiochemical of interest. These chemicals should be compatible with each other in vitro and safe for the patient. In addition, these must not distort the in vivo function of the main chemical. Aluminum breakthrough in a $^{99}$Mo–$^{99m}$Tc generator is an example of potential chemical impurity.

**Sterility** A radiopharmaceutical should be sterile (i.e., free from any microbial contamination) and therefore should be tested to this effect before use in patients. In the case of radiopharmaceuticals labeled with short-lived radionuclides ($^{99m}$Tc and $^{113m}$In), where prior testing of the final product is not feasible, the sterility of the labeling technique should be tested adequately and periodically.

**Apyrogenicity** Even if the preparation is sterile, it may still contain pyrogens that, when intravenously administered to a patient, may cause a reaction. A radiopharmaceutical, therefore, should also be tested for pyrogenicity before use in humans. If this is not feasible, as in the case of short-lived radionuclides, the apyrogenicity of the technique should be ascertained properly and periodically.

# Labeling of Radiopharmaceuticals with Technetium-99m

Because of the very attractive physical characteristics of $^{99m}$Tc, a variety of chemicals have been labeled with this radionuclide, despite the fact that the exact mechanism of technetium labeling with these compounds is often not known. Technetium-99m, in the form of sodium pertechnetate (Na$^{99m}$TcO$_4$), is easily obtained in the laboratory from a $^{99m}$Mo–$^{99m}$Tc generator. The labeling of most chemicals by $^{99m}$Tc is achieved by first reducing the pertechnetate to ionic technetium (mostly Tc4+) and then complexing it with the desired chemical. The common agent used for reducing purposes is stannous chloride (SnCl$_2$). Because the half-life of $^{99m}$Tc is short (6 hours), most labeling has to be performed "in-house." This is greatly simplified by the use of sterile and pyrogen-free kits, in which all the desired chemicals are premixed and held together in a lyophilized state under an inert atmosphere (nitrogen gas), except the radionuclide (hence, quite often referred as "cold kit"). To label a particular chemical compound, it is necessary only to introduce a known amount of sterile and pyrogen-free sodium $^{99m}$Tc pertechnetate into the kit vial; the labeled compound is ready to use within a few minutes.

Three parameters—labeling efficiency, in vitro stability, and in vivo stability—are important considerations in the selection of a kit. Labeling efficiency is defined as the percent of total radioactivity present in the kit that is tagged to the appropriate molecule or compound. For most kits currently in use in nuclear medicine, labeling efficiencies under optimum conditions are in excess of 90%, sometimes even reaching as high as 99%. The remainder of the radioactivity (which is not tagged to the desired compound) is present as radiochemical impurity. In kits that use SnCl$_2$ as the reducing agent, radiochemical impurities are, in general, of two forms: free pertechnetate (which was not reduced) and reduced or hydrolyzed technetium (which was reduced but did not tag to the compound of interest). Reduced or hydrolyzed technetium sometimes forms a colloid with excess tin present in the kit. This is also a radiochemical impurity but in a different form.

The in vitro stability of a labeled compound determines the time it can be stored on the shelf without significant deterioration. A high in vitro stability allows the compound to be labeled once and then used in a number of patients at different times of the day. Both labeling efficiency and in vitro stability of compounds prepared from kits can be maximized by observing a few simple precautions, such as using only oxidant-free sodium pertechnetate solution and ensuring no air (oxygen in air, being an oxidizer, reacts with the reducing agent and thus competes with pertechnetate for the reducing agent) is introduced into the reaction vial during the labeling procedure. The in vitro stability of a kit can also be extended by the use of preservatives in the reaction vial as is done by some manufacturers and/or by storing the labeled material at low temperatures. I should caution here that in vitro stability of a labeled compound is different from in vitro stability of the cold kit or the chemical compound itself.

The in vivo stability of a labeled compound determines how closely the distribution of the radiolabeled compound in the biological system parallels that of the unlabeled compound. The distribution of a labeled compound should be similar to the unlabeled compound at least for the duration of the study.

# Technetium-99m-Labeled Radiopharmaceuticals

The distribution and use of the most common technetium-labeled compounds in nuclear medicine are described below. Most of these compounds can be easily and rapidly prepared from the commercially available kits.

## Technetium-99m Pertechnetate ($^{99m}TcO_4^-$)
This radiopharmaceutical is obtained directly from the $^{99}Mo$–$^{99m}Tc$ generator using saline as the eluting solution. In biological systems, it behaves similarly to iodine. After oral or intravenous administration, it is selectively concentrated in the thyroid, salivary glands, stomach, and choroid plexus. Disappearance of the pertechnetate from plasma is a multiexponential function. About 50% of the compound is rapidly diluted into extravascular spaces within 15 to 20 minutes. The remaining amount disappears from the plasma with a half-life of about 3 hours. About 20% to 30% of the injected dose is excreted eventually in feces at a slow rate.

The stomach, which is the major organ of uptake, contains 20% to 25% of the injected dosage at 4 hours. So much radioactivity remains in the stomach even after 24 hours that it is not advisable to perform imaging of an abdominal organ using $^{99m}Tc$-labeled radiopharmaceuticals (or whose principal $\gamma$ emission is 170 keV or below) on a patient who had imaging performed with $^{99m}Tc$ pertechnetate up to 48 hours before the intended study.

Technetium-99m pertechnetate is presently used for thyroid, salivary gland, and stomach imaging. It is no longer used as a brain imaging agent.

## Technetium-99m-Labeled Sulfur Colloid
This radiopharmaceutical is easily prepared using commercially available kits. Colloids in general are removed from the bloodstream by the reticuloendothelial (RE) cells of the body. The relative distribution of the colloids among the RE cells of the various organs depends on factors such as the size, nature, and amount of colloidal particles; blood supply to the organ; and on other physiologic and pathophysiologic considerations. In the case of colloidal sulfur tagged with technetium-99m (particle size $\sim$0.3 $\mu$m), about 70% to 80% of the injected dosage is localized in the liver within 10 to 20 minutes of intravenous administration. Of the remaining amount, about 3% is deposited in the spleen and about 15% to 20% is localized in the bone marrow. This agent is, therefore, primarily used for liver, spleen, and bone marrow imaging.

Another $^{99m}Tc$-labeled compound sometimes used for liver, spleen, and bone marrow imaging is albumin microaggregates (particle size $\sim$1 $\mu$m).

**Technetium-99m-Labeled Macroaggregated Albumin (99mTc MAA)** This radiopharmaceutical is primarily used in lung imaging. Within a few seconds after intravenous administration of $^{99m}$Tc MAA, 90% to 95% of the injected dosage is trapped in the capillary and precapillary bed of the lungs. For effective lung localization, the albumin macroaggregates must be between 15 and 75 $\mu$m in size. The biological half-life of $^{99m}$Tc MAA in the lungs is about 8 to 12 hours. The $^{99m}$Tc albumin macroaggregates are broken down in smaller (micro) particles that are then taken up by the RE cells of liver and spleen.

**Technetium-99m-Labeled Polyphosphate, Pyrophosphate, and Diphosphonate** These radiopharmaceuticals are primarily used for bone imaging. After an intravenous injection, about 50% to 60% of the injected dosage is localized in the skeleton within 15 to 20 minutes. The remainder of the dose is distributed in soft tissue and plasma from which it is excreted slowly in the urine. About 20% to 30% of the injected dose is either excreted or taken up by the kidneys within 3 hours of the injection. Of these three groups, polyphosphate has the slowest plasma clearance and is therefore the least desirable for bone imaging. Methylene diphosphonate has the fastest plasma clearance of these compounds.

Use of $^{99m}$Tc pyrophosphate and $^{99m}$Tc diphosphonate for the detection of myocardial infarctions is now well established.

**Technetium-99m-Labeled Human Serum Albumin** This radiopharmaceutical is primarily used for blood pool imaging such as heart or placenta. After intravenous administration, it is retained in the plasma for a long period. However, $^{99m}$Tc-labeled albumin is not as stable in vivo as albumin labeled with radioiodine or radiochromium. Therefore, it is not the preferred agent for plasma volume determination.

**Technetium-99m-Labeled Red Cells** Labeling of red cells with radionuclides, in general, is a complex and time-consuming procedure. Recently, however, a simple and expeditious method has been developed to label red cells in vivo with $^{99m}$Tc. This has increased the popularity of $^{99m}$Tc-labeled red cells over that of $^{99m}$Tc-labeled albumin for blood pool scanning, particularly for the heart. In this method, two steps are involved. In step 1, a patient's red cells are coated with stannous ion ($Sn^{2+}$). This is achieved simply by injecting about one-fifth of a "cold" pyrophosphate kit into the patient. A cold kit is a preparation reconstituted using saline only (i.e., without any radioactivity). In step 2, performed about 30 minutes later, the desired amount of the $^{99m}$Tc radioactivity in the form of pertechnetate is administered to the patient as a second injection. The "pretinned" red cells in the patient quickly reduce the pertechnetate to ionic technetium that then readily binds to the red cell surface. Little free pertechnetate or reduced technetium remains in circulation. Most radioactivity (90%) is bound to the patient's red cells.

The second step—tagging of $^{99m}$Tc to the pretinned red cells—can also be performed in vitro by withdrawing pretinned red cells from the patient and incubating them with the desired amount of $^{99m}$TcO$^-_4$. The red cells thus labeled may be heat damaged, if desired, by heating them in a water bath at 50°C for half an hour. Damaged red cells are used to image the spleen, without interference from the liver, which is the case when sulfur or other colloids are used to image the spleen.

**Technetium-99m-Labeled 2,3-Dimercaptosuccinic Acid (DMSA)** This radiopharmaceutical is the agent of choice when morphology of the renal cortex is of interest. After an intravenous administration, this radiopharmaceutical is quickly mixed with the plasma volume from where it is cleared with a half time of about 1 hour. By 2 hours, between 40% and 50% of the injected dosage is taken up by the renal cortex and about 15% is excreted in urine. Because of rapid in vitro decomposition of $^{99m}$Tc-labeled DMSA, it should be stored in a refrigerator and used within half an hour of labeling.

**Technetium-99m-Labeled Diethylenetriamine Pentaacetic Acid (DTPA)** This radiopharmaceutical is used primarily for kidney imaging. After intravenous administration, $^{99m}$Tc DTPA is rapidly cleared by the kidneys. The biological half-life in plasma of DTPA chelates in humans is about 15 minutes. Over 80% of the injected dosage can be recovered in urine between 2 and 3 hours postinjection.

**Technetium-99m-Labeled Glucoheptonate** Biological behavior of this radiopharmaceutical is somewhere between that of $^{99m}$Tc DTPA and $^{99m}$Tc DMSA. Its clearance from plasma is slower than that of $^{99m}$Tc DTPA but faster than $^{99m}$Tc DMSA. Maximum uptake by renal cortex, which is reached at about 1 hour postinjection, is about 25% of the injected dose. Another 25% of the injected dosage is excreted in urine by this time. This radiopharmaceutical is primarily used for renal imaging. Another use of this radiopharmaceutical is in detection of myocardial infarctions at an early stage (within 2–3 days post infarction). At this early stage, $^{99m}$Tc pyrophosphate is not useful for the detection of myocardial infarctions.

**Technetium-99m-Labeled Mertiatide (MAG3)** This compound has recently been introduced to study renal function and serves as a substitute for iodohippuran. After intravenous injection, this compound is rapidly cleared by the kidneys through both active tubular secretion and glomerular filtration. In normal subjects, 90% of the injected dosage can be recovered in urine. This compound, even though bound to plasma proteins, has a fast plasma clearance because of the reversible nature of the binding.

**Technetium-99m-Labeled 2,6-Dimethyl Acetanilide Iminodiacetic Acid (HIDA) and Related Compounds (Diethyl-IDA, PIPIDA, and DISIDA)** These radiopharmaceuticals are used for imaging the hepatobiliary system. In normal subjects, $^{99m}$Tc HIDA is rapidly cleared from blood by hepatocytes. The half time for blood clearance is approximately several minutes. The transit of the radioactivity from the liver through gallbladder to the intestine is also fast. Within an hour after administration, over 70% of the injected dosage is in intestine. About 15% of the injected dosage is excreted in urine during the first hour. The remainder of the activity is eventually excreted in feces. Urinary excretion of diethyl-IDA is smaller than that of PIPIDA or DISIDA.

The transit and excretion of these compounds through the hepatobiliary system is strongly dependent on the patency of this system.

**Technetium-99m-Labeled Sestamibi (Cardiolite)** This compound is primarily used in the imaging of the heart. Its use in tumor imaging (e.g., in the breast) is also being explored. Being a technetium-labeled compound, it has an advantage over thallium for heart imaging in terms of providing higher photon flux for the same radiation dose to the patient. After intravenous injection, it is extracted by the myocardium in proportion to the blood flow. Its first-pass extraction efficiency is slightly less than that for thallous ion, but it does not redistribute and remains in the myocardium up to 3 hours post injection, thus providing a long time for planar imaging and single-photon emission computed tomography (SPECT). The liver and kidneys are other organs of large localization (20% and 14%, respectively). It is excreted intact through the hepatobiliary system and the kidneys.

Lately, it is also finding use in tumor detection, particularly in dense breast where mammography fails to detect these lesions.

**Technetium-99m-Labeled Tetrofosmin (Myoview)** This is the most recent radiopharmaceutical approved for heart imaging. After an intravenous injection, it is rapidly cleared by skeletal muscle, heart (1%), liver (7.5%), and kidneys (6.2%). Less than 5% of the injected dosage remains in blood. Salivary and thyroid glands also show elevated concentrations. Within 48 hours of administration, 75% of the dose is excreted from the body (40% urine and 35% fecal excretion). Excretion, particularly from the skeletal muscle, is increased significantly during exercise. This agent allows the exercise and rest heart scans to be performed on the same day (exercise scan followed 4 hours later with rest heart scan).

**Technetium-99m-Labeled Brain Imaging Agents (Exametazime [Ceretec], Hexamethylpropyleneamine Oxime [HMPAO], and Ethyl Cysteinate Dimer [ECD])** These radiopharmaceuticals cross the blood–brain barrier and therefore actively localize in the brain. Because their uptake is generally a function of regional blood flow, these agents, in conjunction with SPECT, are now being used to measure brain function. After an intravenous injection of Ceretec, the peak uptake (7%) in the brain is reached at 1 minute. The remainder of the dosage is distributed in the whole body, particularly in muscle and soft tissues. It is excreted from the body by way of the gastrointestinal tract and the kidneys in similar amounts.

# Radioiodine-Labeled Radiopharmaceuticals (131I and 123I)

With the advent of technetium-99m-labeled compounds, use of iodine-131-labeled compounds for imaging has declined sharply. However, two radioisotopes of iodine, $^{123}$I and $^{131}$I, are commonly used for diagnosis of thyroid disease. Iodine-131 is also used in the treatment of hyperthyroidism and thyroid cancer. For diagnostic purposes, $^{123}$I (13-hour half-life and 87% 160-keV $\gamma$-ray emission) is the radionuclide of choice because it delivers significantly less radiation dose to the thyroid than $^{131}$I. The two disadvantages of $^{123}$I are its cost and, sometimes, the presence of large amounts of other radioisotopes of iodine such as $^{124}$I. These contaminants not only increase radiation dose but also degrade image quality.

### Iodine-131- or Iodine-123-Labeled Sodium Iodide The radiopharmaceutical, $^{131}$I- and $^{123}$I-labeled, sodium iodide is commercially available as a capsule or solution with high specific activity and is almost carrier free. Because the iodine ion is readily absorbed from the stomach, it is generally administered orally. After an intravenous administration, the iodine ion is very quickly distributed throughout the extracellular water. From there, it is slowly taken up by the thyroid, stomach and intestine, salivary glands, and choroid plexus. A large fraction is filtered into the urine by the kidneys. By 24 hours, about 75% of the injected dose is excreted, 15% taken up by thyroid, 4% to 5% is in the gastrointestinal tract, and 1% to 2% is circulating in the blood. In the thyroid,

iodine is then organified and produces thyroid hormones such as $T_3$ or $T_4$. The distribution of radioiodide can be drastically changed in some disease states, particularly hyperthyroidism or severe kidney malfunctions. In hyperthyroidism, the thyroid can take up to 90% of the administered dosage with practically no excretion, whereas in hypothyroidism, the thyroid takes up little (sometimes less than 1% to 2%) iodide with excretion increased up to 95%.

### Other Iodine-123-Labeled Radiopharmaceuticals Three other $^{123}$I-labeled compounds, $^{123}$I-Hippuran, $^{123}$I-MIBG (metaiodobenzylguanidine, trade name, Androview) and $^{123}$I-BMIPP ($\beta$-methyl-p-[$^{123}$I]-iodophenyl-pentadecanoic acid, trade name, Zemiva), are finding increased use in nuclear medicine. Iodine-123-Hippuran is rapidly cleared by the kidneys and therefore is used to study renal function in the form of renograms that can be obtained either using dual scintillation detector probes or by imaging with a scintillation camera interfaced with a computer. $^{123}$I-MIBG is used for specific detection and localization of neuroendocrine tumors and adrenal medullary hyperplasia. $^{123}$I-BMIPP is a fatty acid analog being used in detecting abnormalities in fatty acid metabolism and is especially useful in heart imaging for acute coronary syndrome.

# Compounds Labeled with Other Radionuclides

### Gallium-67 Citrate This radiopharmaceutical is used in detection of soft tissue tumors and inflammatory diseases. After an intravenous administration, a significant fraction of the gallium in blood (30%) is bound to plasma proteins—in particular to transferrin. The remainder of the gallium quickly diffuses into extracellular spaces and is slowly cleared by the kidneys. By 24 hours, about 15% of the dosage is excreted in urine and about 10% is circulating in the blood. The remainder of the radioactivity is distributed in kidneys, bone, liver, and lymph nodes. The biological half-life of gallium in humans is between 1 and 2 weeks. Therefore, significant amounts of this radionuclide persist in the body even after 2 weeks. Besides excretion in urine (about 25% in

1 week), there is significant (10%) excretion in stool that sometimes interferes in interpretation of images of the abdominal area. The exact mechanism of localization of $^{67}$Ga in tumors or inflammatory lesions is not well established at this time.

**Thallous-201 Chloride** This radiopharmaceutical is primarily used for detection of myocardial infarction and/or ischemia. Thallous ion mimics the biological behavior of potassium, which is avidly localized intracellularly. Like potassium, immediately after intravenous injection thallous ion quickly leaves the circulation ( $T_{\frac{1}{2}} = 4$ minutes) and is taken up by various organs, generally in proportion to the blood supply of the given organ (the brain is one exception where there is almost no accumulation). At about 15 to 20 minutes, 4% of the injected dosage is localized in myocardium, 12% in liver, 4% in kidneys, and the bulk of the remainder is distributed in muscles throughout the body. Biological half-life of thallous ions in humans is about 10 days. Its use for myocardial imaging is based on the fact that its cellular uptake is dependent on blood flow to that region and the integrity of the cells themselves. Therefore, reduced uptake of thallous ion in a region is either a reflection of reduced blood flow (ischemia) or a reflection of damage to the cells (infarction).

**Chromium-51-Labeled Red Cells** These are used to determine the red cell volume and red cell mean life. Because labeling of red cells has to be performed in-house for each patient, this is a complex procedure. First, blood is withdrawn from the patient. It is then incubated with acid dextrose (ACD) and sodium chromate-51 solution at 37°C to 39°C for 10 minutes. Chromate ion readily penetrates the red cell membrane. Inside the cell it is reduced to $Cr^{3+}$, which has high affinity for hemoglobin. Small amounts of chromate ion that do not enter the red cells are then reduced to $Cr^{3+}$ outside the cells by addition of appropriate amounts of ascorbic acid. The blood–ACD–ascorbic acid solution is now ready to be injected back into the patient. Only the labeled red cells remain in circulation. Small amounts of $^{51}Cr^{3+}$ not bound to the cells are quickly excreted in urine by the kidneys.

**Indium-111-Labeled Platelets and Leukocytes** These are used for thrombus and abscess detection, respectively. The technique of platelet or leukocyte labeling with radionuclides is quite involved because it first requires separation of platelets or leukocytes from other components of blood. Once platelets or leukocytes have been separated, they can be labeled with $^{111}$In by incubating them with $^{111}$In oxine at room temperature for 30 minutes. Because of the involved preparation of $^{111}$In-labeled platelets or leukocytes, these have not found widespread use in nuclear medicine.

**Indium-111-Labeled DTPA Pentetreotide (OctreoScan)** This radiopharmaceutical has been recently introduced in clinical nuclear medicine for the detection of somatosin receptor-containing tumors. After an intravenous injection, this is rapidly cleared from blood (30% of the injected dosage in blood at 10 minutes postinjection). It is distributed throughout the soft tissues but has higher concentrations in kidneys, spleen, and liver (7%, 2.5%, and 2% at 4 hours, respectively). Pituitary and thyroid glands also exhibit high concentrations. It is mainly eliminated from the body through urinary excretion (85% in 24 hours). Imaging is performed at 24 hours post injection.

**Radiolabeled Monoclonal Antibodies and Synthetic Peptides** Wide interest exists in the possible use of monoclonal antibodies and their fragments, labeled with different radionuclides, for diagnosis and therapy of cancer and its metastases. Because of the affinity of tumor antibodies for tumor antigens, a high degree of localization occurs in tumors when antibodies labeled with radionuclides are injected into patients. This localization can be used for diagnosis by labeling antibodies with radionuclides such as $^{111}$In and $^{99m}$Tc or for therapy with $^{131}$I. Because antibodies are basically proteins, their blood clearance is generally slow and is similar to radiolabeled human serum albumin. Several such compounds have been approved by FDA for clinical use. These are labeled with either $^{111}$In or $^{99m}$Tc. Examples of $^{99m}$Tc-labeled antibodies for cancer detection are $^{99m}$Tc-labeled CEA-Scan, $^{99m}$Tc-labeled

Verluma, and $^{99m}$Tc-labeled Neotect. Acutect (labeled with $^{99m}$Tc) is used for deep vein thrombosis. Examples of $^{111}$In-labeled antibodies are $^{111}$In-OncoScint and $^{111}$In-ProtaScint. Several antibodies have also been approved for therapy of non-Hodgkin lymphoma. Two of these are Zevlin (labeled with $^{90}$Y) and Bexxar (labeled with $^{131}$I).

## Radioactive Gases and Aerosols

Of all the radioactive gases used in nuclear medicine, $^{133}$Xe has found the most popularity because of its easy availability and useful physiologic properties. It can be used in a gaseous form or as a saline solution. In a gaseous form, it is used for lung ventilation studies; in a saline solution administered intravenously, it is used for lung perfusion studies. When $^{133}$Xe is injected intra-arterially in a saline solution, it can be used to measure the blood flow to the organ supplied by that artery. The biological half-life of xenon in the body is only a few minutes. Only a very small component (~2%), probably the portion that is transferred to fat in the body, has a much longer biological half-life (~10 hours).

Also, use of $^{99m}$Tc DTPA aerosols and $^{99m}$Tc gas (Technegas) for such purposes is now well documented. Commercially available nebulizers produce $^{99m}$Tc-labeled aerosols with particle sizes ranging from 1 to 3 $\mu$m for lung ventilation studies. About 90% of the aerosol remains airborne and the remainder is removed from the lungs rapidly. Equipment to produce Technegas is also easily available. The particle size of Technegas is much smaller than aerosols (in nm) and therefore produces better images.

## Radiopharmeceuticals for Positron Emission Tomography (PET) Imaging

So far our discussion of radiopharmaceuticals has been limited to single photon imaging with a scintillation camera. Positron-emitting radionuclides, even though they emit particulate radiation and the $\gamma$-ray energy is high (511 KeV), are attractive from physiological reasons and may be the only radionuclides available to measure a particular physiological parameter. In this case, coincidence imaging discussed in Chapter 14 provides a better alternative to single photon imaging.

The ideal radionuclide for positron imaging is the one which does not emit $\gamma$-rays, emits positrons only with least amount of energy and is, hopefully, produced by a generator. In addition, it should provide clinically or physiologically important information that is not readily available with single photon imaging. Most of the radionuclides used in single photon imaging ($^{99m}$Tc, $^{67}$Ga, and $^{201}$Tl) are not isotopes of physiologically important elements such as hydrogen, carbon, nitrogen, oxygen, or phosphorus. However, carbon, nitrogen, and oxygen each have only positron emitting isotopes ($^{11}$C, $^{13}$N, and $^{15}$O) that can be used for in vivo imaging. Unfortunately, their half-lives are in minutes only and none of these three is produced by a generator (Table 5.2). As a result, these have to be produced, labeled to a suitable physiologically

| Table 5.2. | Characteristics of Positron Emitting Radionuclides of Interest in Nuclear Medicine | | | |
|---|---|---|---|---|
| Radionuclide | Half-Life (min) | % Positron Emission | $E_{max}$ (MEV) | Range (mm) |
| $^{11}$C | 20.4 | 99 | 0.96 | 0.28 |
| $^{13}$N | 10 | 100 | 1.19 | 0.45 |
| $^{15}$O | 2 | 100 | 1.72 | 1.04 |
| $^{18}$F | 110 | 97 | 0.64 | 0.22 |
| $^{68}$Ga | 68 | 87 | 1.88 | 1.07 |
| $^{82}$Rb | 1.3 | 96 | 3.15 | 1.99 |

interesting molecule, and imaged, depending on the radioisotope, within 10 minutes to an hour of the production. This puts tremendous hurdles in their routine clinical use, even when the cyclotron is at the site of usage. Therefore, their use so far has been limited to clinical research where they are providing a wealth of useful information.

However, another positron emitting radionuclide, $^{18}$F, (as fluoro-deoxy-glucose $^{18}$FDG, 110 minute half-life, see Chapter 2 for the decay scheme), despite it not being an isotope of a physiological important element, is increasingly finding more and more important clinical applications in nuclear medicine. This is in spite of the fact that it is not produced by a generator. Its half-life of about 2 hours (just long enough) and increasing demand make it feasible to produce $^{18}$F-labeled radiopharmaceuticals offsite commercially and supply them to hospitals within a large metropolis at a reasonable price. Even though F is not a physiologically important element, it can be easily substituted for OH group in many physiologically important organic molecules such as glucose, without changing their function in a significant manner. As a result, it provides important information that is not easily available by other methods.

Luckily, several positron emitting radionuclides can be produced with a generator. Of these, two $^{68}$Ga and $^{82}$Rb are finding increasing use in nuclear medicine and their important physical properties are given in Table 5.2. The $^{68}$Ge–$^{68}$Ga generator is now commercially available. A number of $^{68}$Ga-labled compounds are under development. Of these, somatostatin analog, $^{68}$Ga-Dotatoc (DOTA-DPhe1-Tyr 3-Octreotide) is very promising for the detection of a variety of tumors. Another generator is $^{82}$Sr–$^{82}$Rb that produces $^{82}$Rb with half-life of 1.3 minutes. This radionuclide can be used for blood perfusion measurements, and studies can be repeated within few minutes if desired.

### $^{18}$FDG (2-deoxy-fluoro-D-glucose)
$^{18}$FDG (2-deoxy-fluoro-D-glucose) is the work horse of PET imaging. Its applications range a wide gamut. It is used to diagnose a variety of brain diseases, measure regional brain function quantitatively, measure myocardial viability, and diagnose or stage a variety of cancers. Synthesis of $^{18}$FDG, as opposed to labeling with most of the other radiopharmaceuticals, is a complex procedure. However, most of these procedures have been optimized and are now highly efficient, fast, and automated. After the injection, $^{18}$FDG is quickly extracted from blood by tissues. The blood clearance is multiexponential, the fastest component having a half time of about 10 to 15 seconds, the next component having a half time of about 12 minutes. The third component is small and has a long half time. The target to blood ratio becomes optimum from 20 minutes post injection to 90 minutes post injection. As a consequence, most of the imaging is done between these times.

Like glucose, $^{18}$FDG is actively transported from blood through the cell membrane to the cytoplasm where, like glucose again, it goes through phosphorylation by the hexokinase reaction to $^{18}$FDG-6-phosphate. As opposed to glucose-6-phosphate, $^{18}$FDG-6-phosphate is not further metabolized in most tissues (liver, spleen, and kidneys are exceptions) and remains inside the cell for a long time. This is an advantage from the imaging point of view, as well as from quantification perspective, as it simplifies the number of compartments in which $^{18}$FDG is localized.

## Radiopharmaceuticals in Pregnant or Lactating Women

It should be pointed out here that radiopharmaceuticals are, to various degrees, transferred to the fetus from mother through placental crossover and also excreted in mother's milk. Because these transfers are relatively minor as compared to overall distribution of the radiopharmaceutical in mother, this does not affect the imaging procedure. However, as discussed in Chapter 15, it poses potential risk to the fetus or baby if breast feeding. Chapter 7, p 77 discusses the radiation doses to the fetus from common radiopharmaceuticals and Chapter 16, p 178 provides ways to protect a breast feeding baby from potential radiation risk.

## Therapeutic Uses of Radiopharmaceuticals

The main concern of nuclear medicine is diagnostic applications of radionuclides. Here, we briefly discuss some therapeutic uses of radiopharmaceuticals when they are administered internally to a patient.

**Design of a Radiopharmaceutical for Therapeutic Uses** Physiologic and biochemical considerations in designing a radiopharmaceutical for therapeutic purposes are similar to those that apply in designing a radiopharmaceutical for diagnostic uses; the primary objective in both cases is a high target to nontarget ratio. For therapeutic uses, a diseased cell is the target.

Because the objective of therapeutic use of a radiopharmaceutical is to kill diseased cells with radiation, the physical requirements for a radionuclide are the opposite of those desired for diagnostic purposes. The radionuclide should emit only particulate radiation ($\alpha$- or $\beta$-ray) and preferably no penetrating radiation (x- or $\gamma$-ray). However, emission of x- or $\gamma$-ray in the range of 100 to 300 keV is not bad so long it does not contribute more than 10% to the total radiation dose. It can be used to image the distribution of the therapeutic dose in the patient to assess more accurately the radiation dose being delivered.

**Problems and Uses** The main problem arising in the treatment of a patient with internally administered radionuclides is the calculation of the radiation dose (gray or rad) to the target. Accurate calculations of the radiation dose require accurate data about the physical decay characteristics of the radionuclide and its distribution in the body (see Chapter 7). Although accurate data are available with regard to the first parameter, accurate data with regard to the latter are difficult to obtain, particularly in the case of a patient who is about to be treated. Usually, a tracer dose is administered to a patient for this purpose. From the blood disappearance, the urinary and fecal excretion rates, and the relative distribution in the body of this tracer dose, as determined by area imaging or SPECT where possible, estimation is made of the various parameters to be used in the calculation of the radiation dose. Unfortunately, even these parameters may not describe the behavior of the therapy dosage (100–1000 times larger than the trace dosage); therefore, the resulting radiation dose from a therapy dosage may be quite different from that estimated from the trace or diagnostic dosage. Another unpredictable factor in such treatment is the variability of the biological response of different individuals to the same radiation dose.

Despite this inability to deliver the exact number of grays (or rads) to a target by internal administration of the radionuclides, success has been achieved for the treatment of a number

**Table 5.3.**  Therapeutic Uses of Radiopharmaceuticals

| Radionuclide and Chemical Form | Dosage (mCi) and Route of Administration | Dosage (MBq) | Uses |
|---|---|---|---|
| $^{131}$I as iodide | 3–10 oral | 111–370 | Hyperthyroidism |
| $^{131}$I as iodide | 50–200 oral | 1850–7400 | Cancer of thyroid |
| $^{32}$P as orthophosphate | 3–20 intravenous | 111–740 | Polycythemia, bone metastases, and leukemia |
| $^{90}$Sr as strontium chloride | 3–5 intravenous | 111–185 | Bone metastases |
| $^{32}$P, $^{153}$Sm, $^{90}$Y, $^{177}$Lu, and $^{188}$Re in colloidal form, particle size ranging from 0.01 to 50 $\mu$m | 10–150 intravascular, intracavitary, and interstitial | 370–5550 | A variety of malignant diseases and rheumatoid arthritis |
| $^{131}$I antibody (Bexxar) | 5 Intravenous infusion | | Non-Hodgkin lymphoma |
| $^{90}$Y antibody (Zevalin) | 20–30 Intravenous infusion | | Non-Hodgkin lymphoma |

of diseases. Table 5.3 summarizes the present status of the therapeutic uses of internally administered radionuclides. Some of these radionulides are generator produced: $^{188}W-^{188}Re$ and $^{90}Sr -^{90}Y$ are two examples.

# Misadministration of Radiopharmaceuticals

Radiopharmaceuticals, at rare occasions due to human error, can be administered in more amounts, in a different form, or through a different route than prescribed. In either case, the U.S. Nuclear Regulatory Commission (NRC) or comparable state agency, which regulates the use of FDA-approved radiopharmaceuticals and other uses of radionuclides, has defined what constitutes a misadministration. These are divided into three categories: the two radioisotopes, *125I and 131I, in the form of sodium iodide*; all *other diagnostic radiopharmaceuticals*; and all *other therapeutic radiopharmaceuticals*.

1. $^{125}$*I and $^{131}$I, in the form of sodium iodide:* (a) Administration of a dosage greater than 1.1 MBq (30 $\mu$Ci), or to a wrong patient, or through a wrong route and/or (b) whenever the administered dosage exceeds the prescribed dosage by more than 20% and the difference is greater than 1.1 MBq (30 $\mu$Ci).

2. All *other diagnostic radiopharmaceuticals:* (a) Administration of a wrong radiopharmaceutical, or to a wrong patient, or through a wrong route and/or (b) the radiation dose from the administered amount of radioactivity is more than 50 mSv (5 rems) effective dose equivalent or 500 mSv (50 rems) dose equivalent to any individual organ (radiation dose is described in Chapter 7).

3. All *other therapeutic radiopharmaceuticals:* (a) Administration of a wrong radiopharmaceutical, or to a wrong patient, or through a wrong route and/or (b) when the dosage differs from the prescribed dosage by more than 20%.

After the discovery of misadministration, the NRC or appropriate state agency has to be notified no later than the next calendar day. Then a written report has to be submitted within 15 days providing the cause of misadministration and corrective actions taken and proposed.

These regulations are published in Title 10, part 35 of the Code of Federal Regulations (10CFR35) and should be consulted for more details.

## Key Points

1. Radiation dose and the available detection instruments determine the characteristics of an ideal radionuclide to be used in nuclear medicine. An ideal radionuclide emits no particle radiation, emits an x- or $\gamma$-ray of energy in the range of 100 to 300 keV, and has a short half-life.

2. Pharmaceutical principles determine the localization of radiopharmaceuticals in tissues. These are active transport, compartmental localization, simple exchange or diffusion, phagocytosis, capillary blockade, cell sequestration, and receptor binding.

3. Radiopharmaceuticals have to satisfy quality control standards for radionuclidic purity, radiochemical purity, chemical purity, sterility, and apyrogenicity.

4. Commercial kits available for labeling with $^{99m}$Tc should be tested for two chemical impurities: $^{99m}$TcO$_4^-$ and reduced or hydrolyzed $^{99m}$Tc.

5. Labeling with $^{99m}$Tc dominates the radiopharmaceuticals used in nuclear medicine for diagnostic purposes.

6. Positron emitting radiopharmaceuticals such as $^{18}$FDG are also becoming routine in clinical nuclear medicine.

7. The radionuclide $^{131}$I dominates the therapeutic uses.

## Questions

1. List the ideal properties of a radionuclide to be used for diagnostic purposes.
2. Three radionuclides with the following properties are available to you: (a) $T_{\frac{1}{2}}$ = 3 minutes, $\gamma$ emission (70%) of 180 keV; (b) $T_{\frac{1}{2}}$ = 1 day, $\gamma$ emission (100%) of 250 keV, and a small fraction of conversion electrons (5%); (c) $T_{\frac{1}{2}}$ = 2 days, $\gamma$ emission (20%) of 300 keV, $\beta$ emission with a maximum energy of 2.0 MeV. Which one of these is best suited for (a) tumor localization when the optimum tumor uptake occurs at 18 hours post injection, (b) blood perfusion in an organ, and (c) radiation therapy?
3. List the factors that affect the localization of a radiopharmaceutical in tissue.
4. Does strong plasma binding of a radiopharmaceutical (a) help, (b) hinder, or (c) have no effect on the rate of uptake by a tissue?
5. What happens to the radionuclidic purity with time if the half-life of the desired radionuclide is longer than that of the radiocontaminant?
6. What are the two most common radiochemical impurities in a $^{99m}$Tc-labeled radiopharmaceutical?
7. How does the presence of oxygen interface with labeling of a pharmaceutical with $^{99m}$Tc?
8. List the various radiopharmaceuticals that are used for imaging the following organs: liver, bone, bone marrow, myocardium, blood pool, kidneys, lungs, hepatobiliary system, thyroid, spleen, tumors, and brain.
9. What is the main problem in routine use of the $^{11}$C, $^{13}$N, and $^{15}$O radionuclides in nuclear medicine?
10. What is the optimum time for imaging with $^{18}$FDG?
11. Can positron emitting radionuclides be produced by a radionulide generator?
12. What are the ideal properties of a radionuclide to be used for therapy in nuclear medicine?
13. What are the main problems in the use of radionulides for therapy in nuclear medicine?
14. How do the roles of the two agencies, FDA and NRC, differ in regulating the radiopharmaceuticals?
15. What is the maximum time interval between the discovery of misadministration and its written notification to the appropriate agency?

# Interaction of High-Energy Radiation with Matter

Interaction is a fundamental aspect of nature. Our ability to see, hear, smell, and taste is a vivid manifestation of interaction. This chapter, however, focuses on the mechanism of interaction of high-energy radiation with matter. Radiation in this context is used in a general sense. It encompasses both corpuscular radiation (e.g., charged particles and neutrons) and electromagnetic radiation in the form of x- and $\gamma$-rays.

The material presented here is basic to an understanding of the detection and effects (especially biological) of high-energy radiation and of protection against it. Because the subject matter is complex, only the salient features are presented. For ease of presentation and understanding, this chapter has been divided into three sections: (1) interaction of charged particles (with energies of 10 keV to 10 MeV) such as e, e$^+$, p, $\alpha$, and $^2$D; (2) interaction of high-energy photons such as x- and $\gamma$-rays; and (3) interaction of neutrons.

## Interaction of Charged Particles (10 keV to 10 MeV)

**Principal Mechanism of Interaction** When a charged particle passes through a substance (target) it interacts with the negatively charged electrons and positively charged nuclei of the target atoms or molecules. Through the coulomb forces, it tries to attract or repel the electrons or nuclei near its trajectory. As a result of these pushes and pulls (a sophisticated name for these is inelastic collisions), the charged particle loses some of its energy, which is taken up by

the electrons of the target atoms near its trajectory. The absorption of energy by the target atom leads to its ionization or excitation. In this energy range (10 keV–10 MeV), ionization events predominate over excitation events. For this reason, high-energy radiations are sometimes referred to as ionizing radiations, although excitation events are by no means negligible. The probability of inelastic collisions in general is so high that it does not take a material of much thickness to stop the charged particles completely.

**Differences Between Lighter and Heavier Charged Particles** Do all charged particles interact in a similar way? The answer is yes and no. Yes, because inherently the nature of interaction for all charged particles in this energy range is the same (inelastic collisions). No, because the manifestation of these interactions on lighter particles—whose masses are of the order of an electron (e.g., e and e$^+$)—and heavier particles—whose masses are equal to or more than that of a proton (e.g., p and $\alpha$)—is strikingly different. Lighter particles in inelastic collisions with the electrons of the target atoms, besides losing energy, tend to be deflected at larger angles than the heavier particles. This leads to a wide variation in the paths of the two kinds of particles (depicted graphically in Figure 6.1 for an electron and proton). The path of a heavier particle is more or less a straight line, whereas that of a lighter particle is more tortuous (zigzag). Whenever a lighter charged particle is deflected at a large angle, the energy transferred to the target electron is also quite large. As a result, the target electron acquiring this large

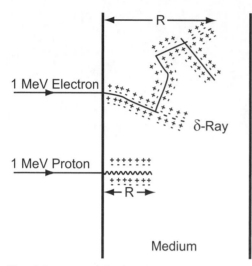

**Fig. 6.1.** Range R of a charged particle. Heavy charged particles (e.g., protons) travel and lose their energy in more or less straight lines. Light charged particles (e.g., electrons) lose their energy in a zigzag fashion. Lighter charged particles can transfer large amounts of energy in a single encounter with an electron of the medium, thus creating what are known as δ-rays. Plus and minus signs represent the ionization of the atoms of the medium. (Figure not to the scale as electrons will travel much farther than protons.)

amount of energy also behaves like a high-energy charged particle, thus creating its own path in the target medium. The paths created by high-energy secondary electrons are known as δ-rays. These are shown by the dotted lines in Figure 6.1. In the case of a proton or other heavier particles, this type of energy transfer is rare.

**Range R of a Charged Particle**  As a charged particle travels farther and farther in a medium,

it loses more and more energy and therefore more and more of the target atoms close to its path become ionized or excited. Eventually, the charged particle loses all its kinetic energy and comes almost to a halt. The average distance traveled by a charged particle in the incident direction is defined as its range R. This definition of range R is strictly valid only for heavy charged particles, such as α particles. For lighter particles, it is difficult to define the range R exactly. For our purpose, it is sufficient to think of the range R of light particles such as electrons or positrons as the minimum thickness of a material that they are just unable to penetrate. The concept of the range of a charged particle is quite useful in radiation protection, design of radiation detectors, and radiation dosimetry.

The range R of the heavier charged particles, because they travel more or less in straight lines, is nearly equal to the average path length of the charged particles in a given medium, whereas the range R for the lighter particles such as electrons, because of their more tortuous paths, is much shorter than the average path length (Fig. 6.1). Table 6.1 lists the ranges of α particles and electrons for various energies and mediums, providing a rough idea of the distances involved.

The concept of range is sometimes used with β-emitting radionuclides in which β particles are emitted with varying amounts of energy up to a maximum, $E_{\beta max}$. In this case, the range is more or less determined by $E_{\beta max}$.

**Factors That Affect Range, R**  The range R of a charged particle depends on various factors. Four of the most important of these are described below.

| | **Range, R (cm)** | | | |
|---|---|---|---|---|
| | **Soft Tissue** | | **Air** | |
| **Energy (keV)** | **e or e$^+$** | **α** | **e or e$^+$** | **α** |
| 10 | $2 \times 10^{-4}$ | $< 10^{-5}$ | $1.6 \times 10^{-1}$ | $1 \times 10^{-2}$ |
| 100 | $2 \times 10^{-2}$ | $1.4 \times 10^{-4}$ | 16 | $1 \times 10^{-1}$ |
| 1000 | $4 \times 10^{-1}$ | $7.2 \times 10^{-4}$ | $3.3 \times 10^{2}$ | $5 \times 10^{-1}$ |
| 10,000 | 5 | $1.4 \times 10^{-2}$ | $4.1 \times 10^{3}$ | 10.5 |

**Table 6.1.**  Approximate Ranges of Charged Particles

**Energy (E)** The range R of a given particle increases with increase in the initial energy E of the particle. For example, the range of a 5-MeV electron is about six times longer than that of a 1-MeV electron. The exact relationship of R to E is complex, but in the energy range of our interest, R is linearly related to the initial energy of the charged particle E, or R = AE + B, where A and B are constants.

**Mass (M)** Lighter particles have longer ranges than heavier particles of the same energy and charge. The range of a 1-MeV positron ($e^+$) is much longer than the range of a 1-MeV proton ($p^+$, 2000 times the mass of an $e^+$). Mass dependence of the range is sometimes expressed as velocity dependence. A 1-MeV positron is traveling at a much higher speed than a 1-MeV proton. The range R of a charged particle increases as the velocity of the charged particle increases.

**Charge (Q)** A particle with less charge travels farther than a particle with more charge. For example, a $_1^3H$ (charge 1; mass 3) particle has a longer range than a $_2^3H$ (charge 2; mass 3) particle of the same energy. The exact relationship is R $\alpha$ ($1/Q^2$). Therefore, a $_1^3H$ particle travels four times the distance of $_2^3H$ particle. The signs of the charge (positive or negative) do not affect the range.

**Density of the Medium (d)** The range R of a charged particle strongly depends on the density of the medium through which it is traversing. The higher the density of the medium, the shorter the range of a charged particle; that is, R is inversely proportional to the density d of the medium or R $\alpha$ (1/d). For this reason, the ranges of charged particles are always much longer in gases than in liquids or solids.

**Bremsstrahlung Production** Besides losing energy through inelastic collisions, charged particles can lose energy through the "bremsstrahlung" process. In this case, when a charged particle in the electric field of a nucleus experiences a sudden acceleration or "de-acceleration," it sometimes emits high-energy photons (x-rays). The probability of such interaction in the energy range of our interest is indeed very small except when electrons and positrons interact with high

atomic-number materials (e.g., lead, steel). The fraction of energy f released as x-rays by electrons of energy E (MeV) in a material with atomic number Z is given approximately by the following equation:

$$f = \frac{Z \cdot E}{1400} \text{ (E is in MeV)}$$

In an x-ray tube with a tungsten target (Z = 74) and electrons with 100-keV incident energy, only 0.5% of the total energy of the electrons is converted into x-rays. The same fraction (0.5%) of the total energy of the electrons is converted into x-rays when a 1-MeV electron passes through water (Z = 7.4), except that the x-ray spectrum (energies of emitted x-rays) in this case is quite different from that produced in the first case (x-ray tube). For the purposes of nuclear medicine, because production of high-energy photons by this mechanism is generally very small, it is therefore ignored.

**Stopping Power (S)** Quite often, instead of using the range R of a charged particle, another parameter known as stopping power S is used. Stopping power is defined as the ratio of the amount of energy lost dE by a charged particle in traversing a small distance dx in a given medium to the distance dx, or

$$S_{medium} = -\frac{dE}{dx}$$

The range R is related to the stopping power in an approximately inverse relationship (i.e., the higher the stopping power of a given medium, the shorter will be the range of a given particle in that medium). Because of this relationship, the stopping power S also depends on the same factors (E, M, Q, and d) on which the range R depends, although the relationships are, approximately, inverse of the range R.

**Linear Energy Transfer (LET)** Linear energy transfer LET is an important parameter in radiation biology. It is defined as the ratio of the amount of energy transferred $dE_{local}$ by a charged particle to the target atoms in the immediate vicinity of its path in traversing a small distance dx to the distance dx, or

$$LET = -\frac{dE_{local}}{dx}$$

**Difference Between LET and Stopping Power S** In discussing stopping power S one is concerned with the total energy lost by the particle, whereas in discussing LET one is concerned with the local (immediate vicinity of the track) deposition of energy by the charged particle. Because of this, S and LET are almost equal for heavier particles. For lighter particles, however, the two quantities differ significantly because of the energy lost in the δ-rays or through the bremsstrahlung process, which does not deposit energy locally. Both stopping power S and LET are measured in the same units (keV/μm).

**Annihilation of Positrons** There is no difference in the way in which an electron or a positron loses energy in a medium. However, a positron, once it has lost its energy, is not stable and is quickly annihilated by combining with an electron. The mass energy of the electron and the positron is converted into two γ-rays of 511 keV that travel in opposite directions as shown in Figure 6.2. Remember that the annihilation of positron occurs only when it has lost almost all of its energy (i.e., near the end of its range in a medium).

# Interaction of X- or γ-Rays (10 keV–10 MeV)

Although a photon does not have any electrical charge, it nevertheless interacts with electrical charges and therefore with matter that is composed of electric charges. The probability of interaction and the modes of interaction of a photon with matter are strongly dependent on the energy of the photon. Here we are interested only in the interaction of high-energy photons (x- or γ-rays) with matter.

The probability of interaction of an x-ray or γ-ray with an atom is, in general, very small compared with that of high-energy charged particles. As a consequence, x- or γ-rays have more penetrating power than high-energy charged particles. Because of this high penetrating power of x- or γ-rays, it is not practical to use concepts such as stopping power or range. Instead, new concepts known as linear attenuation coefficient $\mu$(linear) and the half-value layer (HVL) are commonly used.

**Attenuation and Transmission of X- or γ-Rays** Let us consider a simple experiment in which a parallel beam of x- or γ-rays of a given energy $E_\gamma$ is incident on a thin slab of 1-cm² cross section and x-cm thickness (Fig. 6.3). When a γ-ray passes through this slab, three things may occur: the γ-ray may be completely absorbed by the material, the γ-ray may be deflected (scattered) with some or no loss of energy or the γ-ray may pass through the slab without any interaction. The first two processes together are known as attenuation; the third is known as transmission. The transmission of γ-rays of a given energy $E_\gamma$ through a thickness x in the

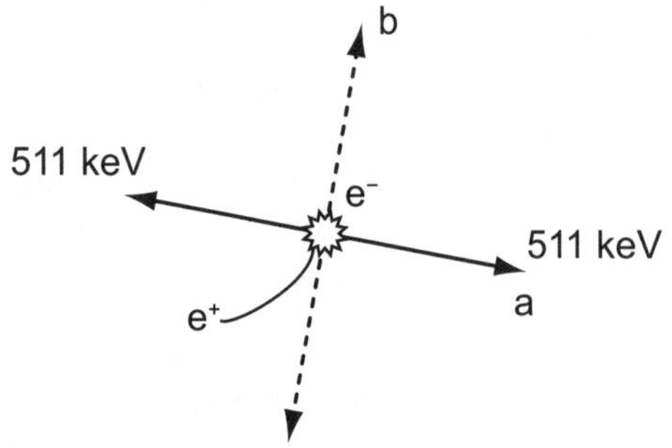

**Fig. 6.2.** Annihilation of a positron occurs when it loses almost all its energy at the end of its range and combines with an electron to produce two γ-rays of 511 keV. The two γ-rays are emitted always in opposite directions as shown in a or b or any other direction but always opposite to each other.

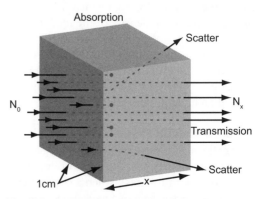

**Fig. 6.3.** Attenuation of γ-rays. When a flux $N_0$ of γ-rays is incident on a substance of x-cm thickness, a smaller flux $N_x$ is transmitted by the substance (shown by the dots). The remaining γ-rays are either absorbed by the substance or scattered out from the incident beam.

above experiment depends only on the nature of the material (density and atomic number) and the thickness x of the slab. For a given material, the dependence on the thickness x can be experimentally determined by measuring the number of $\gamma$-rays (those without any loss of energy or deflection) transmitted through different thicknesses of the slab. The data resulting from such an experiment can be accurately related by the following mathematical expression:

$$\frac{N_x}{N_0} = e^{-\mu(\text{linear})x} \qquad (1)$$

where $N_0$ and $N_x$ are, respectively, the number of $\gamma$-rays incident on the slab and transmitted through a thickness x of the slab. The linear attenuation coefficient, $\mu$(linear), represents in physical terms the probability of the interaction of a $\gamma$-ray passing through a unit area of a material 1-cm thick; $\mu$(linear) strongly depends on the $\gamma$-ray energy $E_\gamma$ and the nature of the material (density and atomic number). Note that equation (1) is mathematically the same as that for radioactivity decay with time (see p. 23, Chapter 3). However, here it is describing a completely different physical process—namely, the transmission of $\gamma$-rays through a thickness x of a given material. The energy dependence of the linear attenuation coefficient of four substances useful for our purpose is shown in Figure 6.4.

Experimentally, it is easier to determine the parameter known as the HVL than to determine $\mu$(linear). HVL is defined as the thickness of a material that attenuates one-half of the incident $\gamma$-rays. Referring to equation (1), when

$$\frac{N_x}{N_0} = \frac{1}{2}, x = \text{HVL}$$

HVL is related to $\mu$(linear) by the following expression:

$$\text{HVL} = \frac{0.693}{\mu(\text{linear})} \qquad (2)$$

which is similar to that for the half-life of a radionuclide $T_{\frac{1}{2}}$ and its decay constant $\lambda$. The parameter $\mu$(linear) is measured in units of $\text{cm}^{-1}$, whereas HVL is expressed in cm. Once HVL or $\mu$(linear) is known, one can easily determine the parallel beam attenuation of $\gamma$-rays through any thickness x of a material using

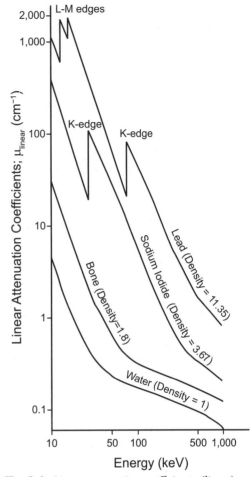

**Fig. 6.4.** Linear attenuation coefficient $\mu$(linear) of water, bone, sodium iodide, and lead as a function of x- or $\gamma$-ray energy.

equation (1) or one of the shortcuts described in Chapter 3 (p. 25) for solving problems involving exponentials.

**Example:**
The half-value layer of a 140-keV $\gamma$-ray in a NaI(Tl) crystal is approximately 0.3 cm. Determine the percentage of $\gamma$-rays transmitted through a 1.2-cm ($\approx$ 1/2 inch) thick NaI(Tl) crystal for a 140-keV $\gamma$-ray parallel beam.

A thickness of 1.2 cm is expressed as $\frac{1.2}{0.3} = 4$ HVL of a 140-keV $\gamma$-ray in a NaI(Tl) crystal. Because for 1 HVL the ratio $\frac{N_x}{N_0} = \frac{1}{2}$, for 4 HVL the ratio will be $\frac{N_x}{N_0} = \left(\frac{1}{2}\right)^2 = \frac{1}{16}$; therefore, the percentage of $\gamma$-rays transmitted is $\frac{100}{16}$ or 6%.

In other words, 94% of the $\gamma$-rays will be attenuated. Here, the thickness x is a multiple of HVL; therefore, it is not necessary to use equation (1).

### Attenuation Through Heterogeneous Medium

Equation (1) describes the attenuation through a homogeneous medium only. When attenuation occurs through a heterogeneous material consisting of layers of different thickness of different materials as shown in (Fig. 6.5), then the attenuation is given by equation

$$I_t = I_0 * e^{(-\mu_1 x_1 - \mu_2 x_2 - \mu_3 x_3)} \tag{3}$$

where the total thickness, $t = x_1 + x_2 + x_3$ If $x_1 = x_2 = x_3$, then

$$I_t = I_0 * e^{-(\mu_1 + \mu_2 + \mu_3)x} \tag{4}$$

In nuclear medicine, one encounters heterogeneous attenuation quite often. For example, during imaging of the heart, the $\gamma$-ray has to pass through different thicknesses of the heart muscle, lungs, and the bones. If not corrected, it introduces significant error in nuclear medicine images.

### Mass Attenuation Coefficient, $\mu$(mass)

Because $\mu$(linear) is dependent on the density of the absorbing material, it is often important to know the mass attenuation coefficient $\mu$(mass) that removes the effect of the density from the linear attenuation coefficient. The mass attenuation coefficient reflects the probability of an interaction with a unit mass of a material. The mass attenuation coefficient is related to the

linear attenuation coefficient by the following expression:

$$\mu(\text{mass}) = \frac{\mu(\text{linear})}{\text{density}}$$

The units for $\mu$(mass) are expressed as $\frac{cm^2}{gm}$.

### Atomic Attenuation Coefficient, $\mu$(atom)

The two probabilities of interaction, $\mu$(linear) and $\mu$(mass), describe the interaction of $\gamma$-rays at the macroscopic level (1 g or 1 cm$^3$). How does one relate these two quantities to those at the atomic level (e.g., the probability of $\gamma$-ray interaction with one atom, $\mu$[atom])? The number of atoms in 1 g of a substance can be determined by dividing Avogadro number $N_{av}$ by the atomic weight A, that is, number of atoms in 1 g $= N_{av}/A$. Then $\mu$(atom) can be determined by dividing $\mu$(mass) by the number of atoms in 1 g of that substance:

$$\mu(\text{atom}) = \mu(\text{mass})/\frac{N_{av}}{A} = \frac{\mu(\text{mass}) \cdot A}{N_{av}}$$

The units for $\mu$(atom) are expressed as cm$^2$.

### Mechanisms of Interaction

We described the attenuation of x- or $\gamma$-rays without, thus far, specifying the mechanisms that cause this attenuation. In this energy range (10 keV–10 MeV), there are three basic processes through which a photon interacts with matter: photoelectric effect, Compton scattering, and pair production. The relative importance of each type of interaction depends on the energy of the photon and the atomic number of the material with which it is interacting.

A salient feature of x- or $\gamma$-ray interaction with matter via any of the above three mechanisms is the production of a high-energy charged particle (electron or positron) that then loses energy in the medium by producing ionizations and excitations as previously discussed. Because of this, x- or $\gamma$-radiation is sometimes known as indirectly ionizing radiation.

### Photoelectric Effect

When an incident photon interacts with a target atom through the photoelectric effect, it transfers all its energy to one of the electrons in the atom (i.e., the photon is completely absorbed by the atom), as shown in Figure 6.6. The absorption of energy by the atom leads to its ionization by the emission of

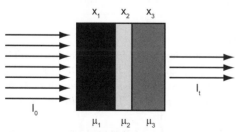

**Fig. 6.5.** Heterogeneous transmission through three layers of different tissues. Three different tissues with thicknesses of $x_1$, $x_2$, and $x_3$, and attenuation coefficients of $\mu_1$, $\mu_2$, and $\mu_3$, respectively, make up the heterogeneous tissue. Total thickness of the tissue is t, and $I_0$ and $I_t$ are the incident and transmitted flux of x- or $\gamma$-rays.

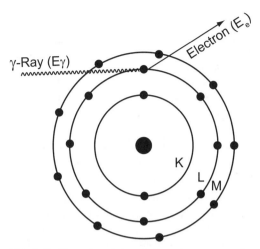

γ-Ray (Eγ)

Electron (E_e)

K
L
M

**Fig. 6.6.** Photoelectric interaction. A γ-ray transfers all its energy to an orbital electron of the absorbing material atom and thereby ionizes the atom. The electron thus released carries an amount of energy Ee that is equal to the γ-ray energy Eγ minus the binding energy of the electron in that orbit. If during ionization the vacancy is created in an inner orbit, a characteristic x-ray or Auger electron will also follow.

an electron, which acquires kinetic energy Ee in an amount equal to that of the photon energy Eγ minus the electron's binding energy (BE) in the shell (; i.e., Ee = Eγ − BE of the electron). The electron can be released from any atomic shell. If it is released from one of the inner shells (e.g., K), a vacancy is created in this shell that is subsequently filled by an electron from one of the higher shells (e.g., L, M), as described in Chapters 1 and 2. This results in the emission of a characteristic x-ray or Auger electron by the atom. If, on the other hand, outer-shell electrons are involved in the photo-electric interaction, the atom is simply ionized. The probability of the photoelectric interaction by an atom τ(atom) strongly depends on two factors: the energy of the photon Eγ and the atomic number Z of the atom involved in the interaction.

***Dependence on Eγ*** The probability of photo-electric interaction τ(atom) decreases sharply with the increase in the x- or γ-ray energy. It is inversely proportional to the cube of γ-ray energy, that is, $\tau(\text{atom}) \, \alpha (1/E_\gamma^3)$. Therefore, the probability of a γ-ray of 45 keV interacting through the photoelectric effect is eight times higher than for a γ-ray of 90-keV energy, that is, $(90^3)/(45^3) = 8$. There is, however, one exception

to this inverse cube law. Whenever the energy of the γ-ray Eγ becomes equal to the binding energies of the electrons in the various atomic shells of an atom, the probability of photoelectric interaction rises sharply. For example, the probability of the photoelectric interaction of a 45-keV γ-ray with a lead atom should be eight times higher than that of a 90-keV γ-ray according to the $1/E_\gamma^3$ rule. However, because the BE of the electrons in the K shell of a lead atom is about 88 keV, the probability of a photoelectric interaction of a 90-keV γ-ray increases to a point where it almost becomes equal to that for a 45-keV γ-ray. The probability of a photoelectric interaction of an 80-keV γ-ray in lead is about six times lower than that of a 90-keV γ-ray, despite the fact that the latter is a higher energy γ-ray. The regions where the $1/E_\gamma^3$ law does not hold are called absorption edges, and their occurrence depends on the atomic number Z of the atom with which the γ-ray interacts. For example, the K absorption edge (where K-shell electrons are involved) occurs at approximately 88 keV in lead but at only 32 keV in iodine (Fig. 6.4).

***Dependence on Z*** The photoelectric probability of interaction τ(atom) also depends strongly on the atomic number of the atom. It is directly proportional to the fourth power of the atomic number; that is, $\tau(\text{atom}) \, \alpha \, Z^4$. For example, the probability of γ-ray of a 50-keV interaction with a lead atom (Z = 82) is 11,000 times higher than that with an oxygen atom (Z = 8) because $[82^4]/[8^4] = 11,000$. Of course, if the γ-ray energy happens to be near one of the absorption edges of that atom, this rule is modified.

**Compton Scattering** In this process, a high-energy photon is scattered in billiard-ball fashion by an electron, as shown in Figure 6.7. The scattered electron gains energy and the incident photon loses energy. The exact amount of the energy gained by the electron or lost by the photon depends on the angle of scatter and the energy of the incident photon Eγ. In general, though, the larger the angle of scatter for a photon, the more energy it loses to an electron. Thus, the maximum transfer of energy from the photon to the electron occurs when the photon is scattered at an angle of 180 degrees (i.e., back-scattered). The energy of the back-scattered

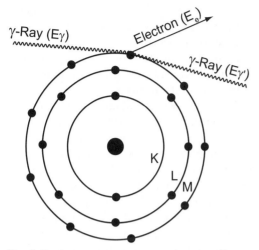

**Fig. 6.7.** Compton interaction. A γ-ray transfers only a partial amount of its energy to an orbital electron (usually the outer shell). The scattered γ-rays carry an energy Eγ′ that is equal to Eγ − Ee, where Eγ is the energy of the primary γ-ray and Ee is the energy carried by the scattered electron.

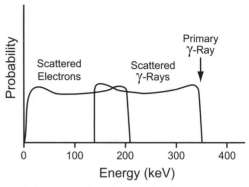

**Fig. 6.8.** Energy distribution of the scattered γ-rays and the scattered electrons in a Compton interaction of a 364-keV γ-ray. The maximum amount of energy that a 364-keV γ-ray can transfer to an electron via this process is 210 keV.

photon (minimum energy of scattered photon) is related to the energy of the incident photon Eγ by the following expression:

$$E\gamma_{minimum} \simeq \frac{E\gamma}{1 + 4E\gamma} (E\gamma \text{ is in MeV})$$

For a 1-MeV incident photon, the minimum energy of the scattered photon is 0.200 MeV; for a 0.360-MeV photon, 0.148 MeV; for a 0.140-MeV photon, 0.090 MeV; and for a 0.080-MeV photon, 0.060 MeV. These values of Eγ$_{minimum}$ are given here as an illustration because of their relevance in γ-ray energy analysis by NaI (Tl) detectors (see Chapter 8). The energies of the scattered photons range from this minimum to that of the incidence photon energy. In Figure 6.8 we show the energy distribution of the scattered photons and scattered electrons for a 360-keV primary photon as a result of Compton interaction.

***Dependence on E*** The probability of Compton interaction σ (atom) initially decreases slowly with the increase in energy E and then falls off more rapidly.

***Dependence on Z*** Because each atom contains Z number of electrons, the probability of

Compton interaction by an atom, σ(atom), is directly proportional to the atomic number, that is, σ(atom) α Z.

**Pair Production** For this interaction to occur, the energy of the γ-ray must be greater than 1.02 MeV. When a γ-ray of energy greater than 1.02 MeV passes through the electric field of a nucleus, it creates an electron and a positron (i.e., part of the γ-ray energy is converted into mass). This process is called pair production and is depicted in Figure 6.9. The excess energy of the γ-ray (Eγ − 1.02 MeV) is shared by e⁻ and e⁺ as kinetic energy.

***Dependence on E*** The probability of pair production κ (atom) is zero below 1.02 MeV. At energies higher than 1.02 MeV, κ (atom) increases with increases in E and in fact becomes the dominant mode of interaction above 10 MeV.

***Dependence on Z*** The probability of pair production κ (atom) for a given atom varies directly as Z².

**Dependence of μ(mass) and μ(linear) on Z** So far we have discussed the dependence of μ(atom) on Z for different processes of interaction. How do the linear and mass attenuation coefficients vary with atomic number? The linear attenuation coefficient μ(linear) and the mass attenuation coefficient μ(mass) depend on

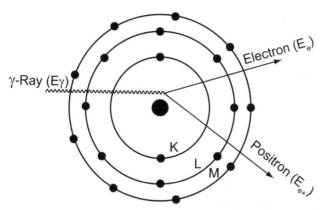

**Fig. 6.9.** Pair production. Under the influence of the positive charge of the nucleus, a γ-ray whose energy Eγ is more than 1.02 MeV annihilates and produces a pair of particles (an electron and a positron) that carry the balance of energy, Eγ − 1.02 MeV. The positron is subsequently annihilated in the manner described on p. 58.

Z as $Z^3$, $Z^0$ (i.e., no dependence on Z), and Z for photoelectric, Compton, and pair production modes of interaction, respectively. In this respect, it is important to remember that when the Compton scattering is the dominant mode of interaction, then each gram of any material (i.e., water, iodine, bone, or lead) attenuates the γ- or x-rays to about the same extent. However, attenuation per $cm^3$ of those materials will still differ, in proportion to their density.

**Relative Importance of the Three Processes** The total interaction probability of an atom $\mu$(atom) then, is the sum of the three probabilities, $\tau$(atom), $\sigma$(atom), and $\kappa$ (atom); that is, $\mu$(atom) = $\tau$(atom) + $\sigma$(atom) + $\kappa$ (atom). Because of the complex and varying dependence of $\mu$(atom) on γ-ray energy Eγ and the atomic number Z of the material, generally one of these processes becomes the dominant mode of interaction for a given γ-ray energy and atomic number of the material. Figure 6.10 shows the relative importance of these processes for the 10-keV to 1 MeV energy range for four materials of great importance in nuclear medicine: water (tissue type), bone, sodium iodide [NaI(Tl)], and lead (Pb). In water or bone, most of the interaction of x- or γ-rays above 50 keV is through the Compton scattering. For

lead, photoelectric interaction is the dominant mode of interaction even up to 1 MeV, although at these energies, Compton interaction does become important. In NaI(Tl), photoelectric effect is the dominant mode of interaction up to 300 keV.

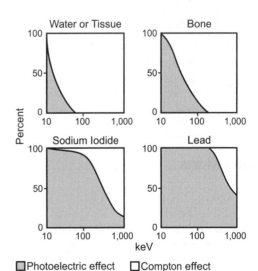

■ Photoelectric effect □ Compton effect

**Fig. 6.10.** Relative contributions of photoelectric and Compton interaction to the total attenuation coefficient of water (tissue), bone, sodium iodide, and lead as a function of energy. In water and bone, almost all interactions above 50 keV are via the Compton scattering, whereas in sodium iodide and lead, the photoelectric effect is the dominant mode of interaction even up to 300 keV.

# Interaction of Neutrons

Because neutrons do not have any electric charge, they do not experience the attractive or repulsive forces experienced by charged particles. Instead, these interact in billiard-ball fashion (direct hit) with the nuclei. When the energy of the neutrons is very low, they can easily enter a nucleus and may form radionuclides. Interaction of neutrons does not play a significant role in nuclear medicine, except in the production of some radionuclides by neutron-capture reactions (see Chapter 4), and therefore is not discussed here.

## Key Points

1. Charged particles interact with matter through inelastic collisions and have a defined range of penetration R.
2. Range R increases with an increase in energy and decreases with an increase in mass and charge of the particle. It decreases with an increase in density of the interacting material. It increases as $Q^2$ but does not depend on the sign of the charge.
3. Linear energy transfer LET of a charged particle is an important parameter that affects biological damage.
4. Electrons and positrons interact in identical fashion except that positrons at the end of their range annihilate by combining with an electron. Annihilation produces two $\gamma$-rays of 511 keV. These $\gamma$-rays travel in opposite direction.
5. Bremsstrahlung is a secondary mechanism of interaction of charged particles. X-rays of various energies are produced when an electron or other charged particle passes in the vicinity of a nucleus.
6. X-rays and $\gamma$-rays do not have a well-defined range of interaction. Instead, half-value layer HVL is used to define a thickness of a substance that attenuates an x- or $\gamma$-ray beam by 50%.
7. For energies of interest in nuclear medicine, three mechanisms, photoelectric (all of the $\gamma$-ray energy given to an electron), Compton ($\gamma$-ray energy shared between an electron and a scattered $\gamma$-ray), and pair production ($\gamma$-ray energy is converted into an electron and positron pair) dominate the interaction of x- and $\gamma$-rays with matter.
8. Photoelectric effect is the dominant interaction for $\gamma$-ray energies up to 500 keV for high-atomic-number materials (>50) such as lead and NaI (Tl).
9. Compton scattering dominates in low atomic number materials such as soft tissue and bone above 100 keV.
10. Pair production is important only at high energies (1022 keV and above).

## Questions

1. Arrange the following radiations in order of their penetrability: 1-MeV x-ray, 1-MeV electron, 1-MeV $\alpha$ particle, 50-keV characteristic x-ray, and 400-keV $\gamma$-ray.
2. List the factors on which the range of a charged particle depends.
3. If you know the range of a charged particle in water, what other information do you need to determine its range in another medium? If you know the linear attenuation coefficient of a $\gamma$-ray in water, will the same information let you determine the linear attenuation coefficient of another medium for the same $\gamma$-ray?
4. When a positron annihilates, what is the result?
5. The linear attenuation coefficients of 300 keV $\gamma$-rays for tissue, sodium iodide, and lead are approximately 0.12, 0.8, and 4.5 cm$^{-1}$, respectively. Determine the half-value layer for each material.
6. Determine the percentage transmission of 50 and 150 keV through 5 cm of tissue if the linear attenuation coefficients are 0.30 and 0.12 cm$^{-1}$, respectively.
7. Determine the percentage transmission of 140 keV through 10 cm heterogeneous layer

of tissue consisting of 3 cm of soft tissue, 5 cm of lung tissue, and 2 cm of bone (linear attenuation coefficient is 0.12 cm$^{-1}$ for soft tissue, 0.21 cm$^{-1}$ for bone, and 0.04 cm$^{-1}$ for lung tissue).

8. The linear attenuation coefficients for lead at 140 and 750 keV are 22.7 and 1.13 cm$^{-1}$, respectively. Determine the percentage transmission through 3 mm lead.

9. Photoelectric effect generally decreases sharply with $\gamma$-ray energy. In what areas (energies) does this law break down?

10. Determine the energy of a back-scattered $\gamma$-ray if the energy of the primary $\gamma$-ray is one of the following: 100 keV, 500 keV, or 1 MeV.

11. What are the relationships among the linear attenuation coefficients of ice, water, and steam?

12. The linear attenuation coefficient of bone for 100-keV $\gamma$-rays is 0.2 cm$^{-1}$. Determine the percentage of 100-keV $\gamma$-rays that will pass through a 2-cm-thick bone without any interaction.

13. If in question 8, 80% of the interactions in bone are due to photoelectric effect and 20% due to Compton scattering, determine the percentage of 100-keV $\gamma$-rays that will interact through photoelectric and Compton interactions, respectively.

14. If a $\gamma$-ray interacts through pair production, what is the minimum energy it must have?

15. Why is LET important?

# Radiation Dosimetry

Radiation is known to produce a number of deleterious effects in a living system. Therefore, it is important to properly assess the benefits and risks to a patient from a given nuclear medicine procedure, ensuring that the benefits outweigh the risks, if any, by a significant margin. One factor that strongly influences the intensity or probability of radiation effects is the energy absorbed by the tissue (radiation dose). Therefore, the assessment of risk can be performed only if one knows the radiation dose that will be delivered to a patient by a particular procedure. This chapter describes the various methods for determining the radiation dose to a patient from internally administered radionuclides or radiopharmaceuticals. However, in the actual risk estimation, two other important factors, the relative biological effectiveness of the radiation and the tissue sensitivity, are also needed; these are discussed in Chapter 15. Radiation exposure and hazard from external radioactive source are discussed in Chapter 16.

## General Comments on Radiation Dose Calculations

In nuclear medicine procedures, it is almost impossible to measure the radiation dose directly using any kind of radiation detector. Instead, this has to be calculated by using a variety of physical and biological data and mathematical equations specially developed for this purpose. It should be emphasized, however, at the outset that the accuracy of these calculations is complicated by several factors. First, even though the physical data needed can be acquired fairly accurately, it is difficult to obtain the biological data needed for these calculations with sufficient accuracy because these are, in practice, extrapolated from animal data or in some cases obtained from limited human data. Second, a variety of assumptions routinely made in these calculations (e.g., uniform distribution, instant uptake of the radiopharmaceutical in the given organ, or single exponential biological elimination) seldom holds true in practice. Third, radiation dose calculations are usually addressed to a hypothetical man known as the "standard man." Various particulars such as the total body weight and weight of various organs of the standard man are given in Appendix E. These may differ appreciably in an actual case. Finally, the calculated dose is obtained by taking an average over a large volume (greater than 1 cm$^3$) and therefore cannot be used to estimate radiation dose at cellular level (microdosimetry).

These factors, when combined, make radiation dose calculations susceptible to large errors. Hence, the radiation dose calculations presented here and elsewhere represent an average dose from a given procedure that may vary by a factor of 2, or even more, in an individual case.

## Definitions and Units

Obviously, to calculate the radiation dose, one should know the meaning of radiation dose and radiation dose rate and their units of measurement.

**Radiation Dose, D** Radiation dose, or, more precisely, radiation absorbed dose, is a measure of the total energy absorbed from the radiation by 1 unit of mass of a substance. In the SI Unit System, absorbed dose is measured in gray (Gy). A gray equals 1 joule of energy absorbed/kilogram of a substance (J/kg). Two commonly used and derived units from gray are centigray ($cGy = 10^{-2}\,Gy$) and milligray ($mGy = 10^{-3}\,Gy$). Its old unit is rad, which is a short notation for the radiation absorbed dose. A rad is defined as 100 ergs of absorbed energy per gram of a tissue or substance. One rad equals 1/100 Gy or equals a cGy and 1 Gy equals 100 rad.

**Radiation Dose Rate, dD/dt** Radiation dose rate, dD/dt, is defined as the amount of energy absorbed per unit time per unit of mass of tissue. Its units may be expressed in various ways, such as mGy (rad) per minute, cGy (rad) per hour, or Gy (rad) per day.

# Parameters or Data Needed

In a typical situation in nuclear medicine, a known amount of radioactivity of a radiopharmaceutical is administered to a patient. A certain fraction f of the radiopharmaceutical is then localized in the organ of interest. One is interested in knowing the radiation dose delivered to this organ and sometimes to various other organs as well. Two types of data are required for these calculations: one related to the decay characteristics of the radionuclide and one to the biological distribution and elimination of the radiopharmaceutical. Table 7.1 lists the various parameters needed for these calculations, together with the units and symbols used here. Some parameters have been defined in Chapters 2 and 3; some are self-evident, and the others are discussed in this chapter. I have retained the old units because a large amount of the data needed in these calculations is still in old units. It is easier to convert the final equations, tables,

| **Table 7.1.** Parameters and Symbols Used in the Calculation of Radiation Dose | | |
|---|---|---|
| **Parameter** | **Symbol** | **Unit** |
| Any given radiation | i | — |
| Total number of radiations | n | — |
| Energy of radiation i | $E_i$ | MeV |
| Frequency of emission of radiation i | $n_i$ | Per decay |
| Equilibrium dose constant for radiation i | $\Delta_i$ | g·rad/$\mu$Ci·h |
| Absorbed fraction | $\phi_i(T \leftarrow S)$ | — |
| Self-absorbed fraction | $\phi_i$ | — |
| Target organ | T | — |
| Source organ | S | — |
| Mass of target organ | M | g |
| Radiation dose rate at time t | dD/dt | rad/h |
| Radiation dose | D | rad |
| Radioactivity in source at time t | A(t) | $\mu$Ci |
| Radioactive dosage at time 0 | $A_0$ | $\mu$Ci |
| Fraction localized in the source | f | — |
| Physical half-life | $T_{\frac{1}{2}}$ | h |
| Biological half-life | $T_{\frac{1}{2}}(Bio)$ | h |
| Effective half-life in the source | $T_{\frac{1}{2}}(eff)$ | h |

or results in the SI units, which I have done here at the appropriate places.

## Calculation of the Radiation Dose

To calculate the radiation dose, one has to determine the average amount of energy absorbed by 1 g of tissue of a target (organ of interest) from the total energy released by the decay of a given amount of radioactivity. Because x- or $\gamma$-rays are more penetrating than particulate radiation, a small x- or $\gamma$-ray emitting source, localized at any site in the body, irradiates practically every organ of the body. For example, an x- or $\gamma$-ray emitting radionuclide localized only in the liver (source S) delivers the radiation dose to all other organs (targets T) of the body in addition to the liver. Thus, if a radiopharmaceutical is localized in multiple organs (sources), the radiation dose from each source to each organ (target) has to be calculated before the final determination of the radiation dose to each organ can be made by adding all contributions. The following four steps are involved in the radiation-dose determinations:

1. Calculation of the rate of energy emission (erg/h) of the various types of radiation emitted by the radionuclide in the source volume.
2. Calculation of the rate of energy absorption from these radiations by the target volume.
3. Calculation of the average dose rate, dD/dt.
4. Calculation of the average dose D.

This method of radiation dose calculation is known as the absorbed fraction method. The first three steps require mainly physical data such as decay characteristics, organ shape and size, and so on, whereas the fourth step requires biological distribution data.

**Step 1: Rate of Energy Emission** Let us first consider a radionuclide that emits only one type of radiation (emission frequency = 1) of energy E (MeV) per decay. One microcurie ($3.7 \times 10^4$ decay/s) of this radionuclide will, therefore, emit energy at a rate of $3.7 \times 10^4 \times$ E MeV/s.

If we change the unit of energy from MeV to erg (1 MeV = $1.6 \times 10^{-6}$ erg) and the unit of time from second to hour (1 h = 3600 s), the rate of energy emission by this radionuclide becomes equal to $3.7 \times 10^4 \times 1.6 \times 10^{-6} \times 3600 \times$ E erg/(h $\cdot$ $\mu$Ci), or 213E erg/(h $\cdot$ $\mu$Ci).

In the case of a radionuclide that emits more than one radiation, say 1, 2, 3, ..., n, with emission frequencies $n_1, n_2, n_3, ..., n_n$ and energies of $E_1, E_2, E_3, ..., E_n$, respectively, the rate of energy emission for each type of radiation will be equal to $213n_1E_1$ erg/(h $\cdot$ $\mu$Ci) for radiation 1, $213n_2E_2$ erg/(h $\cdot$ $\mu$Ci) for radiation 2, and so on.

**Step 2: Rate of Energy Absorption** To calculate the rate of absorption of energy by a target volume T from a radionuclidic distribution in a source volume S, we have to define a new quantity known as the absorbed fraction, $\phi_i$(T←S). The absorbed fraction $\phi_i$(T←S) is defined as the ratio of energy absorbed by a target volume T from a radiation i to the amount of energy released by a radionuclidic distribution in volume S in the form of radiation i. In other words,

$$\phi_i \, (T \leftarrow S)$$
$$= \frac{\text{Energy absorbed in volume T from ratiaton}}{\text{Energy emitted in volume S as radistion i}}$$

In most problems encountered in nuclear medicine, the radioactivity is distributed within the target volume T itself (i.e., T is the same as S). In that case, the absorbed fraction is known as the self-absorbed fraction and is expressed simply as $\phi_i$.

Once $\phi_i$(T←S) is known, the rate of energy absorption by a target volume T is simply obtained by multiplying the rate of energy emission of radiation i (from step 1, $213n_iE_i$) by the absorbed fraction $\phi_i$(T←S), or

Rate of energy absorption by the target volume from radiation i = $213n_iE_i \times \phi_i$(T←S)

$$= 213n_iE_i\phi_i(T \leftarrow S)\text{erg/(h}\cdot\mu\text{Ci)}$$

If there are n radiations, the rate of the total energy absorption will be equal to the sum of the energies absorbed from each radiation, that is,

$$= 213n_1E_1\phi_1(T \leftarrow S) + 213n_2E_2\phi_2(T \leftarrow S) +$$
$$+ ... \, 213n_nE_n\phi_n(T \leftarrow S) \text{ erg/(h} \cdot \mu\text{Ci)}.$$

**Table 7.2.** Self-Absorbed Fraction $\phi_i$ for Different $\gamma$-Ray Energies and Various Organs

| Organ | Energy (keV) | | | | | | |
|---|---|---|---|---|---|---|---|
| | **15** | **30** | **50** | **100** | **200** | **500** | **1000** |
| Bladder | 0.885 | 0.464 | 0.201 | 0.117 | 0.116 | 0.116 | 0.107 |
| Stomach | 0.860 | 0.414 | 0.176 | 0.101 | 0.101 | 0.101 | 0.093 |
| Kidneys | 0.787 | 0.298 | 0.112 | 0.066 | 0.068 | 0.073 | 0.067 |
| Liver | 0.898 | 0.543 | 0.278 | 0.165 | 0.158 | 0.157 | 0.144 |
| Lungs | 0.665 | 0.231 | 0.089 | 0.049 | 0.050 | 0.051 | 0.045 |
| Pancreas | 0.666 | 0.195 | 0.068 | 0.038 | 0.042 | 0.044 | 0.040 |
| Skeleton | 0.893 | 0.681 | 0.400 | 0.173 | 0.123 | 0.118 | 0.110 |
| Spleen | 0.817 | 0.331 | 0.128 | 0.071 | 0.073 | 0.077 | 0.070 |
| Thyroid | 0.592 | 0.149 | 0.048 | 0.028 | 0.031 | 0.032 | 0.029 |
| Total body | 0.933 | 0.774 | 0.548 | 0.370 | 0.338 | 0.340 | 0.321 |

The above expression can be written in a concise form as

$$213 \sum_{i=1}^{n} n_i\, E_i \phi_i(T\leftarrow S)\ \mathrm{erg/hr}\cdot\mu\mathrm{Ci}$$

where $\sum_{i=1}^{n}$ is the sum of all terms when i changes from 1 to n.

How does one determine $\phi_i(T\leftarrow S)$? Determination of the absorbed fraction requires the exact knowledge of the interaction of radiation with matter, discussed in the previous chapter. Computations of $\phi_i(T\leftarrow S)$ for a number of source and target combinations, from these basic mechanisms of interaction of radiation with matter, are quite involved and require the use of large computers. The *Journal of Nuclear Medicine* published a variety of tables listing $\phi_i(T\leftarrow S)$ for different x- or $\gamma$-ray energies and source and target volumes. Table 7.2 lists the absorbed fraction for various organs of a standard man for different x- or $\gamma$-ray energies when the radionuclidic distribution is within the same organ (i.e., T is the same as S). For other combinations, the reader is referred to the original articles.*

## General Comments on $\phi_i(T\leftarrow S)$

The maximum value of $\phi_i(T\leftarrow S)$ can only be 1. This occurs when all emitted energy is absorbed in the target. The minimum value is 0 and

---
* Suppl. No. 1, 1968; Suppl. No. 3, 1969; Suppl. No. 5, 1971.

occurs when there is no absorption of energy in the target.

In the case of particulate radiations such as $\beta$ particles, conversion electrons, or $\alpha$ particles, almost all energy emitted by a radionuclide is absorbed in the volume of distribution itself, provided the source volume is larger than 1 $\mathrm{cm}^3$. Then, $\phi_i(T\leftarrow S) = 0$, unless T and S are the same, in which case $\phi_i = 1$. The same holds true for x- or $\gamma$-radiation with energies less than 10 keV. Thus, these radiations deliver radiation doses only in the volume of distribution and not outside of it.

For x- or $\gamma$-radiations with energies higher than 10 keV, the absorbed fraction $\phi_i(T\leftarrow S)$ strongly depends on the energy of the x- or $\gamma$-ray; the shape and size of the source volume; and the shape, size, and distance of the target volume. In general, $\phi_i$ first decreases with an increase in the energy of the x- or $\gamma$-ray and then eventually levels off. Notice in Table 7.2 that the absorbed fraction, $\phi_i$ drops sharply with energy up to 100 keV but then does not change significantly from 100 to 500 keV for various organs listed.

**Step 3: Dose Rate, dD/dt** If one now divides the rate of energy absorption by the target with its mass M, this will give the rate of energy absorption per gram of tissue, which when divided by 100 (to convert erg/g to rad) yields the dose rate for each microcurie of activity; that is, the dose rate,

$$\frac{dD}{dt} = \frac{2.13}{M} \sum_{i=1}^{n} n_i E_i \phi_i (T \leftarrow S) \ \text{rad/hr} \cdot \mu\text{Ci})$$

By defining $\Delta_i = 2.13 \ n_i E_i$, this reduces to

$$\frac{dD}{dt} = \frac{1}{M} \sum_{i=1}^{n} \Delta_i \phi_i (T \leftarrow S) \ \text{rad/(hr} \cdot \mu\text{Ci)} \quad (1)$$

If the source volume contains $A(t)$ $\mu$Ci at time t, then the dose rate dD from $A(t)$ amount of radioactivity becomes

$$\frac{dD}{dt} = \frac{A(t)}{M} \sum_{i=1}^{n} \Delta_i \phi_i (T \leftarrow S) \ \text{rad/hr} \quad (2)$$

## Step 4: Average Dose, D

The radioactivity $A(t)$ localized in an organ is generally a fraction f of the administered dosage $A_0$ and is being continuously eliminated, with an effective half-life of $T_{\frac{1}{2}}$ (eff); that is,

$$A(t) = f \cdot A_0 \cdot e^{\frac{-0.693t}{T_{\frac{1}{2}}(\text{eff})}} \ \mu\text{Ci} \quad (3)$$

Therefore, the dose rate dD/dt is continuously decreasing with time and eventually becomes zero. How does one compute the total dose to the patient from the time of administration (t = 0) to the time when the dose rate has finally been reduced to zero? For this, one has to integrate the dose rate dD/dt from 0 to $\infty$ time, or $D = \int_0^\infty (dD/dt) \ dt$. This involves integration of $A(t)$ that, for a simple case such as equation (3), leads to the following expression:

$$D(T \leftarrow S) = 1.44 \ T_{\frac{1}{2}}(\text{eff}) \cdot \frac{fA_0}{M} \cdot \sum_{i=1}^{n} \Delta_i \phi_i (T \leftarrow S) \ \text{rad} \quad (4)$$

In the case where the target and source volume are the same, the self-dose D is given by

$$D = 1.44 \ T_{\frac{1}{2}}(\text{eff}) \cdot \frac{fA_0}{M} \cdot \sum_{i=1}^{n} \Delta_i \phi_i \ \text{rad} \quad (5)$$

Note that the factor $(fA_0/M)$ in the above equations is the concentration of the radioactivity in the organ of localization. Therefore, it is the concentration and not the total amount of the radioactivity in an organ that is the primary determinant of the radiation dose.

From these expressions, it is evident *that to minimize the radiation dose to a patient*, smaller amounts of radioactivity ($A_0$), radiopharmaceuticals with shorter $T_{\frac{1}{2}}$ (eff), and radionuclides with smaller absorbed fractions (which means $\gamma$-ray energy higher than 100 keV and no particulate emission as discussed earlier; p. 41) are desired.

## Cumulated Radioactivity

The above equations (4) and (5) assume that the uptake in the organ is instantaneous and the disappearance of the radioactivity from the source can be expressed by a single exponential term, such as in equation (3). This does not have to be so, and often the biokinetics of the radionuclidic distribution is more complex. An example is shown in Figure 7.1. In this case, equation (3) cannot be used to describe the time behavior of the radioactivity in blood or plasma or in organs one and two. For these, the exact time activity curve, $A(t)$, should be used to calculate the cumulated radioactivity Ã, which is defined as $Ã = \int_0^\infty A(t) \cdot dt$. The unit of Ã as used here is h $\cdot$ $\mu$Ci, which means $A(t)$ is measured in $\mu$Ci and time in hours. Because these calculations are more complicated, we shall not go into the details here.

## Simplification of Radiation Dose Calculations Using "S" Factor

Recently, in an attempt to simplify the calculation of radiation dose in routine clinical situations, Snyder and colleagues combined the physical data such as radiations emitted by a radionuclide and the absorbed fractions for various source and target combinations of a standard man into one single term, which they called "S" factor. In fact, S factor is nothing but the dose rate from 1 $\mu$Ci as given by equation (1). Therefore, S is expressed as follows:

$$S(T \leftarrow S) = \frac{dD}{dt} = \frac{1}{M} \sum_{i=1}^{n} \Delta_i \phi_i (T \leftarrow S) \ \text{rad/(hr} \cdot \mu\text{Ci)} \quad (6)$$

Substitution of S factor in equation (4) simplifies it to the following equation:

$$D(T \leftarrow S) = 1.44 \cdot f \cdot A_0 \cdot T_{\frac{1}{2}}(\text{eff}) \cdot S(T \leftarrow S) \ \text{rad} \quad (7)$$

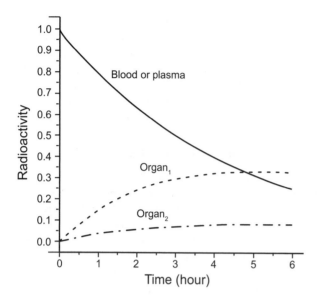

**Fig. 7.1.** Biokinetics of an intravenously administered radiopharmaceutical. Blood or plasma radioactivity decreases with time. A fraction of blood or plasma radioactivity is extracted by organ1, and organ2. Another fraction, not shown here, is excreted. For multicompartmental kinetics such as in this example, none of these curves can be fitted by a monoexponential function given by equation (3). In this case, cumulated activity Ã needed for radiation dose calculations is determined by either graphic methods or multiexponential curve-fitting methods.

In the case of a radiopharmaceutical with complex biokinetics, such as shown in Figure 7.1, cumulated activity A in each organ should be calculated from the actual biokinetic data. Then,

$$D(T \leftarrow S) = \tilde{A} \cdot S(T \leftarrow S) \text{ rad} \qquad (8)$$

S factor depends only on the physical data and is unique for a given radionuclide and a pair of organs of a standard man. Hence, it has to be calculated only once for each radionuclide and each pair of organs (source and target). Snyder and colleagues have calculated these factors for a large number of medically useful radionuclides. These are published as Supplement 11, *Journal of Nuclear Medicine.* Table 7.3 lists some S factors for $^{99m}$Tc for a number of organ pairs of a standard man. For other combinations of pairs and radionuclides, the original reference should be consulted. Unit of S factor is rad/(h · $\mu$Ci). This can be easily converted into SI units, such as Gy/(h · MBq), by dividing the S factors given in Table 7.3 by 3.7.

Knowing S factors, the calculation of the radiation dose is simple. One plugs the values of the radioactivity localized in the source organ (f·A$_0$), the effective half-life, [T$_{\frac{1}{2}}$(eff)], and the S factor in equation (7) to obtain the radiation dose.

*Caution:* The S factor method cannot be applied when the radiation dose is calculated for persons who differ appreciably from a standard man, such as children.

## Some Illustrative Examples

**Problem 1:**
A liver scan is performed on a patient using 2 mCi of $^{99m}$Tc-labeled sulfur colloid. Assuming that 90% of the injected dosage is localized in the liver instantaneously and that the effective half-life, T$_{\frac{1}{2}}$(eff), is equal to 6 hours, calculate the radiation dose delivered to the liver of the patient using the absorbed fraction method [equation (5)].

Calculation: Because mass of the liver is not given in the problem, we shall assume it to be that of a standard man. Therefore, from Appendix E, M = 1800 g. The initial amount of activity localized in the liver, A$_0$(liver) = 0.90 × 2000 $\mu$Ci = 1800 $\mu$Ci (66.6 MBq) and T$_{\frac{1}{2}}$(eff) = 6 hours. Parameters such as n$_i$, E$_i$, and $\Delta_i$ for $^{99m}$Tc and $\phi_i$ for liver for $^{99m}$Tc radiations and the calculations of $\Sigma\Delta_i\phi_i$ are given in Table 7.4. Substituting these values in equation (5) we get Dose (liver) = (1800/1800) × 1.44 × 6 × 0.078 = 0.67 rad (6.7 mGy)

The remaining 10% of the dosage, if not excreted in a short time from the body, will also contribute a radiation dose to the liver. Its contribution, however, will be small and therefore is ignored here. (Actual calculations will be involved. We will have to construct a table similar to Table 7.4.)

**Problem 2:**
Calculate the radiation dose to the liver, red bone marrow, ovaries, and testes using S factors and the data given in problem 1.

**Table 7.3.**  S Factors for $^{99m}$Tc for Various Sources and Targets (rad/h · $\mu$Ci)$^a$

| Target | Source | | | | | | | | | |
|---|---|---|---|---|---|---|---|---|---|---|
| | Bladder Content | Stomach Content | Kidneys | Liver | Lung | Marrow Red | Bone (Av) | Spleen | Thyroid | Total Body |
| Bladder wall | $1.6 \times 10^{-4}$ | $2.7 \times 10^{-7}$ | $2.8 \times 10^{-7}$ | $1.6 \times 10^{-7}$ | $3.6 \times 10^{-8}$ | $9.9 \times 10^{-7}$ | $5.1 \times 10^{-7}$ | $1.2 \times 10^{-7}$ | $2.1 \times 10^{-9}$ | $2.3 \times 10^{-6}$ |
| Bone (total) | $9.2 \times 10^{-7}$ | $9.0 \times 10^{-7}$ | $1.4 \times 10^{-6}$ | $1.1 \times 10^{-6}$ | $1.5 \times 10^{-6}$ | $4.0 \times 10^{-6}$ | $1.1 \times 10^{-5}$ | $1.1 \times 10^{-6}$ | $1.0 \times 10^{-6}$ | $2.5 \times 10^{-6}$ |
| Stomach wall | $2.7 \times 10^{-7}$ | $1.3 \times 10^{-4}$ | $3.6 \times 10^{-6}$ | $1.9 \times 10^{-6}$ | $1.8 \times 10^{-6}$ | $9.5 \times 10^{-7}$ | $5.5 \times 10^{-7}$ | $1.0 \times 10^{-5}$ | $4.5 \times 10^{-8}$ | $2.2 \times 10^{-6}$ |
| Kidneys | $2.6 \times 10^{-7}$ | $3.5 \times 10^{-6}$ | $1.9 \times 10^{-4}$ | $3.9 \times 10^{-6}$ | $8.4 \times 10^{-7}$ | $2.2 \times 10^{-7}$ | $8.2 \times 10^{-7}$ | $9.1 \times 10^{-6}$ | $3.4 \times 10^{-8}$ | $2.2 \times 10^{-6}$ |
| Liver | $1.7 \times 10^{-7}$ | $2.0 \times 10^{-6}$ | $3.9 \times 10^{-6}$ | $4.6 \times 10^{-5}$ | $2.5 \times 10^{-6}$ | $9.2 \times 10^{-7}$ | $6.6 \times 10^{-7}$ | $9.8 \times 10^{-7}$ | $9.3 \times 10^{-8}$ | $2.2 \times 10^{-6}$ |
| Lungs | $2.4 \times 10^{-8}$ | $1.7 \times 10^{-6}$ | $8.5 \times 10^{-7}$ | $2.5 \times 10^{-6}$ | $5.2 \times 10^{-5}$ | $1.2 \times 10^{-6}$ | $9.4 \times 10^{-7}$ | $2.3 \times 10^{-6}$ | $9.4 \times 10^{-7}$ | $2.0 \times 10^{-6}$ |
| Marrows | $2.2 \times 10^{-6}$ | $1.6 \times 10^{-6}$ | $3.8 \times 10^{-6}$ | $1.6 \times 10^{-6}$ | $1.9 \times 10^{-6}$ | $3.1 \times 10^{-5}$ | $6.6 \times 10^{-6}$ | $1.7 \times 10^{-6}$ | $1.1 \times 10^{-6}$ | $1.1 \times 10^{-6}$ |
| Ovaries | $7.3 \times 10^{-7}$ | $5.0 \times 10^{-7}$ | $1.1 \times 10^{-6}$ | $4.5 \times 10^{-7}$ | $9.4 \times 10^{-8}$ | $3.2 \times 10^{-6}$ | $8.5 \times 10^{-7}$ | $4.0 \times 10^{-7}$ | $4.9 \times 10^{-9}$ | $2.4 \times 10^{-6}$ |
| Spleen | $6.6 \times 10^{-7}$ | $1.8 \times 10^{-5}$ | $8.6 \times 10^{-6}$ | $9.2 \times 10^{-7}$ | $2.3 \times 10^{-6}$ | $9.2 \times 10^{-7}$ | $5.8 \times 10^{-7}$ | $3.3 \times 10^{-4}$ | $1.1 \times 10^{-7}$ | $2.2 \times 10^{-6}$ |
| Testes | $4.7 \times 10^{-6}$ | $5.1 \times 10^{-8}$ | $8.8 \times 10^{-8}$ | $6.2 \times 10^{-8}$ | $7.9 \times 10^{-9}$ | $4.5 \times 10^{-7}$ | $6.4 \times 10^{-7}$ | $4.8 \times 10^{-8}$ | $5.0 \times 10^{-6}$ | $1.7 \times 10^{-6}$ |
| Thyroid | $2.1 \times 10^{-9}$ | $8.7 \times 10^{-8}$ | $4.8 \times 10^{-8}$ | $1.5 \times 10^{-7}$ | $9.2 \times 10^{-7}$ | $6.8 \times 10^{-7}$ | $7.9 \times 10^{-7}$ | $8.7 \times 10^{-8}$ | $2.3 \times 10^{-3}$ | $1.5 \times 10^{-6}$ |
| Total body | $1.9 \times 10^{-6}$ | $1.9 \times 10^{-6}$ | $2.2 \times 10^{-6}$ | $2.2 \times 10^{-6}$ | $2.0 \times 10^{-6}$ | $2.2 \times 10^{-6}$ | $6.6 \times 10^{-7}$ | $2.2 \times 10^{-6}$ | $1.8 \times 10^{-6}$ | $2.0 \times 10^{-6}$ |

$^a$To convert to SI unit (Gy/h · MBq), divide these values by 3.7.

Calculation: As in problem 1, $T_{\frac{1}{2}}$ (eff) = 6 hours, $A_0$(liver) = 1800 $\mu$Ci (66.6 MBq), and from Table 7.3,

$$S(liver \leftarrow liver) = 4.6 \times 10^{-5}$$
$$S(marrow \leftarrow liver) = 1.6 \times 10^{-6}$$
$$S(ovaries \leftarrow liver) = 4.5 \times 10^{-7}$$
$$S(testes \leftarrow liver) = 6.2 \times 10^{-8}$$

Substituting these values in equation (7), we get

$$D(liver \leftarrow liver) = 1.44 \times 1800 \times 6 \times 4.6 \times 10^{-5} = 0.72 \text{ rad (7.2 mGy)}$$
$$D(marrow \leftarrow liver) = 1.44 \times 1800 \times 6 \times 1.6 \times 10^{-6} = 0.025 \text{ rad (0.25 mGy)}$$
$$D(ovaries \leftarrow liver) = 1.44 \times 1800 \times 6 \times 4.5 \times 10^{-7} = 0.007 \text{ rad (0.07 mGy)}$$
$$D(testes \leftarrow liver) = 1.44 \times 1800 \times 6 \times 6.2 \times 10^{-8} = 0.001 \text{ rad (0.01 mGy)}$$

This problem illustrates the simplicity of the S factor approach in the calculation of the radiation dose. Without constructing tables like Table 7.4, one is able to calculate radiation doses easily, not for one but several organs. Again we have neglected the contribution to the radiation dose of the 10% radiopharmaceutical dosage not localized in the liver. However, calculation of the radiation doses from this fraction will also be straightforward provided one knows the organ of localization and the effective half-life. Also note that the dose to the liver by this method is slightly higher than that in problem 1. This in part is due to the fact that standard man data used for the calculation of S factors are slightly different than that used to compute the original absorbed fractions, $\phi_i$.

Problem 3:
A patient is treated for hyperthyroidism with 5 mCi of $^{131}$I. Calculate the radiation dose to the thyroid of the patient, assuming that the weight of the thyroid gland is 30 g, the effective half-life is 4 days, and the measured thyroid uptake is 45%.

Calculation: Because the thyroid mass (30 g) is quite different from the thyroid mass (20 g) of the standard man (Appendix E), we cannot use the S factor method here. Thyroid mass M = 30 g. The initial amount of activity localized in the

**Table 7.4.** Calculation of $\Sigma \Delta_i \phi_i$: Problem 1 ($^{99m}$Tc)

| Radiation i | $n_i$ | $E_i$ | $\Delta_i^a$ | $\phi_i$ | $\Delta_i \phi_i$ |
|---|---|---|---|---|---|
| Gamma 1 | — | — | — | — | 0 |
| Conversion electron | 0.986 | 0.002 | 0.004 | 1 | 0.004 |
| Gamma 2 | 0.883 | 0.140 | 0.264 | 0.16 | 0.042 |
| K-conversion electron | 0.088 | 0.119 | 0.022 | 1 | 0.022 |
| L-conversion electron | 0.011 | 0.138 | 0.003 | 1 | 0.003 |
| M-conversion electron | 0.004 | 0.140 | 0.001 | 1 | 0.001 |
| Gamma 3 | | | | | |
| Conversion electron | 0.01 | 0.122 | 0.003 | 1 | 0.003 |
| K($\alpha$) x-ray | 0.064 | 0.018 | 0.003 | 0.88 | 0.0026 |
| K($\beta$) x-ray | 0.012 | 0.021 | — | 0.87 | — |
| KLL Auger electron | 0.015 | 0.015 | — | 1 | — |
| LMM Auger electron | 0.106 | 0.002 | — | 1 | — |
| MXY Auger electron | 1.23 | 0.0004 | — | 1 | — |
| | | | | $\Sigma \Delta_i \phi_i = 0.078^b$ | |

$^a\Delta_i = 2.13 n_i E_i$.
$^b$Sum of all $\Delta_i \phi_i$.

thyroid, $A_0$(thyroid) = 0.45 × 5000 $\mu$Ci = 2250 $\mu$Ci (83.25 MBq), and $T_{\frac{1}{2}}$(eff) = 4 days = 4 × 24 hours = 96 hours. Parameters such as $n_i$, $E_i$, and $\Delta_i$ for $^{131}$I; $\phi_i$ for thyroid for $^{131}$I radiations; and the calculations of $\Sigma\Delta_i\phi_i$ are given in Table 7.5. Substituting these values in equation (5),

$$D(\text{thyroid}) = (2250/30) \times 1.44 \times 96 \times 0.433 \text{ rad}$$
$$= 4489 \text{ rad } (44.89 \text{ Gy})$$

The important thing to note here is that if we had used only the particulate radiations of $^{131}$I in our calculations (Table 7.5), the radiation dose would have been 4043 rad [i.e., 90% of the radiation dose to the thyroid by $^{131}$I is delivered by particulate (mainly $\beta^-$) radiations]. This is the reason why $^{131}$I is a good radionuclide for use in therapy and not diagnosis.

# Radiation Doses in Routine Imaging Procedures

Table 7.6 lists the average radiation doses delivered to an adult patient from a number of radiopharmaceuticals commonly used in nuclear medicine. Although an internally administered radiopharmaceutical delivers a radiation dose to practically each and every organ in the body, only the total body and critical organ (the one that receives the highest radiation dose) radiation doses are used to illustrate the extent of the radiation doses routinely delivered to the patients. To assess the actual risk from these procedures, one has to calculate the radiation doses for all organs as described above and from them then calculate the effective dose as described in

| **Table 7.5.** Calculation of $\Sigma\Delta_i\phi_i$: Problem 3 ($^{131}$I) | | | | | |
|---|---|---|---|---|---|
| **Radiation i** | $n_i$ | $E_i$ | $\Delta_i$ | $\phi_i$ | $\Delta_i\phi_i$ |
| Beta 1 | 0.016 | 0.070 | 0.002 | 1 | 0.002 |
| Beta 2 | 0.069 | 0.095 | 0.014 | 1 | 0.014 |
| Beta 3 | 0.005 | 0.143 | 0.001 | 1 | 0.001 |
| Beta 4 | 0.905 | 0.192 | 0.369 | 1 | 0.369 |
| Beta 5 | 0.006 | 0.286 | 0.004 | 1 | 0.004 |
| Gamma 1 | 0.017 | 0.080 | 0.003 | 0.035 | — |
| K-conversion electron Gamma 2 | 0.029 | 0.046 | 0.003 | 1 | 0.003 |
| Conversion electron | 0.004 | 0.129 | 0.001 | 1 | 0.001 |
| Gamma 3 | 0.047 | 0.284 | 0.029 | 0.03 | 0.001 |
| K-conversion electron | 0.002 | 0.250 | 0.001 | 1 | 0.001 |
| Gamma 4 | 0.002 | 0.326 | 0.001 | 0.03 | — |
| Gamma 5 | 0.833 | 0.364 | 0.646 | 0.03 | 0.019 |
| K-conversion electron | 0.017 | 0.330 | 0.012 | 1 | 0.012 |
| L-conversion electron | 0.003 | 0.359 | 0.002 | 1 | 0.002 |
| Gamma 6 | 0.003 | 0.503 | 0.003 | 0.03 | — |
| Gamma 7 | 0.069 | 0.637 | 0.093 | 0.03 | 0.003 |
| Gamma 8 | 0.016 | 0.723 | 0.025 | 0.03 | 0.001 |
| K ($\alpha$) x-rays | 0.038 | 0.030 | 0.002 | 0.15 | — |
| | | | | $\Sigma\Delta_i\phi_i = 0.433$[a] | |

[a]Sum of all $\Delta_i\phi_i$.

**Table 7.6.**   Radiation Doses in Common Imaging Procedures

| Radiopharmaceutical | Radioactivity Dosage | | Radiation Dose (Total Body) | | Radiation Dose (Critical Organ) | | Critical Organ |
|---|---|---|---|---|---|---|---|
| | mCi | MBq | rad | mGy | rad | mGy | |
| 99mTc-labeled | | | | | | | |
| Pertechnetate | 10 | 370 | 0.15 | 1.5 | 2.5 | 25 | Stomach |
| Glucoheptonate | 20 | 740 | 0.15 | 1.5 | 4.5 | 45 | Bladder |
| Phosphate, etc. | 10 | 370 | 0.1 | 1 | 1.5 | 15 | Bladder |
| Sulfur colloid | 3 | 111 | 0.05 | 0.5 | 0.9 | 9 | Liver |
| MA albumin | 3 | 111 | 0.05 | 0.5 | 1 | 10 | Lungs |
| DMSA | 6 | 222 | 0.1 | 1 | 4.0 | 40 | Kidneys |
| DTPA | 20 | 740 | 0.1 | 1.2 | 3.5 | 35 | Bladder |
| Red cells | 20 | 740 | 0.4 | 4 | 0.4 | 4 | Total body |
| HIDA, etc. | 5 | 185 | 0.05 | 0.5 | 1.6 | 16 | Small intestine |
| Mertiatide (MAG3) | 10 | 370 | 0.07 | 0.7 | 4.8 | 48 | Bladder |
| Sestamibi (Cardiolite) | 30 | 1110 | 0.5 | 5 | 5.4 | 54 | Upper large intestine |
| Tetrofosmin (Myoview) | 30 | 1110 | 0.4 | 4 | 3.6 | 36 | Gallbladder wall |
| Exametazime (Ceretec) | 20 | 740 | 0.3 | 3 | 5.2 | 52 | Lacrimal glands |
| 67Ga citrate | 5 | 185 | 1.3 | 13 | 4.5 | 45 | Lower large intestine |
| 111In-Pentetreotide (OctreoScan) | 3 | 111 | 0.5 | 5 | 74 | 7.4 | Spleen |
| 123I-Iodide | 0.1 | 3.7 | 0.004 | 0.04 | 2.2 | 22 | Thyroid |
| 123I-MIBG | 10 | 370 | 0.3 | 3 | 3.5 | 35 | Bladder wall |
| 133Xe | 10 | 370 | 0.001 | 0.01 | 0.3 | 3 | Lungs |
| 201Tl-thallous chloride | 3 | 111 | 0.7 | 7 | 4.5 | 45 | Kidneys |
| 18FDG | 10 | 370 | 0.6 | 7 | 7 | 70 | Bladder Wall |

DMSA, 2, 3-dimercaptosuccinic acid; DTPA, diethylenetriamine pentaacetic acid; and HIDA, (2,6-dimethylacetanilide)iminodiacetic acid.

Chapter 15. It is the effective dose that determines the risk from radiation exposure.

**Radiation Doses in Children** In children, the radiation doses from the adult radiopharmaceutical dosage (as listed in Table 7.6 can be higher by an order of magnitude depending the age of the child. Younger the child, higher will be the radiation dose. Hence, the radiopharmaceutical dosage in children is always proportionally reduced to account for the smaller surface area or weight of a child as compared with an adult. As a result, similar concentrations (radioactivity/g) are localized in both cases. Still, because of the smaller size of organs, the radiation doses in children will be slightly different (some higher and some lower) from the adult radiation doses. Also, as discussed in Chapter 15, children are at a higher risk than an adult for the same radiation dose.

**Radiation Dose to a Fetus** Because a fetus is more sensitive to radiation than an adult, it is not generally advisable to administer radiopharmaceuticals to a pregnant patient. However, there are occasions when, either because of strong medical reasons or inadvertently, a pregnant patient may receive radiopharmaceuticals. In these cases, it is essential to estimate the radiation dose to the fetus. The radiation dose to the fetus in these circumstances is derived from two sources: the radionuclide distributed in the mother's body and the radionuclide distributed in the fetal body due to the placental crossover. For most $^{99m}$Tc-labeled radiopharmaceuticals (except pertechnetate), there is little placental crossover, and therefore most of the radiation dose is derived from distribution in the mother's body. In these cases, the estimated radiation dose to the fetus is between 100 and 400 mrad (2–4 mGy) from 10 mCi (370 MBq) of the administered radioactivity.

Radionuclides such as $^{131}$I, $^{67}$Ga, $^{201}$Tl, and $^{18}$FDG cross the placenta and therefore, depending on the stage of pregnancy, can deliver a relatively large radiation dose. In early pregnancy (first trimester) when the placental crossover is small, the radiation dose to the fetus from diagnostic dosages of $^{67}$Ga, $^{201}$Tl, and $^{18}$FDG given in Table 7.6 is between 1 and 2 rad (10–20 mGy). However, in case of $^{131}$I, because of relatively small dosage (0.05 mCi) is only about 30 mrad (0.3 mGy). These doses increase up to a factor of three in later stages of pregnancy.

## Key Points

1. Radiation absorbed dose is an important physical parameter that determines biological effect.
2. The SI unit is gray and is defined as 1 joule of energy absorbed/kilogram of a substance. One gray equals 100 rad, the older unit of the absorbed dose.
3. Calculation of radiation dose involves four steps: rate of energy emission, rate of energy absorption, dose rate, and dose.
4. Radiation dose increases with an increase in dosage of the radiopharmaceutical and effective half-life in the tissue. It also depends on the mass of the tissue and the energies of radiations emitted by the radionuclide.
5. Routine radiopharmaceuticals deliver radiation doses under 1 cGy (1 rad) to the total body and under 10 cGy (10 rad) to the critical organ.

## Questions

1. Convert the following radiation doses into SI units: (a) 350 rad, (b) 120 mrad, (c) 5 rad.
2. Calculate the average radiation dose to liver if 1.6 kg of liver tissue of a patient absorbs 0.12 J of energy from a radiopharmaceutical.
3. Calculate the average radiation dose to (a) an adult (70 kg weight) who absorbs a total of 98 J of energy from a nuclear medicine procedure, and (b) a child (15 kg weight) who absorbs 30 J of energy from the same procedure.

4. List the major factors on which the radiation dose from a radiopharmaceutical depends.

5. What is the largest source of error in the radiation dose calculations?

6. A $\beta$ emitter is distributed with uniform concentration in (a) a sphere, (b) a cylinder, and (c) a cube of the same volume. Is the radiation dose the same or different in the three cases?

7. What if the radionuclide in problem 6 is a pure $\gamma$ emitter?

8. On what factors does the absorbed fraction, $\phi_i$, depend?

9. For a monoexponential decay [equation (3)], what is the relationship between the cumulated radioactivity $\tilde{A}$ and f, $A_0$, and $T_{\frac{1}{2}}(\text{eff})$.

10. How does the S factor simplify the radiation dose calculations? What are its limitations? Can this method be used to calculate a radiation dose for a given patient?

11. Calculate the radiation dose to lungs of a patient from 100 MBq of $^{99m}$Tc-MAA, given that all radioactivity is uniformly localized in the lungs, $T_{\frac{1}{2}}(\text{eff}) = 3$ hours and S factor $= 1.4 \times 10^{-5}$ Gy/MBq·h.

12. A $\gamma$ emitter is localized in a patient's liver. Can it deliver a radiation dose to his or her brain, thyroid, lungs, spleen, testes, or ovaries? If yes, which of these organs will receive the maximum and minimum dose?

13. What nuclear medicine procedure delivers the largest radiation dose to the total body?

# Detection of High-Energy Radiation

When high-energy radiation interacts with matter, it produces certain physical or chemical changes in matter. These changes, which can be either transitory or permanent, are the basis for detection of high-energy radiation (referred to as radiation, for conciseness, in this chapter). However, these changes generally are too minute to be directly detected by our senses. Therefore, highly complex methods have been developed to detect radiation. Here I describe the various detectors used in nuclear medicine. However, two relevant questions, what properties of radiation and what properties of detectors are important in nuclear medicine, are addressed first.

## What Do We Want To Know About Radiation?

Basically, we are interested in knowing one or more of the following.

**Simple Detection** Is radiation present? This question usually does not arise in nuclear medicine because one always administers a known radionuclide to the patient. In special circumstances, however, such as contamination of surroundings or personnel, one may be faced with this question. Of course, any presence of radiation will lead to the next question.

**Quantity of Radiation** How much radiation or radioactivity is present? In any use of radiation in nuclear medicine, one must answer this basic question, if not in absolute terms, then in relative terms (i.e., with respect to a standard). In dynamic studies, this question is modified as how much radiation or radioactivity is present at a given time? This requires measurement of radioactivity or counting rate as a function of time.

**Energy of the Radiation** In nuclear medicine, unlike nuclear physics, one is not interested in knowing the energy of the radiation per se. From practical considerations, however, it is helpful in two ways: to discriminate against undesired events such as scattered $\gamma$-rays that may be identified by energy measurement and to identify two radionuclides that may be used simultaneously.

**Nature of Radiation** In general, in nuclear medicine one knows the kind of radiation with which one is involved. However, again in cases of contamination, one may be faced with the task of identifying the type of the radiation.

Not every detector can answer all of these questions. One type of detector can measure each radiation interacting with it individually but not the energy of the radiation [e.g., Geiger–Mueller (GM) counters]. Scintillator detectors can measure both the energy and the individual interaction of the radiation. Ionization chambers cannot be used as counters or to measure energy of radiation but are still useful under many circumstances, such as measurement of radiation "exposure." Exposure depends on both the energies and the number of radiations interacting in the detector and is a useful concept in radiation protection from external x- or $\gamma$-ray emitting radiation sources (see Chapter 16).

# What Makes One Radiation Detector Better Than Another?

The answer to this complex question primarily depends on the use one wishes to make of the radiation detector. However, the following properties of a detector are of significance in radionuclidic imaging, which is the primary activity in nuclear medicine.

**Intrinsic Efficiency or Sensitivity**  Intrinsic efficiency $E_i$ of a detector is the measure of its ability to detect radiation and is generally defined as the ratio of the number of rays of a given radiation ($\alpha$, $\beta$, or $\gamma$) detected to the number of rays incident on the sensitive volume of the detector:

$$E_i = \frac{\text{Number of rays detected by the detector}}{\begin{array}{c}\text{Number of rays incident}\\\text{on the sensitive volume}\\\text{of the detector}\end{array}}$$

A value of 0.5 (50%) for the intrinsic efficiency means that only one-half of the rays incident on the sensitive volume of the detector is detected and the other half passed without any interaction within the sensitive volume. The higher the intrinsic efficiency of a detector, the better it is for use in nuclear medicine. Higher intrinsic efficiency allows a shortened imaging time, a reduced radiation dose to patients, or both. Intrinsic efficiency of a detector primarily depends on the linear-attenuation coefficient, $\mu$(linear), and the thickness of the sensitive volume.

**Dead Time or Resolving Time**  Dead time or resolving time (used interchangeably here) is a measure of the ability of a detector to function accurately at high count rates encountered when large amounts of radioactivities are used. For any detector, there is a small but finite interval between the time when a ray interacts with a detector and the time when the detector responds and the event is recorded. This interval is known as "dead time" or resolving time of the detector. What happens if a second ray arrives and starts interacting with the detector while it is still processing the first ray? The response of a detector under such circumstance is broadly

described under two categories: paralyzable and nonparalyzable. Both mechanisms may be operative in the same detector.

In the paralyzable situation when the second ray arrives within the dead time of the detector, the detector becomes insensitive for another time interval equal to the time of arrival of the second ray. For example, if the dead time of a detector is 100 $\mu$s and the second ray arrives after 30 $\mu$s of the arrival of the first, the detector becomes insensitive for a total of 30 + 100 = 130 $\mu$s, provided, of course, no third ray arrives within this interval. In that case, the interval will be extended further depending on the time of arrival of the third ray and so on. Thus, depending on the count rate, which determines the average time interval between the arrivals of two successive rays, in the paralyzable case a large number of rays can be lost without registering in the detector.

In the nonparalyzable case, the insensitive period of the detector is not affected by the arrival of the second ray. The second ray or others arriving in this insensitive period are lost. Figure 8.1 shows the effect of dead time on various count rates for a paralyzable and nonparalyzable detector. For a nonparalyzable detector, the detector

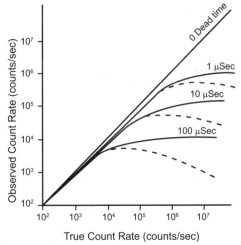

**Fig. 8.1.**  Observed count rate versus true count rate for detectors with different dead times. Solid lines are for nonparalyzable detectors; broken lines, paralyzable detectors. If both components, paralyzable and nonparalyzable, contribute to the dead time, the response will be in between the two extremes. Note that as the dead time of a detector increases, the usable count-rate range (linear portion) becomes smaller.

response (observed count rate) at first increases linearly with the true count rate but then reaches a plateau. On the other hand, for a paralyzable detector, the initial part of the response is the same, but after reaching a peak, the observed count rate actually starts decreasing with an increase in the true count rate. In other words, for paralyzable-type counters, the same observed count rate is obtained with two different true count rates (or radioactivities), one low and one high; this is a serious pitfall to be aware of.

Ideally, the detector should have as short a dead time as possible because it will detect very high count rates without significant losses. For the count rates encountered in nuclear medicine from the routine dosage of the current radio-pharmaceuticals, a system dead time of about 10 $\mu$s is acceptable. However, for fast dynamic imaging of the heart where higher count rates are desirable, system dead time shorter than 10 $\mu$s (2–3 $\mu$s) are essential.

**Energy Discrimination Capability or Energy Resolution** The ability of a detector to distinguish between two radiations of different energies (e.g., two $\gamma$-rays of different energies) is known as its energy discrimination capability or energy resolution. Full-width at half-maximum (*FWHM*) is commonly used as a measure of energy resolution and is defined later in this chapter. It represents the minimum difference

necessary between the energies of two $\gamma$-rays if they are to be identified as having different energies. If the *FWHM* of a detector is 20 keV, then two $\gamma$-rays with a difference in energy less than 20 keV cannot be distinguished by this detector. A lower value of *FWHM* indicates a better energy discrimination capability. Another way to look at *FWHM* is to consider it as a measure of error in the energy determination of an x- or $\gamma$-ray by a detector. The lower this error is, the more accurate the detector will be in measuring $\gamma$-ray energy and therefore in detecting smaller changes in the energy of x- or $\gamma$-rays.

**Other Considerations** Because most detectors use electronic components whose behavior quite often is susceptible to change with fluctuations in line voltage and environment temperature, detectors whose response is not appreciably affected by these fluctuations are preferred. Detectors should also be portable (depending on their desired use), simple to operate, and, of course, inexpensive.

## Types of Detectors

With this background in mind, various types of radiation detectors are discussed: gas-filled detectors, scintillation detectors, and semiconductor detectors. Their main characteristics and uses are summarized in Table 8.1.

**Table 8.1.**    Some Characteristics of Common $\gamma$-Ray Detectors

| Detector | Intrinsic Efficiency | Dead Time | Energy Discrimination | Uses in Nuclear Medicine |
|---|---|---|---|---|
| Ionization chambers | Very low | —a | None | Dose calibrators |
| Proportional counters | Very low | $\sim$ ms | Moderate | Rarely used |
| Geiger–Mueller counters | Moderate | $\sim$ ms | None | Radiation survey work |
| NaI(T1) scintillation counters | High | $\sim \mu$s | Moderate | Most widely used detector, well counters, scintillation camera |
| Semiconductor Ge(Li) counters | Moderate | $<1\ \mu$s | Very good | Neutron activation analyses |
| Cd Te and CZT detectors | High | $<\mu$s | Very good | Surgical probes and SPECT |

aCannot be used as a counter.

# Gas-Filled Detectors

As discussed in Chapter 6, the first action of high-energy radiation on matter is the production of ionization. In general, it is not possible to measure the amount of ionization produced in matter except in gases and some solids, known as semiconductors. The measurement of the amount of ionization produced by radiation in a small gas volume is the basis of three types (i.e., ionization chambers, proportional counters, and GM counters) of gas-filled detectors.

**Mechanism of Gas-Filled Detectors** To explain the mechanism of detection of gas-filled detectors, let us consider what happens when ionization is produced by a ray or particle in a gas volume enclosed between two electrodes with an applied voltage V (Fig. 8.2). When the applied voltage V between the two electrodes is zero, the ion pairs produced by the radiation recombine to form neutral atoms or molecules, and no current flows in the circuit. However, under the influence of the electric field that exists between the two electrodes when V is greater than zero, some ion pairs reach the electrodes and a transient current (current pulse) is produced in the circuit. The amount of current produced depends on several factors, such as the applied voltage V; distance between the two electrodes; type of gas; volume, pressure, and temperature of the gas; and geometry and shape of the electrodes. The most important parameter, however, is the applied voltage V between the two electrodes. The amount of the current produced by a single radiation in a typical gas-filled detector as a function of voltage V is shown in Figure 8.3. The dependence of the current on voltage is

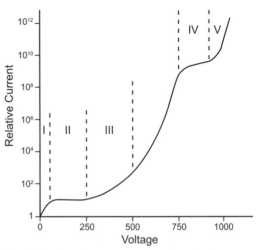

**Fig. 8.3.** Plot of current as a function of voltage V applied to the two electrodes of Figure 8.2. Origin of the five regions marked I, II, III, IV, and V is explained in the text. Region I, ion-pair recombination; region II, ionization chambers operate in this region; region III, proportional counters; region IV, GM counters. The unmarked region between regions III and IV is of no practical importance.

complex. There are five distinct regions that need explanation. Keep in mind that if no ionization is produced by the radiation in the gas volume, the current will be zero irrespective of the voltage applied.

***Region I or Recombination*** The voltage is low so that some ion pairs produced by a ray or particle (called primary ion pairs) are still able to recombine and form neutral atoms or molecules. In other words, there is an incomplete collection of the primary ion pairs by the electrodes. As the voltage increases, more primary ion pairs are collected by the electrodes and more current flows.

***Region II or Ionization Plateau*** The voltage is now sufficiently high to attract all primary ion pairs produced by a ray or particle to the electrodes, and there is little recombination. The amount of the current does not change appreciably with an increase in the voltage because all primary ion pairs produced by the radiation have been collected. The amount of current produced by a single ray or particle (total number of primary ion pairs) is still small and cannot be detected unless integrated for interaction of many rays or particles.

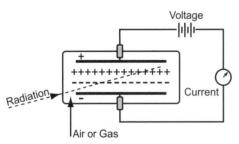

**Fig. 8.2.** Schematic of gas-filled radiation detector. The two electrodes collect the ion pairs produced in the gas by radiation.

*Region III or Proportional Region* The voltage is even higher. This is not only enough to attract all primary ion pairs to the electrodes but is also sufficient to provide enough energy to some primary ion pairs that now produce secondary ion pairs through collisions with neutral atoms and molecules of the gas. The amount of secondary ion pairs produced depends on the energy acquired by the primary ion pairs, which depends on the voltage. As a result, the amount of current produced by a radiation increases with increase in voltage. The current is now sufficiently high for detection in response to a single ray or particle interaction in the gas volume. It is also proportional to the energy of the radiation. However, as the voltage increases further (unmarked region between III and IV), this relationship with energy becomes nonlinear.

*Region IV or GM Plateau* The voltage is so much higher that the primary ion pairs produced by a ray or particle acquire large energy to produce a large number of secondary ion pairs and excitations, which then strike the metallic electrodes and more neutral gas molecules to produce more ionizations and excitations. The deexcitation of the molecules produces ultraviolet light, which produces more ionization. The result is that the total gas volume is in a temporary state of discharge and the amount of current produced is more or less independent of the voltage and the energy of the radiation.

*Region V* The voltage is so high that radiation is not necessary to produce discharge. Under the influence of such a high electric field, the electrons are pulled out from the atomic shells, the atoms and molecules become ionized, and a discharge may be established even without radiation.

**Ionization Detector (Chamber)** Ionization detectors are one of the earliest types of gas-filled detectors used for radiation measurement. The operating voltage in these detectors lies in region II of Figure 8.3. In this region, small fluctuations in the applied voltage do not affect the current significantly. As a result, ionization chambers are highly stable and reliable. These can be made in a variety of shapes and sizes and are relatively inexpensive. Their main disadvantages are a poor

intrinsic efficiency for x- or $\gamma$-rays and a lack of energy discrimination. Because the amount of current produced in response to a single ray or particle is small, these cannot be used as counters. Therefore, their principal use is in the measurement of radiation exposure such as that encountered in diagnostic and therapeutic radiology. They are principally used in nuclear medicine as "dose calibrators" to measure radioactivity in the microcurie-to-curie range. Occasionally, these may be used to measure exposure to individual radiation workers in the form of "pocket dosimeters," as discussed in Chapter 16.

*Dose Calibrator* Dose calibrators are, generally, cylindrically shaped ionization chambers filled with a rare gas such as argon at high pressure ($\sim$20 atmospheres). High pressure increases the density of the gas, which increases the intrinsic efficiency of the ionization chamber. There is a small hole along the axis of the cylinder so that the radioactive sample whose radioactivity is to be measured can be inserted close to the center of the ionization chamber (Figs. 8.4 and 8.5). This type of geometric arrangement increases the overall sensitivity of a detector and is known as $4\pi$ arrangement (see Chapter 9). The outside walls of the chamber are appropriately shielded to minimize the interference from radioactive sources outside the chamber.

The principle and operation of a dose calibrator are simple. The current produced in the ionization chamber by a given radioactive source in a given geometric arrangement is directly proportional to the amount of the radioactivity of the source. However, different radionuclides with the same amount of radioactivity produce different amounts of current. This difference in current produced by the same radioactivities of different radionuclides arises mainly from the differences in emission frequency $n_i$ and the energy $E_i$ of $\gamma$-rays emitted by them. Therefore, before an ionization chamber can be used as a dose calibrator, it needs to be calibrated for the desired radionuclides individually. The initial calibration is performed by measuring the amount of current produced for 1 mCi of a given radionuclide. This process is repeated for all desired radionuclides. Sources of known radioactivity (to a 5% or less accuracy) can be obtained from the National

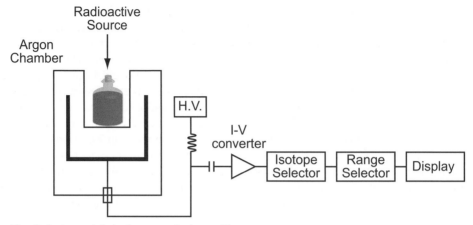

**Fig. 8.4.** A simplified schematic of a dose calibrator.

Bureau of Standards, who determines the radio-activity of these sources accurately by complex and time-consuming methods. Once the calibration factors are known, the unknown radioactivity of a given radionuclide is easily obtained by dividing the current produced by the unknown radioactivity with the calibration factor for that radionuclide.

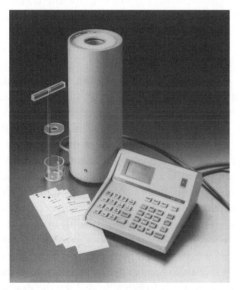

**Fig. 8.5.** A commercial dose calibrator. Shown are the shielded well-type ionization chamber, the electronic console, and the plastic syringe and vial holder (Reproduced from Bushberg JT, Siebert JA, Leidholdt EM Jr, et al. *The Essential Physics of Medical Imaging*, 2nd ed. Philadelphia: Lippincott Williams & Wilkins; 2002, with permission).

In commercial dose calibrators (Figs. 8.4 and 8.5), the ionization chamber is connected to a digital current meter and the calibration factors for a number of radionuclides are predetermined and stored so the results of the unknown radioactivity are directly displayed in microcurie, millicurie, or curie (or MBq, etc.) when the appropriate button for the given radionuclide is selected. With these calibrators, however, it should be remembered that when we press a button labeled "$^{99m}$Tc," all we are doing is recalling the calibration factor of $^{99m}$Tc. We are not discriminating against other radionuclides. A $^{99m}$Tc source in a dose calibrator will display radioactivity at other radionuclidic settings, but these will not be correct radioactivity of the $^{99m}$Tc sample. As a result, dose calibrators cannot be used to determine the radioactivity of a mixed (containing more than one radionuclide) sample except as described under $^{99}$Mo Breakthrough Measurement.

***Quality Assurance:*** To ensure the proper operation of a dose calibrator, its linearity (i.e., the current is proportional to the radioactivity for a given radionuclide) and accuracy should be measured yearly. Accuracy should be better than 10%. For routine assurance, a constancy check should be performed daily by measuring the radioactivity of a standard source consisting of a long-lived radionuclide such as $^{137}$Cs or $^{57}$Co. The measured radioactivity should not vary more than 10% from the radioactivity of the standard source, corrected for the decay. It must also be noted that the calibration factors are valid only for a given geometric setup, source volume, and source container. If the shape or type of the source container or the volume of the source is changed appreciably, the calibration factor will change and therefore should be measured again.

***$^{99}$Mo Breakthrough Measurement:*** Although a dose calibrator cannot measure accurately the radioactivities of two radionuclides when present simultaneously in a sample, it can be used to measure the radioactivity of $^{99}$Mo breakthrough in the $^{99m}$Tc eluate obtained from a generator by using an ingenious method. It involves the use of a lead container of a wall thickness sufficient to attenuate essentially all γ-rays (140 keV) emanating from a typical $^{99m}$Tc radioactivity obtained from a generator. This thickness of lead is not enough to attenuate high-energy $^{99}$Mo γ-rays (740 and 778 keV) to any great extent (question 8, chapter 6 illustrates this point). Lead containers of appropriate thickness are usually provided by the manufacturers of dose calibrators. To measure $^{99}$Mo breakthrough, two measurements are made on the vial containing $^{99m}$Tc eluate: on the $^{99m}$Tc setting without the lead container, which gives the $^{99m}$Tc radioactivity; and at the $^{99}$Mo setting with the vial in the lead container, which, when multiplied by the attenuation factor for $^{99}$Mo γ rays (provided by the manufacturer), yields the $^{99}$Mo radioactivity. Because the $^{99m}$Tc radioactivity in the eluate is typically 1000 times the $^{99}$Mo radioactivity (parent breakthrough), error in the $^{99m}$Tc radioactivity in the presence of a small amount of $^{99}$Mo radioactivity is small and therefore neglected. Division of the $^{99}$Mo radioactivity (in microcurie) by the $^{99m}$Tc radioactivity (in millicurie) yields the $^{99}$Mo breakthrough in the appropriate unit.

**Proportional Detector (Counter)** These detectors operate in region III of Figure 8.3, where there is a built-in amplification (~$10^6$) of the primary ionization through the production of secondary ionization. A sufficient amount of current is produced by a single ray for it to be counted, and the current is directly proportional to the energy of the radiation. Hence,

a proportional detector, unlike the ionization chamber, can be used to count individual events and to determine the energy of the radiation. Proportional counters require a sufficient amount of expertise in their construction and use. Their stability, with time and voltage fluctuations, is not as good as that of the ionization chambers. Proportional counters are rarely used in nuclear medicine.

**Geiger–Mueller Detector (Counter)** The operating voltage of GM detectors is in the region IV of Figure 8.3. The incoming particle in this case causes a discharge in the gas, and the amount of the current produced is more or less independent of the energy of the radiation and of the voltage. Once the discharge is established in the gas by a ray, how does one stop the process so that the detector is ready for the next ray? This is accomplished chemically. Small amounts of halogens or their organic compounds are introduced in the gas as impurities. These impurities, known as chemical quenchers, absorb the ultraviolet light produced during the discharge and the energy from the secondary ion pairs. Absorption of energy by the quencher molecules causes the discharge to stop but leads to their dissociation. However, within a short time, most quencher molecules are able to recombine to form the original molecule. Therefore, there is little depletion of the quencher. It takes from about 50 to 200 μs to quench the discharge. During this time, the GM counter does not respond to another radiation; therefore, this is approximately the dead time of the detector and is nonparalyzable. The maximum usable count rate for a typical GM counter is 60,000 counts/min. GM detectors are the most sensitive of the gas-filled detectors.

A typical commercial GM counter or survey meter is shown in Figure 8.6. GM counters can be made in any shape and size, are easy to operate, and are quite stable in reference to temperature and voltage fluctuations; however, they cannot measure the energy of a radiation. For the detection of β-rays, there is a small window made of thin aluminized Mylar either at the end or one side of the GM tube. For the detection of x- or γ-rays, this window is generally closed. Also, because the interaction of x- or γ-rays in the gas

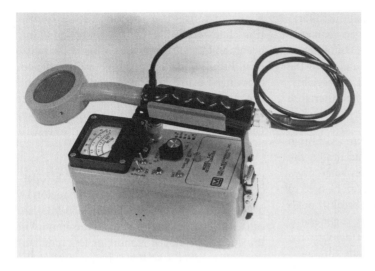

**Fig. 8.6.** A typical GM counter. The handheld probe detaches from the meter for easy radiation survey or contamination check (Reproduced from Bushberg JT, Siebert JA, Leidholdt EM Jr, et al. *The Essential Physics of Medical Imaging*, 2nd ed. Philadelphia: Lippincott Williams & Wilkins; 2002, with permission).

volume itself is minimal, the detection of these radiations is primarily through the photo- and Compton-electrons generated in the inner walls of the GM tube. These are rugged, portable, and comparatively inexpensive detectors. The principal use of GM detectors in nuclear medicine is in radiation protection work for surveying the contamination of surroundings and personnel from x- and γ-ray emitting radionuclides.

## Scintillation Detectors (Counters)

A variety of substances known as phosphors scintillate (produce light) under the influence of high-energy radiation. This property is used for the detection of radiation by instruments known as scintillation detectors. However, for the detection of the light generated in a material, it should be able to be transmitted out of the material itself. In liquids, it poses no serious problem. For solids, only single crystals or glasses can be used because in powders (microcrystals), light is absorbed and scattered at the boundaries of the microcrystals, thereby causing significant and variable loss of light before its detection.

Two other types of substances, thermoluminescent and photoluminescent, are also used as radiation detectors. These substances do not produce light immediately after interacting with radiation but can store some of the energy given by the radiation for a long time. The stored energy is released in the form of light at a later

time by either heating (thermoluminescent) the irradiated substance or exposing it to laser light (photoluminescent). Thermoluminescent detectors are used in radiation monitoring and are discussed in Chapter 16. Photoluminescent detectors have not found use in nuclear medicine but are finding uses in diagnostic radiology, particularly in digital radiology.

A typical scintillation counter is shown schematically in Figure 8.7. It consists of a scintillator, photomultiplier PM tube to detect the light, preamplifier, amplifier, and assorted electronics such as a pulse-height selector and a count-rate meter or scaler for automatic data collection and analysis. The following section outlines the mechanism of a typical scintillation counter used in the detection of γ-rays. Liquid scintillation counters used in the detection of high-energy charged particles (i.e., $\alpha$ and $\beta$) are described in Chapter 9.

**Scintillator** The number of scintillating substances (scintillators) is large. Anthracene, naphthalene, various plastics, alkali halide crystals doped with or without impurities such as NaI(Tl) or CsF, lead tungstate, bismuth germanate, lanthanum bromide, and aromatic compounds such as terphenyl and 2,5-diphenyloxazole have all been used as scintillators.

*Mechanism of Light Production* Because the mechanism of light production in a substance under the influence of radiation is complex and

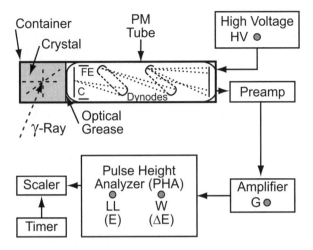

**Fig. 8.7.** Schematic of a scintillation counter. The four controls denoted by HV (high voltage), G (gain of the amplifier), LL or E (lower level or energy), and W or $\Delta$E (window width or energy width) are important in the operation of a scintillation counter. In the PM tube, C stands for photocathode, FE for focusing electrode, and A for anode.

not well understood, there are no theoretical laws to predict the behavior of a given substance in this regard. Briefly, a $\gamma$-ray loses its energy in a scintillator through the photoelectric, Compton, or pair-production mechanisms. The electrons thus generated then lose their energy within short distances through ionization and excitation of the scintillator molecules. The ion pairs thus produced then combine among themselves or with other atoms or molecules of the scintillator and produce certain excited states that, during their subsequent decay, emit light. The nature and quantity of these excited states determine the amount, color, and phosphorescent decay time of light.

***Properties of Scintillator*** A scintillator is primarily characterized by intrinsic efficiency, amount of light produced per unit of absorbed energy (light conversion efficiency), and the time in which emission of light takes place (phosphorescent decay time). The intrinsic efficiency of a scintillator for a $\gamma$-ray of a given energy depends on its linear attenuation coefficient, which in turn depends on the atomic number and the density of the material (see Chapter 6). The amount of light produced per unit of absorbed energy, which in effect determines the energy resolution of these detectors, and the phosphorescent decay time, which is an important parameter for the dead time of these detectors, vary from substance to substance.

Light in a scintillator is produced in a very small volume, mainly determined by the range

of photoelectrons or Compton recoil electrons produced in the scintillator. For energies of x- or $\gamma$-rays less than 1 MeV, this range does not exceed more than a millimeter in a NaI(Tl) crystal or other scintillators used in PET. From this small volume of production, light travels in all directions, as shown in Figure 8.7. The direction of most of the light toward the PM tube is achieved by coating the outside surface of the scintillator, except the side facing the PM tube, with a light reflector such as magnesium oxide. The coupling of the crystal assembly to the PM tube is also important because of possible light loss at the interface of the crystal and PM tube. This loss is generally minimized by the use of optical grease.

***Scintillator for Scintillation Camera, NaI(Tl)*** Of all the known scintillators, sodium iodide crystals doped with small amounts of thallium, NaI(Tl), are most widely used in nuclear medicine, particularly in the scintillation camera. Its moderate density (d = 3.67 g/cm$^3$) and effective atomic number ($Z_{eff}$ = 45) make it very efficient for the detection of x- or $\gamma$-rays in the energy range of 30 to 500 keV. The amount of light produced per unit of absorbed energy in a NaI(Tl) crystal is one of the highest, despite the fact that sodium iodide crystals without thallium doping do not produce much light. The presence of small amounts of thallium (one part in 10$^6$) enhances the light output by a factor of 10 or more. The phosphorescent decay time, which eventually determines the dead time of a scintillation detector, is ~0.23 $\mu$s and is adequate for the amounts of radioactivities presently used in nuclear medicine. In addition, the technology required to grow these crystals in large sizes and various shapes is well advanced, making their use more economical compared with many other scintillators.

Sodium iodide crystals are hygroscopic and have to be hermetically sealed, usually in thin-walled aluminum or steel containers. Thin aluminum or steel walls attenuate high-energy $\gamma$-rays only to a small degree. These crystals should not be subjected to abrupt temperature changes (no more than 10°C/h change), even when these are not in use (e.g., during shipment or storage). Such changes can produce severe mechanical stresses in the crystal, causing them to crack. Also, the amount of light produced in these crystals is somewhat dependent on ambient temperature. As a result, the response of these detectors changes slightly with change in room temperature.

A newer scintillator, lanthanum bromide, $LaBr_3(Ce)$ has been recently developed that has superior characteristics than NaI(Tl) scintillator as can be seen in Table 8.2. It has better attenuation properties, produces more light and has faster phosphorent decay time than NaI. It is one of prime candidates to replace NaI detectors in future.

*Scintillators for PET* Because in PET, the energy of the radiation to be detected is very high, 511 keV as opposed to 140 keV for $^{99m}$Tc, NaI(Tl) is not a good choice as a scintillator material as its detection efficiency drops off rapidly with

the energy of $\gamma$ ray. Instead, another scintillator, Bismuth Germanate, commonly known as BGO, has been the scintillator of choice. BGO has a big advantage over NaI(Tl) in the detection efficiency at 511 keV. However, its light output/keV of absorbed energy, which determines its energy resolution, is very low (1/7 that of NaI) and therefore it has poor energy resolution compared to a NaI(Tl) detector. Poor energy resolution means poor scatter rejection (Chapter 10). Also, its phosphorent decay time is slightly longer than NaI, making its dead time slightly longer than that of the NaI(Tl) detector.

Because of these shortcomings, BGO is being replaced by a new and recently developed scintillator, Lutetium Oxyorthosilicate or LSO. The new scintillator LSO has almost the same detection efficiency for 511 keV as BGO, but also has five times higher light output than BGO and its decay time is only 40 ns as opposed to 300 ns for BGO. Higher light output produces better energy resolution. Better energy resolution allows better rejection of the scattered radiation (Chapter 10). Shorter decay time means shorter dead time. Shorter dead time allows the detectors to operate at high count rates without loss. As a result of these, LSO scintillator is replacing BGO in most of the PET instrumentation. The slight disadvantage of LSO is that lutetium has a long-lived (39 billion year half-life) radioisotope $^{176}$Lu, naturally present at about 2.6% concentration. The decay of $^{176}$Lu causes the background radiation for these detectors to increase significantly. However, with the amount of radioactivity that one uses in PET procedures, the background radiation is still insignificant in relation

**Table 8.2.** Characteristics of Common Scintillators Used in Nuclear Medicine

| Material | Density (g/cm3) | Effective Atomic No. | Light Output Relative to NaI | Phosphorent Decay Time ($\mu$s) |
|---|---|---|---|---|
| Sodium Iodide, NaI(Tl) | 3.67 | 46 | 1 | 0.23 |
| Lanthanum Bromide, $LaBr_3$:Ce | 5.3 | 47 | 1.6 | 0.025 |
| Bismuth Germinate, $Bi_4Ge_3O_{16}$ (BGO) | 7.13 | 74 | 0.15 | 0.30 |
| Lutetium oxyorthosilicate, $Lu_2SiO_4O$ (LSO) | 7.4 | 66 | 0.75 | 0.04 |

to the counts originating from the radioactive patient by an order of magnitude and therefore poses little problem. Table 8.2 summarizes the important properties of these materials.

## Associated Electronics

*PM Tube* The amount of light produced in NaI(Tl) crystals or any other scintillator is quite small relative to that which the human eye can easily detect. Even if we could observe individual scintillations occurring in the scintillator with the naked eye, it is not practical to count light flashes in this way. A PM tube is a light-sensitive device that converts light into measurable electronic pulses. It consists of a photocathode facing the window through which light enters, a series of metallic electrodes known as dynodes arranged in a special geometric pattern, and an anode—all enclosed in vacuum in a glass tube. When the light photon hits the photocathode, it produces an electron of low energy (0.1–1 eV) through photoelectric interaction. This photoelectron is then accelerated toward a dynode by the application of a voltage (between 50 and 100 V) to that dynode. As a result of this acceleration, the electron acquires sufficient kinetic energy (50–100 eV) to produce a number of secondary electrons when it collides with the dynode. The number of secondary electrons produced varies between 1 and 10. These secondary electrons are then accelerated toward a second dynode (at two times the voltage applied on the first dynode) where a similar multiplication in the number of electrons occurs. Eventually, at the last dynode (generally the tenth), there are between $10^5$ and $10^8$ electrons for each of the photoelectrons produced. These electrons generate a current pulse of a few microamperes in amplitude and less than a microsecond in duration at the anode.

The voltage to different dynodes is supplied from a single high-voltage source (500–1500 V) by using a voltage divider. The gain of a PM tube (the multiplication of electrons) strongly depends on the voltage applied to dynodes; therefore, small changes in the high voltage can change the output of these detectors significantly. The crystal and the PM tube are generally combined in a single light-tight unit. This prevents ambient light from reaching the PM tube.

*Preamplifier* The electric pulses arriving at the anode of a PM tube are small (microampere) and therefore require amplification to several volts before they can be further analyzed or processed. The output of a PM tube, however, cannot be directly fed into an amplifier because of the wide difference in the output impedance (an important electronic parameter) of a PM tube and the input impedance of an amplifier that results in signal distortion and attenuation. A preamplifier is a device that solves the problem of impedance mismatch. It is located next to the PM tube because long connecting cables at this stage also attenuate the signal. Output of the preamplifier, however, can be sent many feet away from the detector assembly without attenuation.

*Linear Amplifier* A linear amplifier amplifies the incoming pulses in a direct proportion. The ratio between the amplitudes of the outgoing and incoming pulses is known as amplifier gain. The amplification can be changed by adjusting the gain control G specifically provided for this purpose.

*Pulse-Height Analyzer or Single-Channel Analyzer* A pulse-height analyzer (PHA) or single-channel analyzer (SCA) is an electronic device that accepts the pulses whose voltage (height) lies between a preselected range and rejects the pulses whose voltage lies outside this range. An SCA is provided with two controls known as lower level and window that determine the range of the pulses to be selected. For example, if pulses with voltages varying from 1 to 10 are being produced by a linear amplifier in response to an x- or $\gamma$-ray, to select pulses whose voltage lies between 5 and 6, it is necessary to set the lower level of SCA at 5 V and the window at 1 V. The SCA will produce an output pulse only when the input pulses lie in this range.

In many instruments, the two controls, lower level and window, have been replaced by peak voltage and percent window. In this terminology, if we wish to select pulses that fall between 5 and 6 V, peak voltage will be set at 5.5 V (center of the range) and % window = (window width ÷ peak voltage) × 100, which in this case equals (1 V ÷ 5.5 V) × 100 or 18%. Alternatively, a 20% window at 1.40 peak voltage will be

0.2 × 1.40 = 0.28 V wide. In this case, the window is set symmetrically on each side of the peak voltage. Thus, the pulses selected will be in the range from 1.40 – (0.28 ÷ 2) to 1.40 + (0.28 ÷ 2) or 1.26 – 1.54 V. As described later, pulse height can be related to the energy of a γ-ray. As a result, the two controls, peak voltage and % window, quite often are directly labeled in terms of energy E and %ΔE. This, of course, assumes that the volt-to-energy calibration factor does not change with time.

***Multichannel Analyzer*** A PHA or SCA selects only one range of pulse-height distribution. In a multichannel analyzer, there are many PHAs (1000 or more) that can simultaneously separate the pulses into multiple ranges; therefore, the whole spectrum of pulse-height distribution can be measured at one time.

***Scaler and Timer*** These devices comprise an electronic counter used for counting the pulses coming from an amplifier or SCA either for a specific time interval or until a predetermined number of counts has been collected. In either case, both the number of counts and the time during which they are collected are obtained.

***Rate Meter*** This is a device that, instead of giving the number of counts and the time period in which the counts were collected, yields directly the count rate (counts/min). With the ubiquitous use of computers, rate meters are now rarely used in nuclear medicine instruments.

### Response to Monochromatic (Single-Energy) γ-RAYS

***Production of Pulse-Height Distribution*** Let us now review the steps leading to the production of the voltage pulse in a scintillation detector. A γ-ray interacts within the crystal through the photoelectric, Compton, or pair-production mechanism. In each case, either a high-energy electron or electron–positron pair is produced that deposits all its energy within a small volume of the site of production. Some energy deposited by the electron or electron–positron pair is converted into light. Light triggers an electric pulse in the PM tube that is then amplified by the linear amplifier.

The height (amplitude or voltage), v, of the pulse coming out of the amplifier is directly proportional to four parameters: amount of energy deposited by a γ-ray ($E_d$), light conversion efficiency of the scintillator ($L_{eff}$) that is constant for a given scintillator, PM tube gain ($G_{pm}$), and amplifier gain (G). In other words,

$$v = \text{constant} \times E_d \times L_{eff} \times G_{pm} \times G$$

The variable $G_{pm}$ depends on high voltage applied to the PM tube. If one keeps $G_{pm}$ and G constant, then the pulse height v in a given scintillator detector depends only and linearly on the energy deposited ($E_d$) by a γ-ray. As $E_d$ increases, so does the pulse height v. The linear relationship between v and $E_d$, in essence, is the source of the energy-measuring ability of a scintillation detector.

A γ-ray of energy Eγ, however, does not deposit the same amount of energy $E_d$ each time it interacts with a crystal. Absorbed energy $E_d$ depends on the type of interaction (e.g., photoelectric, Compton, or pair production). In photoelectric events, all γ-ray energy is deposited in the crystal, that is, $E_d$ = Eγ. In Compton and pair-production events, $E_d$ is always less than Eγ, and there is no simple relationship that relates Eγ to the pulse height v. Therefore, to perform energy measurement with a scintillation detector, one has to select only the photoelectric events. This is done with the help of a PHA or SCA.

***Pulse-Height Spectrum*** Figure 8.8 shows pulse-height distribution (spectrum) produced by a NaI(Tl) detector for a monochromatic γ-ray (<1 MeV) as a result of individual interaction in the crystal of several thousand γ-rays. Here, only photoelectric and Compton interactions are important. The spectrum is divided into two regions, a and b.

Region a, is known as the Compton plateau, and pulses in this region originate as a result of Compton interaction. Depending on the amount of energy given to the Compton electron, a pulse of different amplitude is produced. Because in Compton interaction a γ-ray does not transfer all its energy to an electron, the maximum transfer of energy to the electron

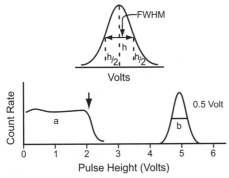

**Fig. 8.8.** Pulse-height distribution produced by a NaI(Tl) scintillation detector in response to γ-rays of single energy. The distribution is divided into two distinct areas, a and b. Area a (Compton plateau) results primarily because of the Compton interaction of γ-rays in the NaI(Tl) crystal. The edge of the Compton plateau (indicated by arrow) is produced when a γ-ray transfers maximum energy possible in a Compton interaction to an electron. Area b (photo peak) is produced when γ-rays interact in the crystal via photoelectric effect. The narrowness or width of the photo peak is indicative of the energy-resolving capability of a detector. Quantitatively, energy-resolving capability is measured by *FWHM*. *FWHM* is depicted in the inset (top) where h is the height of the photo peak.

takes place when the γ-ray is back scattered (see Chapter 6, p. 62). When such an event occurs, it corresponds to the Compton edge indicated by the arrow in Figure 8.8.

Region b, a bell-shaped curve, is known as the photo peak. Pulses in this region are primarily produced through photoelectric interaction. A few pulses in this region may also arise as a result of a single or multiple Compton interaction followed by a photoelectric interaction. Thus, total energy of the γ-ray is deposited through multiple interactions rather than a single interaction in the crystal. Multiple interactions from a single γ-ray are much less probable than single photo or Compton interactions. The photo peak is also called total absorption peak.

Because these two regions are generally separated by a valley, the photoelectric events can be easily selected by using a PHA. The lower level and window of a PHA are set to just encompass

the photo peak. In Figure 8.8, these may be set at 4.5 and 5.5 V, respectively. A good rule of thumb to select a window width for a γ-ray is for it to be about two times the energy resolution (discussed below) of the detector for the energy of the γ-ray. Similar pulse-height spectra are generated by other scintillators.

***FWHM and Energy Resolution*** Production of light in a crystal and electron multiplication in a PM tube are both statistical processes similar to radioactive decay. As a result, a NaI(Tl) detector or any other scintillator does not produce pulses of constant voltage (height) V, even for photoelectric interactions where the same amount of energy $E_d$ is absorbed each time. Instead, the pulse heights are distributed as a bell shape (Gaussian) in the photo peak. The pulse-height distribution in the photo peak determines the energy-discriminating ability of a detector. The narrower the distribution, the better is the energy-discriminating ability of a detector. *FWHM* is used as a measure of the energy-discriminating ability or energy resolution of a detector. It is expressed as,

$$\% \text{ energy resoluation} = \frac{(\text{FWHM} \times 100)}{(\text{peak voltage})}$$

In Figure 8.6, *FWHM* = 0.5 V and the peak is at 5 V; therefore, % energy resolution = (0.5 × 100) = 5.0 = 10%.

Because the amount of light produced in the crystal for the photo peak increases linearly with γ-ray energy and more light has less statistical variation, energy-resolution depends on the energy of a γ-ray. The higher the energy of a γ-ray, the better is the energy resolution, although these are not linearly related. Another factor on which energy resolution depends to a slight extent is the size and shape of the sodium iodide crystal. For a well-type crystal, energy resolution is poorer than a cylindrical crystal. Typical energy resolution for a 662-keV γ-ray of $^{137}$Cs varies between 8% and 10%. At 140 keV ($^{99m}$Tc γ-ray), it ranges from 11% to 14%. Of course, energy resolution for other scintillators such as BGO or LSO are worse than NaI(Tl).

Periodic (yearly) measurement of energy resolution is used to diagnose slow deterioration of the crystal due to moisture leaks in the crystal

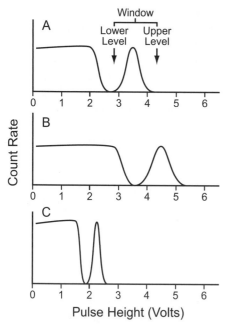

**Fig. 8.9.** Effect of changes in high voltage (or amplifier gain) on pulse-height distribution. An increase in high voltage from that of A produces a pulse-height distribution shown in B, whereas a decrease in high voltage, produces a pulse-height distribution shown in C. In these extreme cases (B and C), the photo peak moves out of the selected PHA range completely, thereby reducing the count rate drastically. In practice, small variations in high voltage or amplifier gain can result in appreciable changes in the count rate obtained with a preset PHA setting.

housing and/or the PM tube weakening. Energy resolution gets worse with time as a result of any of these problems.

**Response to Change in Amplifier Gain or High Voltage** An increase or decrease in high voltage or amplifier gain increases or decreases the pulse-height distribution accordingly, as shown in Figure 8.9. If one has already set the lower level and window of a PHA to encompass the photo peak, then a small change in amplifier gain or high voltage can move the photo peak outside the window. Therefore, it is important that the high voltage and the amplifier gain are stable with time, ambient temperature, and line-voltage fluctuations.

**Energy Calibration** Because by arbitrarily increasing the high voltage and/or amplifier gain one can produce a pulse of any desired height v

for a given energy γ-ray, how does one calibrate pulse height to γ-ray energy? This is done by using standard source of a radionuclide, which emits a single γ-ray of known energy and is long-lived. An example of such a source is $^{137}$Cs, which emit γ-rays of 662- keV energy, only.

A calibration scheme, universally used in nuclear medicine, is that a 100-keV γ-ray produces a photo peak centered at 1.00 V. To achieve this, one adjusts and readjusts the PM tube high voltage in such a manner that the $^{137}$Cs photo peak is centered at 6.62 V. Once this calibration has been achieved, neither the amplifier gain nor the high voltage should change. Because high voltage drifts with time, energy calibration should be checked daily.

**Response to γ-Rays of Two Energies** In this case, the pulse-height distribution is the sum of the two individual pulse-height distributions of γ1 and γ2, as shown in Figure 8.10. The photo peak of the high-energy γ-ray γ2 is still isolated, and the low-energy γ-ray γ1 causes no interference in its detection. However, the photo peak of γ1 lies in the Compton plateau of γ2 and there is no way to avoid the Compton pulses of -γ2 from being counted in the PHA window set for the photo peak of γ1. The Compton contribution (leakage) of γ2 in γ1 photo peak, however, can be determined by using a source that emits a γ-ray of single energy very close to that of γ2. With this source, two measurements are made, first at the photo peak setting of γ2 and the second at the photo peak setting of γ1. The second count is the Compton contribution from γ2 at the photo peak of γ1. This is expressed as a percentage of the first count. From this, one is able to correct for Compton leakage in the lower energy peak from the higher energy peak.

**Secondary Peaks** Quite often, besides the photo peak and Compton plateau, additional but much smaller peaks can be recognized in a γ-ray spectrum. These should not be confused with the presence of some weaker γ-rays in the radionuclide emissions. Rather, these have well-defined characteristics and causes as described below.

**7.** Na(Tl) crystal is the most common scintillator used in nuclear medicine. It possesses high intrinsic efficiency and produces a pulse-height spectrum in response to a monochromatic $\gamma$-ray. However, for PET imaging, BGO and LSO are better choices.

**8.** The photo peak voltage is directly proportional to energy of a $\gamma$-ray. Energy resolution of a good NaI(Tl) detector is about 10% at 662 keV energy.

**9.** These should be calibrated daily.

**10.** Semiconductor detectors have superior energy-resolution (1%) when used at low temperatures. Semiconductor detectors operating at room temperature (CZT) have problems relating to defect-free production in large sizes and are expensive. Their energy resolution for $^{99m}$Tc is about 6%.

## Questions

**1.** List the factors on which intrinsic efficiency of a detector depends. Why is this important in nuclear medicine?

**2.** Is the dead time of a detector related to the maximum detectable count rate directly, inversely, or with some other power?

**3.** Which gas-filled detector can measure energy of an x- or $\gamma$-ray?

**4.** Why can an ionization chamber not be used as a counter?

**5.** What is the maximum count rate for a typical GM counter?

**6.** Which detector discussed here is appropriate for the following applications? (a) For surveying the extent of contamination when a technologist, during an injection of a radiopharmaceutical, spilled some radioactive material on the patient's bed and his own clothing. (b) To determine a small amount (0.01 $\mu$Ci) of radioactivity in a sample. (c) To determine large amounts of radioactivities such as those given to patients. (d) To characterize different radionuclides in a mixture of radionuclides.

**7.** List the properties of the NaI(Tl) detector that make it so attractive for use in a scintillation camera.

**8.** Why is BGO a better choice than NaI(Tl) for PET?

**9.** Why is LSO even a better choice than BGO for PET?

**10.** What is the function of a pulse-height analyzer?

**11.** If a PHA is set on the photo peak, what effect will making the window narrower have on the observed count rate?

**12.** Three NaI(Tl) detectors have *FWHMs* of 18, 20, and 22 keV for a 140-keV $\gamma$-ray. What is the percent energy resolution of these detectors and which one should you select?

**13.** Why is CZT detector better than NaI(Tl) detector?

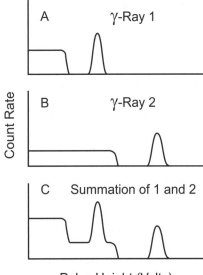

**Fig. 8.10.** Pulse-height distribution produced in response to $\gamma$-rays consisting of two distinct energies, 1 and 2. As shown in C, this is an exact sum of the pulse-height distributions produced by $\gamma$-rays of energy 1 and energy 2 independently, as shown in A and B, respectively. Low-energy $\gamma$-rays do not produce pulses with enough height to cause any interference in the photo peak of the higher energy grays. However, high-energy $\gamma$-rays produce pulses with a height corresponding to the photo peak pulses of lower energy $\gamma$-rays. Therefore, a correction has to be applied whenever a low-energy $\gamma$-ray radionuclide is being counted in the presence of a higher energy $\gamma$-ray radionuclide. This is not so in the opposite case.

***K Escape Peak*** This barely visible peak, mostly observed when the energy of a $\gamma$-ray lies between 50 and 150 keV, lies about 28 keV below the photo peak of a $\gamma$-ray. In this energy range (50–150 keV), most x- or $\gamma$-interactions are through the photoelectric effect in the K shell of iodine atoms and most of these interactions are close to the crystal surface (within a few millimeters). Therefore, the K x-ray produced when the vacancy in the K shell of the iodine atoms is filled has a finite chance of escaping from the crystal without depositing its energy. Thus, in many cases, the energy deposited by the $\gamma$-ray, even when the interaction is through photoelectric effect, is not the entire energy of the $\gamma$-ray E$\gamma$ but equals E$\gamma$ – E$_{k\ x\text{-ray}}$. The energy of the K x-ray for an iodine atom is about 28 keV;

hence, the escape peak is 28 keV below the photo peak of a $\gamma$-ray.

***Summation Peak*** With radionuclides emitting multiple-energy $\gamma$-rays, sometimes additional peaks corresponding to the sum of individual $\gamma$-ray energies are encountered even though no $\gamma$-ray with such energy is emitted by the radionuclide. As the name implies, these peaks originate because of the summation of the energies of two different grays in the crystal. Summation of energies occurs only when two $\gamma$-rays simultaneously or almost simultaneously (within 0.25 $\mu$s) interact within the crystal. Summation peaks are more pronounced for radionuclides that emit several $\gamma$-rays within a microsecond or less of each other and for well-type scintillation detectors (see Chapter 9). Some examples of this type of radionuclide are $^{125}$I (28 K x-ray followed by another 28 K x-ray) and $^{111}$In (173- and 247-keV $\gamma$-rays). If a spectrum is plotted for these radionuclides using a well-type scintillation detector, besides the 28-keV x-ray of $^{125}$I, another peak at 28 + 28 = 56 keV is also observed, although $^{125}$I does not emit any x- or $\gamma$-ray of 56-keV energy. Similarly in $^{111}$In, a summation peak at 173 + 247 = 420 keV is observed, although $^{111}$In does not emit a $\gamma$-ray with this energy. For summation to occur, two $\gamma$-rays do not have to interact through the photoelectric effect only. The interaction may occur through the Compton scattering as well. Then, the summated pulse, which is also called "pile-up" pulse, will equal the sum of the energies deposited by each $\gamma$-ray. At high count rates, pile-up pulses result accidentally, even when the radionuclide emits single-energy $\gamma$-rays only.

***Back-Scattered Peak and Lead X-ray Peak*** These peaks originate from the environment or surroundings of the NaI(Tl)) detectors. Because the detectors are generally shielded by lead from all sides except one to reduce the background radiation, the $\gamma$-rays interacting with the lead shield produce scattered $\gamma$-rays and lead K x-rays of about 80 keV. Some of these secondary radiations can be detected by the crystal. Of the scattered $\gamma$-rays from the shield, only those that are scattered more or less in the backward direction have a chance to interact with the crystal. The energy of these back-scattered $\gamma$-rays is determined by the expression given on p. 62. The back-scattered γ rays are not of a single energy but are distributed in a broad range. As a rule, the sum of the back-scattered peak energy and the Compton-edge energy in the spectrum of a monochromatic γ-ray equals the photo peak energy.

## Semiconductor Detectors

It is not generally possible to measure the amount of ion pairs produced by ionizing radiation in a solid, as is possible in a gas. However, under certain conditions and for a class of solid substances known as semiconductors, it is possible to measure the amount of such ion pairs produced. The physical arrangement is similar to that of an ionization chamber except that instead of gas, there is a small cylindrical or rectangular prism-shaped piece of semiconductor between the two electrodes (Fig. 8.11). In a semiconductor, the ion pairs produced are electrons and holes (it behaves like an electron with positive charge; however, it is not a positron). Without the electric field between the two electrodes,

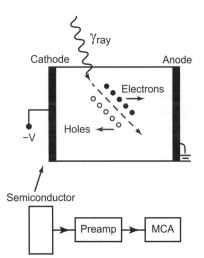

**Fig. 8.11.** Schematics of a semiconductor detector. Energy deposited by a γ-ray is converted into electron-hole pairs. Under the influence of the electric field generated by the two electrodes, holes and electrons produce current pulse that can be detected by associated electronics. Current produced is directly proportional to the energy deposited by γ-ray and thus produce a spectrum similar to that produced in a NaI(Tl) detector. MCA (multichannel analyzer) directly records this spectrum.

these electron-hole pairs recombine among themselves or with impurities or crystal defects present in the detector material. However, under the influence of electric field, current is generated. The amount of the current depends upon the energy deposited in the semiconductor material, thickness of the detector, and the temperature. Also, the purity and defect-free growth of the single crystals of these materials, particularly in large sizes, is an important consideration that sometimes becomes a major hurdle in their wide use.

In general, the number of electron-hole pairs generated for the same amount of energy deposited is many times more than the light photons generated in a scintillation detector. As a result, the energy resolution of these detectors is much better than scintillator detectors. Depending on the use, these detectors can be made as small as 1 mm in size. The intrinsic efficiency of these detectors depends on the same parameters as other detectors, namely linear attenuation coefficient ($Z_{eff}$ and density) and the thickness of the detector. The dead time of these detectors is in nanoseconds.

The two most successful semiconductor detectors so far, use germanium and silicon crystals doped with a small amount of lithium, Ge(Li) and Si(Li). However, for their optimum performance these have to be cooled at liquid nitrogen ($77^0$ K). Si(Li) detector, because of its low atomic number ($Z = 14$), is primarily used for the detection of corpuscular radiation, whereas Ge(Li) detector with its slightly higher atomic number ($Z = 32$) is used for the detection of x- or γ-rays.

The principal advantage of a Ge(Li) detector over a scintillation detector is its excellent energy resolution. A typical Ge(Li) detector can easily yield a 1% energy resolution for $^{137}$Cs γ-rays compared with 10% using a NaI(Tl) detector. The main drawbacks of Ge(Li) detectors, severely limiting their application in nuclear medicine, are their low sensitivity (because of lower atomic number, $Z = 32$, compared to $Z_{eff} = 50$ for NaI), the necessity of maintaining them at a low temperature of 77 K that makes them bulky (room temperature is about 300 K), and their unavailability in larger sizes. A spectrum produced by a $^{60}$Co source and obtained with a Ge(Li) detector is shown in Figure 8.12, where it is also compared with a NaI(Tl) detector.

In recent years, tremendous progress has been made in the development of room temperature semiconductor detectors that do not require bulky cooling apparatus, to the point, that they are commercially viable and finding increasing use in Nuclear Medicine. Two successful materials are Cadmium Tellurium (CdTe) and Cadmium Zinc Tellurium (CZT). Their atomic number are very close to that of NaI(Tl) but the densities are higher than that of NaI(Tl). As a result, for a given thickness of the detector, their linear attenuation coefficient, μ(linear) is slightly higher than that of NaI(Tl). They have better sensitivity than NaI(Tl). Their energy resolution (6% vs. 10% and further development can improve it by a factor of 2) and dead time (ns vs. μs) are also superior to that of NaI(Tl). In addition, as there is no PM tube needed, the assembled size of these detectors is much smaller (as small as a mm) than that of a NaI(Tl) detector. To form large-size detectors, one arranges them in two-dimensional arrays consisting of a large number of detectors. Of the two, CdTe and CZT, CZT detectors have better semiconductor properties and performance. Therefore, these are finding increased uses in Nuclear Medicine and have a better potential to replace NaI(Tl) detectors completely from Nuclear Medicine once the technical problems in the development of large-size detector assemblies are solved. Their current uses are discussed in Chapter 14.

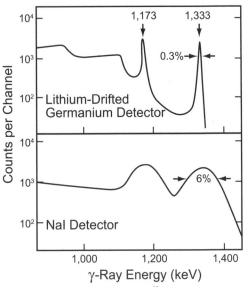

**Fig. 8.12.** γ-ray spectrum of a $^{60}$Co source (two γ-rays with 1173 and 1333 keV energy each) taken with a Ge(Li) semiconductor detector and a NaI(Tl) detector, respectively. With the Ge(Li) detector, the two photo peaks are narrow and clearly resolved. With the NaI(Tl) detector, the two photo peaks are broad and barely resolvable. The energy resolution for a 1333-keV γ-ray is 0.3% for the Ge(Li) detector and 6% for the NaI(Tl) detector. If a third γ-ray with an intermediate energy of about 1250 keV was also present in the $^{60}$Co emissions, a NaI(Tl) detector would have been unable to resolve the three γ-rays, whereas a Ge(Li) detector would have identified them clearly.

## Key Points

1. Three important properties of a radiation (x- and γ-rays) detector for use in nuclear medicine are its intrinsic efficiency, dead time, and energy resolution.
2. Of these, intrinsic efficiency is the most important. It depends on the linear attenuation coefficient of the detector material and the thickness of the detector.
3. Gas-filled detectors detect ionization produced by radiation in a gas. Ionization chambers, proportional counters, and GM counters are all gas-filled detectors.
4. Ionization chambers are used in dose calibrators because of their stability, although their intrinsic sensitivity is low compared with other radiation detectors. Dose calibrators have to be monitored daily for constancy check and annually for accuracy.
5. GM counters are used in contamination detection and general-purpose radiation-level monitoring. These are portable, inexpensive, and stable devices and should be calibrated annually.
6. Scintillator detectors produce light in response to radiation and are used to detect radiation in conjunction with a photomultiplier tube and associated electronics.

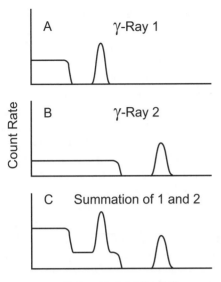

**Fig. 8.10.** Pulse-height distribution produced in response to γ-rays consisting of two distinct energies, 1 and 2. As shown in C, this is an exact sum of the pulse-height distributions produced by γ-rays of energy 1 and energy 2 independently, as shown in A and B, respectively. Low-energy γ-rays do not produce pulses with enough height to cause any interference in the photo peak of the higher energy grays. However, high-energy γ-rays produce pulses with a height corresponding to the photo peak pulses of lower energy γ-rays. Therefore, a correction has to be applied whenever a low-energy γ-ray radionuclide is being counted in the presence of a higher energy γ-ray radionuclide. This is not so in the opposite case.

***K Escape Peak*** This barely visible peak, mostly observed when the energy of a γ-ray lies between 50 and 150 keV, lies about 28 keV below the photo peak of a γ-ray. In this energy range (50–150 keV), most x- or γ-interactions are through the photoelectric effect in the K shell of iodine atoms and most of these interactions are close to the crystal surface (within a few millimeters). Therefore, the K x-ray produced when the vacancy in the K shell of the iodine atoms is filled has a finite chance of escaping from the crystal without depositing its energy. Thus, in many cases, the energy deposited by the γ-ray, even when the interaction is through photoelectric effect, is not the entire energy of the γ-ray Eγ but equals $E\gamma - E_{k\ x\text{-}ray}$. The energy of the K x-ray for an iodine atom is about 28 keV;

hence, the escape peak is 28 keV below the photo peak of a γ-ray.

***Summation Peak*** With radionuclides emitting multiple-energy γ-rays, sometimes additional peaks corresponding to the sum of individual γ-ray energies are encountered even though no γ-ray with such energy is emitted by the radionuclide. As the name implies, these peaks originate because of the summation of the energies of two different grays in the crystal. Summation of energies occurs only when two γ-rays simultaneously or almost simultaneously (within 0.25 μs) interact within the crystal. Summation peaks are more pronounced for radionuclides that emit several γ-rays within a microsecond or less of each other and for well-type scintillation detectors (see Chapter 9). Some examples of this type of radionuclide are [125]I (28 K x-ray followed by another 28 K x-ray) and [111]In (173- and 247-keV γ-rays). If a spectrum is plotted for these radionuclides using a well-type scintillation detector, besides the 28-keV x-ray of [125]I, another peak at 28 + 28 = 56 keV is also observed, although [125]I does not emit any x- or γ-ray of 56-keV energy. Similarly in [111]In, a summation peak at 173 + 247 = 420 keV is observed, although [111]In does not emit a γ-ray with this energy. For summation to occur, two γ-rays do not have to interact through the photoelectric effect only. The interaction may occur through the Compton scattering as well. Then, the summated pulse, which is also called "pile-up" pulse, will equal the sum of the energies deposited by each γ-ray. At high count rates, pile-up pulses result accidentally, even when the radionuclide emits single-energy γ-rays only.

***Back-Scattered Peak and Lead X-ray Peak*** These peaks originate from the environment or surroundings of the NaI(Tl)) detectors. Because the detectors are generally shielded by lead from all sides except one to reduce the background radiation, the γ-rays interacting with the lead shield produce scattered γ-rays and lead K x-rays of about 80 keV. Some of these secondary radiations can be detected by the crystal. Of the scattered γ-rays from the shield, only those that are scattered more or less in the backward direction have a chance to interact with the crystal. The energy of these back-scattered γ-rays is determined by the expression given on p. 62. The back-scattered γ rays are not of a single energy but are distributed in a broad range. As a rule, the sum of the back-scattered peak energy and the Compton-edge energy in the spectrum of a monochromatic γ-ray equals the photo peak energy.

## Semiconductor Detectors

It is not generally possible to measure the amount of ion pairs produced by ionizing radiation in a solid, as is possible in a gas. However, under certain conditions and for a class of solid substances known as semiconductors, it is possible to measure the amount of such ion pairs produced. The physical arrangement is similar to that of an ionization chamber except that instead of gas, there is a small cylindrical or rectangular prism-shaped piece of semiconductor between the two electrodes (Fig. 8.11). In a semiconductor, the ion pairs produced are electrons and holes (it behaves like an electron with positive charge; however, it is not a positron). Without the electric field between the two electrodes,

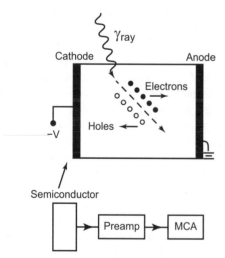

**Fig. 8.11.** Schematics of a semiconductor detector. Energy deposited by a γ-ray is converted into electron-hole pairs. Under the influence of the electric field generated by the two electrodes, holes and electrons produce current pulse that can be detected by associated electronics. Current produced is directly proportional to the energy deposited by γ-ray and thus produce a spectrum similar to that produced in a NaI(Tl) detector. MCA (multichannel analyzer) directly records this spectrum.

these electron-hole pairs recombine among themselves or with impurities or crystal defects present in the detector material. However, under the influence of electric field, current is generated. The amount of the current depends upon the energy deposited in the semiconductor material, thickness of the detector, and the temperature. Also, the purity and defect-free growth of the single crystals of these materials, particularly in large sizes, is an important consideration that sometimes becomes a major hurdle in their wide use.

In general, the number of electron-hole pairs generated for the same amount of energy deposited is many times more than the light photons generated in a scintillation detector. As a result, the energy resolution of these detectors is much better than scintillator detectors. Depending on the use, these detectors can be made as small as 1 mm in size. The intrinsic efficiency of these detectors depends on the same parameters as other detectors, namely linear attenuation coefficient ($Z_{eff}$ and density) and the thickness of the detector. The dead time of these detectors is in nanoseconds.

The two most successful semiconductor detectors so far, use germanium and silicon crystals doped with a small amount of lithium, Ge(Li) and Si(Li). However, for their optimum performance these have to be cooled at liquid nitrogen ($77^0$ K). Si(Li) detector, because of its low atomic number (Z = 14), is primarily used for the detection of corpuscular radiation, whereas Ge(Li) detector with its slightly higher atomic number (Z = 32) is used for the detection of x- or γ-rays.

The principal advantage of a Ge(Li) detector over a scintillation detector is its excellent energy resolution. A typical Ge(Li) detector can easily yield a 1% energy resolution for $^{137}$Cs γ-rays compared with 10% using a NaI(Tl) detector. The main drawbacks of Ge(Li) detectors, severely limiting their application in nuclear medicine, are their low sensitivity (because of lower atomic number, Z = 32, compared to $Z_{eff}$=50 for NaI), the necessity of maintaining them at a low temperature of 77 K that makes them bulky (room temperature is about 300 K), and their unavailability in larger sizes. A spectrum produced by a $^{60}$Co source and obtained with a Ge(Li) detector is shown in Figure 8.12, where it is also compared with a NaI(Tl) detector.

In recent years, tremendous progress has been made in the development of room temperature semiconductor detectors that do not require bulky cooling apparatus, to the point, that they are commercially viable and finding increasing use in Nuclear Medicine. Two successful materials are Cadmium Tellurium (CdTe) and Cadmium Zinc Tellurium (CZT). Their atomic number are very close to that of NaI(Tl) but the densities are higher than that of NaI(Tl). As a result, for a given thickness of the detector, their linear attenuation coefficient, $\mu$(linear) is slightly higher than that of NaI(Tl). They have better sensitivity than NaI(Tl). Their energy resolution (6% vs. 10% and further development can improve it by a factor of 2) and dead time (ns vs. $\mu$s) are also superior to that of NaI(Tl). In addition, as there is no PM tube needed, the assembled size of these detectors is much smaller (as small as a mm) than that of a NaI(Tl) detector. To form large-size detectors, one arranges them in two-dimensional arrays consisting of a large number of detectors. Of the two, CdTe and CZT, CZT detectors have better semiconductor properties and performance. Therefore, these are finding increased uses in Nuclear Medicine and have a better potential to replace NaI(Tl) detectors completely from Nuclear Medicine once the technical problems in the development of large-size detector assemblies are solved. Their current uses are discussed in Chapter 14.

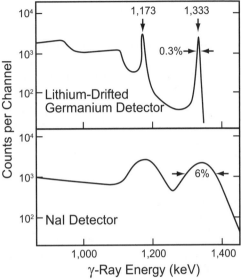

**Fig. 8.12.** $\gamma$-ray spectrum of a $^{60}$Co source (two $\gamma$-rays with 1173 and 1333 keV energy each) taken with a Ge(Li) semiconductor detector and a NaI(Tl) detector, respectively. With the Ge(Li) detector, the two photo peaks are narrow and clearly resolved. With the NaI(Tl) detector, the two photo peaks are broad and barely resolvable. The energy resolution for a 1333-keV $\gamma$-ray is 0.3% for the Ge(Li) detector and 6% for the NaI(Tl) detector. If a third $\gamma$-ray with an intermediate energy of about 1250 keV was also present in the $^{60}$Co emissions, a NaI(Tl) detector would have been unable to resolve the three $\gamma$-rays, whereas a Ge(Li) detector would have identified them clearly.

## Key Points

1. Three important properties of a radiation (x- and $\gamma$-rays) detector for use in nuclear medicine are its intrinsic efficiency, dead time, and energy resolution.

2. Of these, intrinsic efficiency is the most important. It depends on the linear attenuation coefficient of the detector material and the thickness of the detector.

3. Gas-filled detectors detect ionization produced by radiation in a gas. Ionization chambers, proportional counters, and GM counters are all gas-filled detectors.

4. Ionization chambers are used in dose calibrators because of their stability, although their intrinsic sensitivity is low compared with other radiation detectors. Dose calibrators have to be monitored daily for constancy check and annually for accuracy.

5. GM counters are used in contamination detection and general-purpose radiation-level monitoring. These are portable, inexpensive, and stable devices and should be calibrated annually.

6. Scintillator detectors produce light in response to radiation and are used to detect radiation in conjunction with a photomultiplier tube and associated electronics.

7. Na(Tl) crystal is the most common scintillator used in nuclear medicine. It possesses high intrinsic efficiency and produces a pulse-height spectrum in response to a monochromatic γ-ray. However, for PET imaging, BGO and LSO are better choices.

8. The photo peak voltage is directly proportional to energy of a γ-ray. Energy resolution of a good NaI(Tl) detector is about 10% at 662 keV energy.

9. These should be calibrated daily.

10. Semiconductor detectors have superior energy-resolution (1%) when used at low temperatures. Semiconductor detectors operating at room temperature (CZT) have problems relating to defect-free production in large sizes and are expensive. Their energy resolution for $^{99m}$Tc is about 6%.

## Questions

1. List the factors on which intrinsic efficiency of a detector depends. Why is this important in nuclear medicine?

2. Is the dead time of a detector related to the maximum detectable count rate directly, inversely, or with some other power?

3. Which gas-filled detector can measure energy of an x- or γ-ray?

4. Why can an ionization chamber not be used as a counter?

5. What is the maximum count rate for a typical GM counter?

6. Which detector discussed here is appropriate for the following applications? (a) For surveying the extent of contamination when a technologist, during an injection of a radiopharmaceutical, spilled some radioactive material on the patient's bed and his own clothing. (b) To determine a small amount (0.01 μCi) of radioactivity in a sample. (c) To determine large amounts of radioactivies such as those given to patients. (d) To characterize different radionuclides in a mixture of radionuclides.

7. List the properties of the NaI(Tl) detector that make it so attractive for use in a scintillation camera.

8. Why is BGO a better choice than NaI(Tl) for PET?

9. Why is LSO even a better choice than BGO for PET?

10. What is the function of a pulse-height analyzer?

11. If a PHA is set on the photo peak, what effect will making the window narrower have on the observed count rate?

12. Three NaI(Tl) detectors have *FWHMs* of 18, 20, and 22 keV for a 140-keV γ-ray. What is the percent energy resolution of these detectors and which one should you select?

13. Why is CZT detector better than NaI(Tl) detector?

# *In Vitro* Radiation Detection

In many nuclear medicine procedures, such as the Schilling test, blood volume determinations, protein and fat absorption studies, ferrokinetics, and various radioimmunoassays, it is necessary to determine the amount of radioactivity in a given sample as compared with a standard. In some of these tests (e.g., Schilling test), a radioactive substance is administered to a patient; in others, such as various radioimmunoassays, no radioactive compound is given to the patient. In both cases, however, the choice of the radiation detector and the geometric setup for the measurement of a given radioactive sample is of great importance and is primarily dictated by the overall efficiency (sensitivity) of a particular setup. An increased overall efficiency in these studies allows one to reduce either the radiation dose to a patient or the count time for a given standard deviation error.

This chapter describes the various techniques used for the in vitro detection of the radioactivity of both $\beta$-ray and $\gamma$-ray emitting radionuclides.

## Overall Efficiency E

The overall efficiency E of a given device for the measurement of radioactivity depends on the geometric efficiency of the physical setup $E_g$ and the intrinsic efficiency $E_i$ of the detector. Thus, the overall efficiency can be expressed as

$$E = E_g \times E_i$$

**Intrinsic Efficiency** The intrinsic efficiency $E_i$ (see Chapter 8) is defined as

$$E_i = \frac{\text{Number of radiations detected by the detector}}{\text{Number of radiations incident on the sensitive volume of the detector}}$$

It depends primarily on the linear attenuation coefficient $\mu$(linear) of the material of which a detector is made and on the thickness of the detector.

In a scintillation counter, when one restricts oneself to the photo peak counts only, the resulting intrinsic efficiency is known as the photo peak efficiency.

**Geometric Efficiency** Geometric efficiency $E_g$ can be understood as follows. Let a small sample of radioactive compound be located at a distance from a detector with a cross-sectional radius r as shown in Figure 9.1 (top). Because there is no preferred direction for the emission of radiation from a radionuclide, the radiations ($\alpha$, $\beta$, or $\gamma$) from a radioactive sample will be emitted with equal probability in all directions. Therefore, of the total number of nuclear radiations emitted in all directions, only a fraction of these will be incident on the sensitive volume of the detector (Fig. 9.1 top). Geometric efficiency $E_g$, then, is defined as the ratio of the number of radiations incident on the detector from a radioactive sample to the total number of radiations emitted by the sample, or

$$E_g = \frac{\text{Number of radiations incident on detector}}{\text{Number of the total radiations emitted by source}}$$

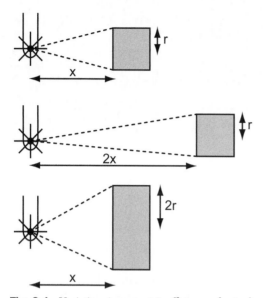

**Fig. 9.1.** Variations in geometric efficiency of a single radiation detector in three different geometric arrangements (top, center, and bottom). A radioactive source emits radiations in all directions. Only those radiations that travel in the direction enclosed by the dotted lines reach the detector. The geometric efficiency, which is a measure of the number of $\gamma$-rays that reach the detector, depends on the distance x between the source and the detector and the radius of the detector as $1/x^2$ and $r^2$. Thus, the geometric efficiency of center arrangement is one-fourth of top arrangement; the geometric efficiency of bottom arrangement is four times that of top arrangement. In such an arrangement, however, geometric efficiency can never be higher than 50%.

The geometric efficiency $E_g$, for the device shown in Figure 9.1 (top), depends on two factors: the distance x between the source and the detector and the radius r of the cross-sectional area of the detector. For distances that are sufficiently larger than the radius of the detector (i.e., $x \gg r$), the geometric efficiency varies as $1/x^2$ and $r^2$, respectively, with the distance x and the radius r; that is, if one increases the distance between the sample and the detector twofold, the geometric efficiency is reduced fourfold (Fig. 9.1center). If the radius of the detector is doubled, the geometric efficiency will be increased fourfold (Fig. 9.1bottom).

When the sample is very close to the detector (i.e., $x \ll r$), the above relationship $E_g \propto (1/x^2)$ does not hold true. The exact relationship between $E_g$ and the distance x, in this case, is of no practical

concern to us here except to know that the maximum obtainable geometric efficiency is achieved when x = 0 (i.e., the source is directly against the face of the detector). In this case, $E_g$ approaches 50%, because even in this situation, one-half of the radiations are emitted away from the detector.

To increase $E_g$ to more than 50%, one has to either use more than one detector or somehow surround the sample from all sides by the detector. The second approach is used in well-type NaI(Tl) scintillation detectors (well counters) and liquid scintillation detectors described below and is also used in dose calibrators as is described in Chapter 8.

## Well-Type NaI(Tl) Scintillation Detectors (Well Counters)

In terms of its operation and associated electronics, the well-type NaI(Tl) scintillation detector (well counter) is exactly the same as the NaI(Tl) scintillation detector described in Chapter 8, except that in a well counter, a small cylindrical hole is constructed in the NaI(Tl) crystal to allow a radioactive sample to be positioned very close to the center of the crystal (Fig. 9.2). In this type of detector, only a small fraction (<5%) of the radiations emitted by the sample, escapes

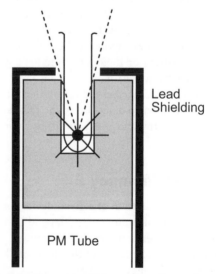

**Fig. 9.2.** Geometric efficiency of a well-type detector. The NaI crystal is shown in grey color. Only a small fraction of radiations that are emitted in the direction enclosed by two dotted lines miss the detector. In such an arrangement, geometric efficiency is close to 95%.

from the sensitive volume of the crystal. Thus, $E_g$ approaches 95%. The intrinsic efficiency of a NaI(Tl) detector is dependent on the size of the crystal—the larger the crystal, the higher the intrinsic efficiency for a given energy $\gamma$-ray. Well counters are available commercially in various sizes. The so-called standard well counter (1.75 inch diameter, 2 inches in height with a hole 0.75 inches in diameter and 1.5 inches deep) enjoys the most popularity in nuclear medicine. For high-energy $\gamma$-rays ($>$500 keV), however, one achieves a far better count rate with a 3 $\times$ 3-inch well counter than with the standard model. Table 9.1 lists the intrinsic efficiencies of standard and 3 $\times$ 3-inch well counters for various $\gamma$-ray energies. It can be seen from columns 2 and 3 that at higher energies, one gains a factor of 1.5 in intrinsic efficiency by using a 3 $\times$ 3-inch rather than a standard well counter. For many procedures, one is interested only in the photo peak counts (i.e., one rejects $\gamma$-ray interactions via the Compton scattering). In this case, the advantage of a 3 $\times$ 3-inch over a standard well counter for higher energy $\gamma$-rays becomes even greater (see columns 4 and 5 in Table 9.1).

The overall efficiency of a well counter can be easily calculated. The geometric efficiency for a small radioactive sample ($<$1 mL) is approximately 95%; the intrinsic efficiencies for various $\gamma$-rays are given in Table 9.1. For a $\gamma$-ray with an energy of 140 keV, a standard well counter will have an overall efficiency E equal to 0.95 $\times$ 0.94 = 0.89 (i.e., 89%); the overall photo peak efficiency will be simply 0.95 $\times$ 0.88 = 0.84 (84%). One can now also determine the count rate for the photo peak of $^{99m}$Tc (140 keV) for a $\mu$Ci sample. A $\mu$Ci sample of $^{99m}$Tc emits a total of 3.7 $\times$ $10^4$ $\times$ 0.88 $\gamma$-rays per second with energy of 140 keV; 0.88 is the number of 140 keV $\gamma$-rays per disintegration of $^{99m}$Tc, $n_i$ (see Chapter 2, p. 18). Therefore, the photo peak count rate obtained by a standard well counter will be 3.7 $\times$ $10^4$ $\times$ 0.88 multiplied by the overall photo peak efficiency (84%), or

$$\begin{aligned} \text{Photo peak count rate} &= 3.7 \times 10^4 \times 0.88 \times \\ & \quad 0.84 \text{ counts/s} \\ &= 2.73 \times 10^4 \text{ counts/s} \\ &= 1.6 \times 10^6 \text{ counts/min} \end{aligned}$$

In these calculations, we ignored the absorption effects of the thin aluminum container of the crystal and the self-absorption in the solution and the absorption by the walls of the test tube

| Table 9.1. | Efficiency of a Well Counter | | | |
|---|---|---|---|---|
| | **Intrinsic Efficiency** | | **Photo Peak Efficiency** | |
| **Energy (keV)** | **Standard Well** | **3 $\times$ 3-inch Well** | **Standard** | **3 $\times$ 3-inch Well** |
| 80 | 97[a] | 98[a] | 97[a] | 98[a] |
| 140 | 94 | 98 | 88 | 96 |
| 280 | 61 | 80 | 49 | 70 |
| 320 | 51 | 73 | 36 | 59 |
| 360 | 48 | 68 | 31 | 50 |
| 410 | 43 | 66 | 24 | 45 |
| 510 | 38 | 59 | 17 | 36 |
| 660 | 32 | 51 | 12 | 25 |
| 880 | 29 | 46 | 8 | 17 |
| 1110 | 28 | 45 | 7 | 16 |
| 1170 | 25 | 42 | 6 | 15 |
| 1270 | 24 | 40 | 5 | 14 |

[a]Attenuation in sample and sample holder will reduce these numbers slightly.

containing the sample. In practice, therefore, one will obtain a count rate slightly less than the one calculated above. However, for the present, assuming the overall efficiency as $1.6 \times 10^6$ counts/min, 10 pCi ($10^{-5}$ $\mu$Ci) will yield 16 counts/min. This is a realistic lower limit for the detection of $^{99m}$Tc radioactivity by a well detector and clearly demonstrates the high sensitivity of this device. The actual lower limit of detection, however, will depend on the room background and the availability of the time for a given measurement.

The above discussion about overall efficiency pertains only to small sample volumes (<1 mL). How does the overall efficiency vary with the volume of a sample? This can be ascertained from Figure 9.3, where the variation in the overall efficiency of a well counter is shown in relationship to the change in the sample volume (keeping the total activity constant). The addition of 1 mL of dilutant to successive samples progressively reduces the geometric efficiency. Because the intrinsic efficiency remains constant, the overall efficiency behaves in a fashion similar to the geometric efficiency with the increase in sample volume. The overall efficiency for the same amount of radioactivity in a 4-mL volume as compared with 1-mL volume is about 88% of the latter. Therefore, for a given amount of radioactivity, it is preferable to have the volume of a sample smaller than 2 mL.

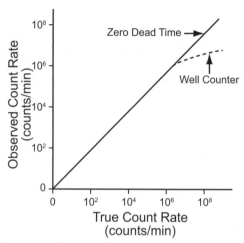

**Fig. 9.4.** Effect of the dead time of the scintillation detector on the count rate.

The other important parameter of a well counter is the dead time, which limits the maximum amount of radioactivity that can be measured without significant (<5%) count loss. Figure 9.4 shows the relationship of the true count rate to the observed count rate for a typical standard well counter. A good rule of thumb to avoid counting loss due to dead time in a well counter is to keep the total (not just the photo peak) count rate below 1 million counts per minute. This corresponds to roughly 1 $\mu$Ci of radioactivity for the common radionuclides, such as $^{131}$I or $^{99m}$Tc. Hence, any sample containing more than 1 $\mu$Ci of radioactivity should not be counted inside the well unless one has taken into account the dead time loss. In that case, a simpler alternative to the correction of dead time loss is either to dilute the sample, using a small aliquot of it for counting, or to use another geometric technique such as counting the sample outside the well.

## Liquid Scintillation Detectors

Six elements—hydrogen, carbon, nitrogen, oxygen, phosphorus, and sulfur—make up more than 97% of the total human body weight. There is, therefore, considerable interest in the radioisotopes of these elements for both research and clinical use. The number of radioisotopes of these elements that are easily available and

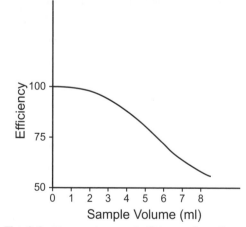

**Fig. 9.3.** Geometric or total efficiency of a well-type detector as a function of the sample volume (keeping the amount of radioactivity constant).

have half-lives long enough for their routine and widespread use is, however, limited to four: $^3$H, $^{14}$C, $^{32}$P, and $^{35}$S. These radionuclides emit only $\beta$-rays ($\beta^-$); they emit no x- or $\gamma$-rays. The detection of charged particles ($\beta$ particle, conversion electron, or $\alpha$ particle) is much more complicated than the detection of x- or $\gamma$-rays because charged particles have short ranges in solids and liquids, leading to their absorption in the radioactive sample itself and in the walls or window of the detector before detection. To avoid this problem, it is necessary either to prepare an extremely thin sample and use a detector with a very thin window or to somehow mix the detector and the radioactive source together so that the absorption problem does not arise. This latter alternative is the basis of liquid scintillation counting of $\beta$ or other charged particles. Liquid scintillation counting, because of its ease and versatility compared with other methods, is the preferred method for $\beta$-particle detection, in particular for $^3$H and $^{14}$C, which emit relatively low-energy $\beta$ particles.

**Basic Components** A liquid scintillation detector (Fig. 9.5) consists of two basic parts: a sample detector vial and a photomultiplier (PM) tube and its associated electronics (see also in Figure 8.7). Because the latter was discussed in detail in Chapter 8, we restrict ourselves here to

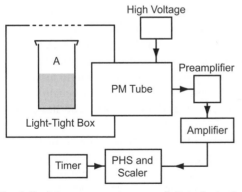

**Fig. 9.5.** Schematic presentation of a liquid scintillation detector. The electronics used in this case are identical to those used in a NaI(Tl) scintillation detector. However, in a liquid scintillation counter, the radioactive sample and the scintillator are mixed together with the help of a solvent in a sample detector vial (A).

a description of the sample detector vial. This vial consists of the radioactive sample and a suitable scintillator dissolved in a common solvent to form a solution as colorless as possible. The scintillator molecules in this solution act as a radiation detector. Homogeneous mixing of the radioactive sample and detector in this manner has two advantages: Because each radio atom of the sample is practically surrounded from all directions by scintillator molecules, the geometric efficiency of such a device is close to 100% and there is little material between the radiation source and the detector (scintillator) to cause the loss of some $\beta$ particles except for the presence of solvent molecules, which in this case aids in the transfer of energy to the scintillator molecules. Because most effective scintillators are solids, a solvent is essential to achieve a homogeneous mixture of the scintillator and radioactive sample.

The interaction of $\beta$ particles in the solution with the scintillator, and with solvent molecules, results in the loss of energy, some of which is then converted into light by the scintillator molecules. The amount of light produced in this case, as in a NaI(Tl) scintillator, is directly proportional to the amount of energy lost. Because a $\beta$-ray has a short range in liquids and loses all its energy in the solution, the amount of light produced is proportional to the energy of the $\beta$-ray. The voltage of the pulse produced by a PM tube in turn is directly related to the amount of light incident on the PM tube. Consequently, the voltage of the pulse produced is directly proportional to the energy of the $\beta$-ray. Pulse-height analysis of the pulses produced then allows the simultaneous use of two or more radionuclides with differing $\beta$-energy spectra in the same sample (e.g., $^3$H and $^{14}$C).

The sample detector vial and the PM tube are enclosed in a light-tight compartment to exclude the room and other stray light from reaching the PM tube. In modem liquid scintillation counters, the sample-detector vial is viewed from opposite sides by two PM tubes rather than one. In this arrangement, using coincidence circuits, electronic noise can be reduced significantly, thus enhancing the sensitivity of low-energy $\beta$ particles that otherwise will be lost in the electronic noise.

**Preparation of the Sample Detector Vial** The main problem in the use of a liquid scintillation detector lies in the proper preparation of the sample detector vial. This requires a careful selection of the scintillator and the solvent.

**Selection of Scintillator** A good scintillator should have high light-conversion efficiency, be sufficiently soluble in the solvent of choice, and be chemically stable under a variety of environmental conditions (temperature, humidity, or room lighting). Among the common scintillators used in liquid scintillation counting, 2,5-diphenyloxazole, ap-terphenyl, and 2,5-bis-2(5-t-butylbenzoxa-zolyl)-thiophene enjoy the most popularity. Usually, a small amount of another chemical known as a secondary scintillator is added to the primary scintillator in the solution. The purpose of a secondary scintillator is to absorb light photons emitted by the primary scintillator in the short-wave length regions (ultraviolet and violet) and to re-emit them at longer wave lengths (blue, green, or yellow) that can then be more efficiently detected by a PM tube. The compound 1,4-bis-2(5-phenyloxazolyl)benzene is widely used as a secondary scintillator.

**Selection of Solvent** The choice of a solvent is dictated by the following requirements: energy deposited in the solvent must be efficiently transferred to the scintillator molecules, the solvent must be transparent to the light produced by the scintillator, and the solvent should be able to dissolve a variety of compounds and be usable at a wide range of temperatures. Toluene, xylene, and dioxane fulfill these requirements and are therefore widely used as solvents. However, because of their hazardous nature, these have been now replaced by safer and better solvents such as di-isopropyl naphthalene. The commercial availability of premixed scintillator and solvent (e.g., Ultima Gold) in a readily usable form has considerably eased the problems in liquid scintillation counting.

**Problems Arising in Sample Preparation** The problems connected with liquid scintillation counting do not end with the proper selection of a scintillator and a solvent. The sample, generally a biological tissue, has to be processed in such a way that an almost colorless solution is produced when mixed with the scintillator and solvent. This is achieved either by digesting the tissue in a solubilizing agent such as hyamine (a quaternary amine) or by the more involved technique of combustion and oxidation to produce $^{14}CO_2$, $^{3}H_2O$, and $^{35}SO_2$ that are then easily absorbed or dissolved in a suitable scintillator solvent system. Although the hyamine method has the advantage of relative ease over the combustion and oxidation method, it entails additional problems due to a phenomenon known as "quenching."

**Quenching** Quenching can be described as any process that interferes with the production or transmission of light from the sample detector vial. This can happen either by chemical quenching or by color quenching.

In chemical quenching, the presence of trace amounts of certain chemicals (generally present in the tissue or biological sample) interferes with the transfer of energy from $\beta$-rays to the scintillator molecules. Transfer of energy from $\beta$-rays to the scintillator is mediated by short-lived chemical species known as radicals. Chemicals causing chemical quenching also react with these radicals but in a non–light-producing manner, thereby reducing the amount of light produced. In color quenching, the presence of various colored substances in the sample vial reduces by absorption the amount of light produced, hence lowering the amount of light transmitted to the PM tube.

The end result of this loss of light due to quenching is the diminution in the overall efficiency of the system. This diminution in efficiency varies from one sample to another, depending on the degree of quenching present. For quantitative work, one has to take into account this variation in the overall efficiency. This can be done by counting the various samples first and then recounting them after the addition of a known amount of a standard radioactive substance. The effect of quenching can also be corrected by the use of an external $\gamma$-ray source and what is known as the channel ratio method. The details of this method are out of the scope of this book.

**Photo- and Chemiluminescence** Two other effects that may interfere with the efficiency of liquid scintillation detectors are photoluminescence and chemiluminescence. Because of the property of certain molecules that lets them absorb light and re-emit it at a later time, the sample detector vial continues to emit light for a short time even when it has been placed in a dark room. This phenomenon is called photoluminescence. "Dark adapting" the samples for several hours before counting generally, eliminates this problem.

In chemiluminescence, when two chemicals are mixed or involved in a reaction, some light may be produced, depending on the nature of the two chemicals involved. Many biological samples, when mixed with toluene or other solvents, produce chemiluminescence. The only way to avoid the production of light through this effect is to wait for the chemical reaction to be completed (which may take up to several days) before counting.

## Key Points

1. In counting, besides the intrinsic efficiency, geometric efficiency is another important consideration.
2. Geometric efficiency depends on distance x between the radioactive sample and the detector, and area A of the detector. It varies as the inverse square of x and is directly proportional to A or as $r^2$ for a circular detector.
3. Well-type detectors have close to 100% geometric efficiency.
4. A well-type NaI(Tl) detector has very high overall (geometric × intrinsic) efficiency for x- or $\gamma$-rays used in nuclear medicine.
5. Liquid scintillator detectors are the detectors of choice for $\beta$-emitting radionuclides, such as $^3$H, $^{14}$C, $^{32}$P, and $^{35}$S.
6. In a liquid scintillator, the radioactive sample and the scintillator are mixed together in a sample vial. Light produced in the vial is detected with a PM tube and associated electronics.

## Questions

1. How can one increase the geometric efficiency of a detector? Does it depend on the type of the detector being used? What are the advantages of $4\pi$ geometry?
2. Why do the decay rate of a sample and the observed count rate generally differ? Which one of the two is generally greater?
3. A radioactive sample containing 5 $\mu$Ci of $^{51}$Cr produces $1.5 \times 10^6$ counts in 3 minutes. Calculate the overall efficiency of the counting setup.
4. A sample contains 2 $\mu$Ci of radioactivity. Calculate the average count rate it will produce if the overall efficiency is 0.15 and the emission frequency for the $\gamma$ ray being counted, $n_i = 0.25$.
5. Calculate the overall efficiency if the intrinsic efficiency = 0.75 and the geometric efficiency = 0.90.
6. A detector is 10 cm away from the radioactive sample. The measured count rate for this sample is 5000/min. What is the expected count rate if the sample is moved to 20 cm from the sample?
7. A radioactive sample (1 mL volume) is counted in a well-type scintillator detector. It gives $3 \times 10^3$ counts in 1 minute. Four milliliters of water is added to the sample and it (5 mL) is counted again for a minute. What is the expected count rate for this diluted sample? Assume that efficiency/volume curve is that given in Figure 9.3.
8. Will the thickness of a sample affect the determination of its radioactivity?
9. Why is the determination of radioactivity of a pure $\beta$ emitter sample more problematic than a $\gamma$ emitter?
10. What is the geometric efficiency in a liquid scintillation detector?

# *In Vivo* Radiation Detection: Basic Problems, Probes, and Rectilinear Scanners

*In vivo* detection of radioactivity using external detectors constitutes a major concern of nuclear medicine. This involves a variety of studies that can be divided into two subgroups, organ uptake and organ imaging. In organ uptake studies, we are interested in the uptake of radioactivity by an organ as a whole, either at a given time (static) or as a function of time (dynamic). Some examples of organ uptake studies are radioiodine uptake by the thyroid, renograms, cardiac output measurements, and blood flow determinations. In organ imaging studies, we are not interested in the uptake of radioactivity by an organ as a whole, but in the relative distribution of radioactivity in the organ either at a given time (static) or as a function of time (dynamic). For example, in liver imaging, one is interested in the distribution of radiolabeled colloid in various parts of the liver rather than the total uptake of colloid by the liver. Other examples of this group are bone, brain, heart, lung, spleen, kidney, and thyroid imaging.

Although uptake and imaging studies have quite different aims, some problems of in vivo detection are common to both and the same radiation detector, a NaI(Tl) scintillation detector, is used in both. Therefore, in this chapter, I first discuss the common problems encountered in in vivo detection. I then briefly touch on the specialized instruments (probes) for organ uptake measurement and follow with a brief description of a rectilinear scanner, which is used for organ imaging. Both instruments are rarely used in practice but form an important link in the historical development of nuclear medicine instrumentation.

## Basic Problems

The use of external detectors for in vivo measurement of radioactivity automatically excludes the use of radionuclides, which do not emit penetrating radiation. Therefore, radionuclides that emit x- or $\gamma$-radiation must be used. Three types of problems arise in the in vivo detection of such radionuclides: collimation, scattering, and attenuation. All three factors, coupled with the fact that a detector has to be a certain distance away from a radioactive source (the source being in vivo), reduce the geometric efficiency in in vivo detection by two to three orders of magnitude as compared with the in vitro case (see Chapter 9). This is one of the reasons why millicurie (MBq) amounts are used in in vivo studies as compared with only microcurie or less (kBq) in in vitro studies.

**Collimation** Because one is interested in the detection of radioactivity present in a small area or volume (e.g., an organ or part of an organ), it is important to exclude all x- or $\gamma$-rays originating outside the area or volume of interest from reaching the radiation detector. This is achieved by the use of a collimator, a device that limits the field of view (FOV) of a radiation detector. A variety of collimators are available for different purposes. These are usually made of lead, which is inexpensive and possesses both a high-density and a high-attenuation coefficient for the x- or $\gamma$-rays whose energies are of particular interest in nuclear medicine ($<$500 keV). A diagram of a simple collimator is shown in Figure 10.1. Note that simple collimation does not allow full discrimination

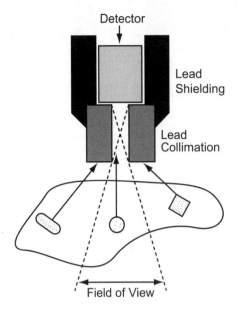

**Fig. 10.1.** A simple collimator. The collimator restricts the field of view of a radiation detector. Of the three sources, oblong, circular, and rectangular, only those γ-rays that originate from the circular radioactive source can reach the detector, whereas all γ-rays originating from the oblong and rectangular radioactive sources are blocked by the collimator. The field of view of this type of collimator increases with distance from the collimator, as shown by the dotted lines.

against the radioactivity underlying or overlying the volume of interest. Also, the FOV of such a collimator is determined by two parameters: the length and the radius of the opening (hole) in a collimator. By reducing the radius or increasing the length, one can reduce or narrow the FOV of a collimator to any desired size.

The FOV of a single-hole collimator is related to the spatial resolution and sensitivity of the collimator. Increasing the FOV degrades the spatial resolution and improves the sensitivity and vice versa (Chapter 12). The FOV also increases with depth; therefore, spatial resolution also gets worse with depth—a troublesome feature to be dealt with when accurate quantification of radioactivity is desired [i.e., single-photon emission computed tomography (SPECT); Chapter 14].

**Scattering** The γ- and x-rays emitted by radionuclidic sources embedded in a mass of matter experience, during interaction with that

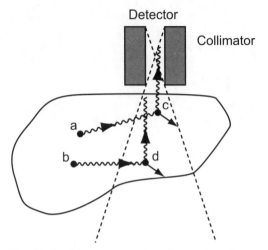

**Fig. 10.2.** Compton scattering of γ-rays interferes with the function of a collimator. γ-rays originating outside the field of view from points a and b are able to reach the detector as a result of Compton scattering at points c and d, respectively. The only effective way to reject such events is by the use of pulse-height analysis. The solid arrows at points, c and d, represent the Compton-scattered electrons. The dotted lines show the field of view of the collimator.

material, scattering via the Compton process. In Compton scattering (see Chapter 6), an interacting γ- or x-ray loses some of its energy and changes its direction. The change in the direction of many γ-rays that originate outside the FOV of the collimator causes them to be scattered toward the radiation detector, thus defeating the purpose of this device (Fig. 10.2).

Depending on the angle of scattering, an x- or γ-ray loses different amounts of energy during Compton scattering. As a result, x- or γ-rays emerging from a monochromatic source embedded in a tissue volume are no longer monochromatic but are polychromatic, as shown in Figure 10.3A. In the case of a 140-keV γ-ray, the energies of scattered γ-rays range from 90 to 140 keV. This assumes that a γ-ray is scattered only once in the tissue. In the case of double or triple Compton scattering, which are generally negligible but become more probable as the tissue volume embedding the source increases, the lower limit of scattered γ-ray energy (90 keV) becomes even lower. In diagnostic x-ray imaging, scattered x-rays are reduced by using grids. In nuclear medicine, this can be accomplished by using energy

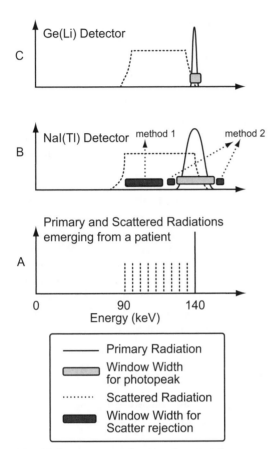

**Fig. 10.3.** Scattering of γ-rays in tissues of a patient. (A) Monochromatic γ-rays of 140 keV energy from a source embedded in tissue, because of Compton scattering in the tissue, become polychromatic (energy of γ-rays emerging from a patient range from 90 to 139 keV for the scattered radiation and 140 keV for the primary radiation). (B) A NaI(Tl) detector, because of its poor energy resolution, detects a significant fraction of scattered radiation in a typical window width used in clinical imaging. Narrowing the window, results in loss of sensitivity. Methods 1 and 2 as discussed in text are good solutions to this dilemma. (C) A Ge(Li) detector, because of its better energy resolution, detects little scattered radiation in a typical window width used for such detectors but suffers from low intrinsic sensitivity.

discrimination. Efficiency of scatter rejection with energy discrimination depends on the energy resolution of a detector. When using a NaI(Tl) detector (Fig. 10.3B), pulse-height analyzer (PHA) controls, E and $\Delta E$, are set to accept only those pulses whose height corresponds to the photo peak of the

unscattered γ-ray. For an effective job of energy discrimination, the energy resolution of a detector should be very good. For a 140-keV γ-ray, NaI(Tl) scintillation detectors possess moderate energy discrimination capability with full-width at half-maximum (*FWHM*) of 15 to 20 keV as compared with Ge(Li) semiconductor detectors (Fig. 10.3C) with *FWHM* of 1 to 2 keV. As a result, a Ge(Li) detector is capable of rejecting almost all scattered radiation, whereas a NaI(Tl) detector does only a partial job. However, despite their better energy discrimination capability, Ge(Li) detectors are seldom used in nuclear medicine, primarily because of their very low sensitivity compared with a NaI(Tl) scintillation detector. The newer detector, CZT has energy resolution in between the two, NaI(Tl) and Ge(Li) and therefore better scatter rejection ability than NaI. It also has better sensitivity than NaI(Tl) detector (see Chapter 8). That is why it is a prime candidate to replace NaI detector in nuclear medicine, once the technical problems in growing good quality CZT crystals have been overcome.

The amount of scattered radiation rejected by a NaI(Tl) detector depends on the width of the PHA window. The narrower the window, the more scattered radiation is excluded. But narrowing the window to reject scattered radiation exacts a price in terms of reduced sensitivity because more of the primary radiation also is rejected. There are two better ways to reject scattered radiation. One way is the simultaneous use of one more (second) window at a lower energy as shown in Figure 10.3B. The counts or a fraction of counts in the second window are subtracted from the window set at the photo peak. Another way is the simultaneous use of two more windows (second and third) that are only a few keV in width and set just below and above the photo peak as shown in Figure 10.3B. Here, the average of the counts from these two windows is subtracted from the window set at the photo peak. Both methods are better than narrowing the photo peak window because primary radiation is not lost. However, these methods by no means reject scatter completely and accurately or as much as a Ge(Li) detector does as shown in Figure 10.3C.

**Attenuation** Because the depth, shape, and size of an organ containing the radioactive substance

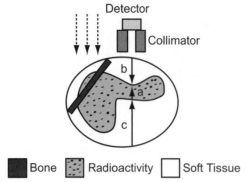

Detector

Collimator

b

a

c

■ Bone  ▦ Radioactivity  □ Soft Tissue

**Fig. 10.4.** Attenuation of radioactivity in in vivo imaging is difficult to correct because the area or volume of radioactive distribution in the field of view of the collimator is unknown (shown by arrow a) and the thickness of the underlying or overlying tissue is unknown (arrows b and c). Point-to-point variations (e.g., at dotted arrows) in these two parameters cause the uniform distribution of radioactivity (per gram or per cubic centimeter of liver) to give different counts at different locations of the detector. Tissues with different attenuation (e.g., bone, soft tissue, or lungs) further complicate the situation.

are unknown beforehand, the attenuation of x- or γ-rays (absorption through the photoelectric effect and the Compton scattering) in the organ and the tissue overlying or underlying the organ is another serious hurdle in the in vivo determination of radioactivity. As can be seen in Figure 10.4, the distribution of radioactivity varies throughout the cross section, and x- or γ-rays emitted by a radioactive source, depending on its location, pass through different thicknesses and often different types of underlying or overlying tissue and therefore are attenuated by different amounts. As a result, a uniform distribution of radioactivity produces different counts at different locations of the organ, not a desirable feature in any imaging.

It is possible to minimize attenuation loss by the use of high-energy x- or γ-rays. The attenuation coefficient for x- or γ-rays in tissue drops sharply with an increase in γ-ray energy up to about 100 keV and levels off with the increase in γ-ray energy above 100 keV. Therefore, radionuclides emitting x- or γ-rays with energies above 100 keV are preferred. Because the sensitivity of NaI(Tl) detectors and the collimators used in scanning decreases with the increase in x- or

γ-ray energy, the optimum range of energies for in vivo use is between 100 and 300 keV (see p. 41 and Figure 6.4 p. 59).

In organ uptake studies such as thyroid uptake of radioiodine, in addition to the use of high-energy γ-rays, attenuation effects are taken care of by measuring a known amount of radioactivity in a standard phantom that reflects the average size, shape, and depth of an organ in a standard man.

In organ imaging studies, generally, attenuation is considered a fait accompli and is taken into account only when interpreting a scan. However, newer imaging instruments fitted with computers can compensate for some attenuation effects by taking images from two opposite sides and then forming a geometric mean image. Geometric mean G of two images or numbers, $N_1$ and $N_2$, is defined as $G = \sqrt{N_1 \times N_2}$. Methods of attenuation correction in SPECT are discussed in Chapter 14.

## Organ Uptake Probes

An uptake probe consists of two basic parts: a NaI(Tl) detector and a collimator.

**NaI(Tl) Detector**  In in vivo studies, the size of the crystal in a NaI(Tl) detector is an important consideration. Crystal size is determined by the energy of the γ-ray to be detected and the sensitivity requirements of a particular study. For thyroid uptake studies using $^{131}I$, the International Atomic Energy Agency recommends that a crystal less than $1 \times 1$ inch should not be used. A $1.5 \times 1$-inch crystal is generally adequate for thyroid uptake measurements of $^{131}I$ and also serves as a multipurpose instrument in the nuclear medicine laboratory.

**Collimator**  The design of a collimator for uptake studies is dictated by its intended application. However, the following general requirements apply in most cases:

1. To keep the radiation burden to the patient to a minimum, the overall efficiency should be as high as possible;
2. The FOV of the collimator should be well defined but flexible enough to take into account the varying size of a particular

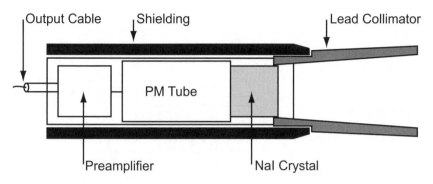

Fig. 10.5. A typical NaI(Tl) crystal collimator assembly (probe) used for thyroid uptake of $^{131}$I.

organ in different patients while at the same time excluding any radioactivity present in other organs;

3. Because the distribution of radioactivity within the organ and its size, shape, and depth are not known, the overall efficiency or sensitivity should be uniform across the FOV of the collimator and throughout the thickness of the organ.

Because requirements 1 and 3 oppose each other to some extent, one should make the best of a given situation. A typical collimator used in thyroid uptake measurement is shown in Figure 10.5. The overall sensitivity within the FOV of such a collimator varies inversely as the square of the distance between the source and the detector but the uniformity across the organ improves as the distance from the detector is increased. For thyroid uptake, a distance of 30 cm is considered optimum.

## Miniature Surgical Probes

These probes are used to detect the radioactive uptake in surgical procedures called intraoperative lymphatic mapping or sentinel lymph node biopsy, a minimally invasive technique for evaluating the potential spread of cancer to lymph node tissues and organs. They consist of a small detector (5 to 15 mm diameter and 2 to 5 mm thickness) and a collimator with a narrow FOV or resolution (3 mm to 1.5 cm). Because of surgical requirements, these probes have to be small and sterile. As a result, either semiconductor detectors, CdTe or CZT, or scintillator detec-

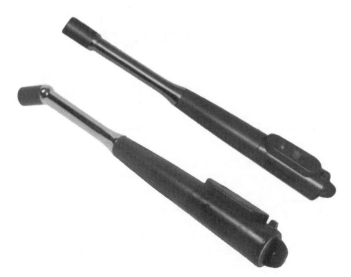

Fig. 10.6. Wireless miniature surgical probes (From Neoprobe, Dublin, Ohio, with permission)

tor, BGO with a photodiode instead of a PM tube, are used in these probes. Recently, wireless probes have been introduced to make their use even simpler during surgery (Fig. 10.6).

## Organ Imaging Devices

Administration of a particular radiopharmaceutical results in its selective localization in the organ or organs of interest in a patient. The distribution of the radiopharmaceutical in an organ may vary within the organ itself, particularly as a result of some focal disease. A diseased or abnormal area in the organ may be hotter (more radioactivity) or colder (less radioactivity) than the adjacent normal tissue. The purpose of organ scanning or imaging is to unravel this relative distribution of the radioactivity present in an organ. Ideally, we should delineate this distribution in all three dimensions (volume), but because of various technical problems, this is not routinely feasible. Instead, a two-dimensional or areal distribution of radioactivity, which is very useful clinically, is obtained. The lack of three-dimensional information in this case is somewhat compensated for by determining the area distribution from multiple directions, generally four: anterior, posterior, right, and left laterals. A two-dimensional record of the distribution of the radioactivity present in an organ is called a scan or an image.

A scanner or imager consists of four elements: a collimator, radiation detector, device to give the location (i.e., x, y coordinates) of the radioactivity, and a system to display the relative distribution in a manner easy to comprehend. Depending on how the x, y coordinates, or information about the location of the radioactivity, are obtained, imaging devices can be grouped into two classes: rectilinear scanners and scintillation cameras (γ cameras). Only the rectilinear scanner is discussed here. The scintillation camera is discussed in the next chapter.

**Rectilinear Scanner** Rectilinear scanners were the first instruments used in Nuclear Medicine. These are no longer in use and are discussed briefly for historical reasons. In a rectilinear scanner, a NaI(Tl) scintillation detector

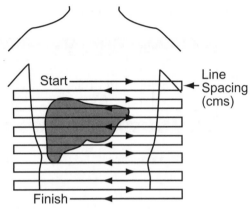

**Fig. 10.7.** Path of a detector head in rectilinear scanning of an organ.

with an appropriate collimator (detector head) is moved over the organ of interest in a straight line with the help of an electric motor. After traversal of a specified distance, the detector head either steps up or steps down a small distance and then continues the straight line motion in the opposite direction. This back-and-forth motion of the detector head (Fig. 10.7) continues until the area occupied by the organ has been fully scanned. The FOV of the collimator in this case is narrow,

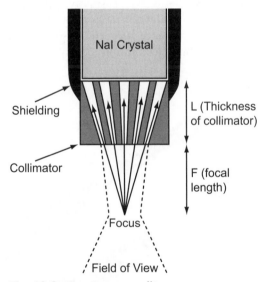

**Fig. 10.8.** Focusing-type collimator. γ-rays can reach the detector only through the narrow channels as shown by the solid arrows. The field of view of such a collimator (dotted lines) is in general narrow and is narrowest (about 1 cm) in the focal plane. It becomes wider above or below the focal plane.

and the rectilinear motion of the detector head over the organ generates the span point by point.

The detector head assembly consists of a collimator, NaI(Tl) crystal and associated electronics. The collimator used in a rectilinear scanner is known as a multihole focusing type collimator and is shown in Figure 10.8. It consists of a lead cylinder with a number of tapered holes formed to converge at a single point outside the collimator, known as the focus. The information gathered by the detector head regarding the amount of radioactivity at a given location is continuously relayed to a photographic system, where a small cathode-ray tube, with a fast phosphor screen and well-collimated light spot that exposes an x-ray film, is moved in a light-tight box in synchronization with the detector head. At the completion of the scan, the x-ray film is developed portraying the distribution of radioactivity in the organ.

## Key Points

1. Three problems, collimation, attenuation, and Compton scattering, make in vivo detection of radiation difficult.
2. Collimation is needed to exclude detection of radiation emitted outside the area of interest. FOV of a collimator is determined by the size of the area of interest. FOV is related to the resolution and sensitivity of a collimator. Collimators are primarily made of lead, an inexpensive, high–atomic-number, and high-density material.
3. Compton scattering in the FOV of a collimator of γ-rays emitted outside the FOV allows some γ-rays to be detected from outside the FOV. The scattered radiation can be reduced (but not eliminated) with a narrow window set on the primary γ-ray energy in a NaI(Tl) detector.
4. Other methods of reducing the contribution of scattered γ-rays in a clinical situation use two or three windows as described in the text.
5. Attenuation by the overlying tissue is the main source of error in quantification of radioactivity in vivo. In routine imaging, this is taken into consideration while interpreting the images.
6. Organ uptake probes are used to determine radioactivity in a whole organ (e.g., thyroid). Miniature uptake probes are used during surgery to detect small lesions.
7. Rectilinear scanners were the earliest instruments to determine the radioactive distribution within an organ. However, their inability to detect the radionuclidic distributions at a fast rate made them obsolete.

## Questions

1. List the problems that make quantification of in vivo radioactivity difficult.
2. How does pulse-height analysis help in the detection of in vivo radioactivity?
3. What is the ideal detector from the scatter rejection point of view?
4. What is the effect of narrowing the PHA window on the scattered counts and the sensitivity of a NaI detector?
5. Attenuation is a problem in in vivo detection of radioactivity. Which of the following organs poses the most challenge in this regard: brain, heart, or kidneys?
6. How does one obtain a geometric mean image?
7. What is the primary function of a collimator? Why are collimators made of lead? Can other materials be used instead of lead?
8. Why is there an optimum range of distance between the patient's thyroid and the probe when measuring the radioiodine uptake?
9. What are miniature surgical probes are used for?
10. Why is the rectilinear scanner no longer in clinical use?

# *In Vivo* Radiation Detection: Scintillation Camera

A gamma camera, in particular a scintillation camera, occupies a central place in every nuclear medicine department. In a gamma camera, as opposed to a rectilinear scanner where an organ is scanned point by point, the whole organ or a large part of the body is imaged simultaneously. In this respect, a gamma camera behaves similarly to a photographic camera, although the two types of cameras are entirely different in construction and operation. Unlike light rays, x- or γ-rays cannot be reflected or refracted by using mirrors, lenses, or prisms. Therefore, the general principles of light photography cannot be applied to imaging of objects emitting x- or γ-rays. Instead, the selective attenuation and transmission of x- and γ-rays by different materials, such as lead and air, forms the basis of imaging with a gamma camera.

The simultaneous visualization of an entire organ or organs by a gamma camera is its single most important quality that made rectilinear scanners obsolete. This feature makes the study of rapid dynamic processes possible. Dynamic studies with 10 to 20 images/s are now routinely obtained to determine cardiac output and ejection fraction.

Of a variety of approaches attempted in research laboratories for the development of gamma cameras, the scintillation camera developed by Anger has emerged as a superior choice in clinical nuclear medicine. Since its commercial introduction in 1966, the modem scintillation camera has gone through several waves of technologic innovations, from improved photomultiplier (PM) tubes and collimators, nonuniformity correction modules, to all digital cameras of the present. It is now almost a new instrument. The only constant element is the scintillator material, which is still a NaI(Tl) crystal. However, CZT detector with further improvement is a serious threat to NaI(Tl) detector. Dedicated gamma camera using CZT detectors for small field of view for cardiac studies (discussed in Chapter 14) and mammography using radiopharmaceuticals (LumaGem) are already available.

## Scintillation Camera

In a scintillation camera, a large disc- or rectangular-shaped NaI(Tl) crystal is viewed from one side by an array of PM tubes. Such an array of PM tubes not only determines the total amount of light produced by a γ-ray interaction, as is common in a scintillator detector and discussed in Chapter 8, but also the location of light production in the crystal. The other side of the crystal is attached to a collimator that acts like a lens of a photo camera.

Physically, a scintillation camera is divided in two parts. The detector head contains the collimator and the NaI(Tl) crystal with PM tubes and associated electronics and is mounted on a stand where it can be easily moved up or down or rotated in any desired position with handheld controls or automatically under the direction of a computer (Fig. 11.1). Recently, two or even three detector heads have become popular, particularly with single-photon emission computed

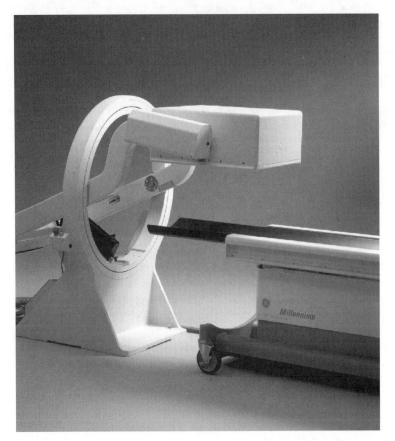

**Fig. 11.1.** A single head detector mounted on a stand. It can be easily positioned for imaging at any angle to a patient lying on the bed. (From General Electric, with permission.)

tomography (SPECT, Chapter 14). Increased geometric efficiency is the obvious advantage of multiple detector heads. The second part is the console, which houses the power supplies and operational controls of the scintillation camera, including the display module and quite often an integrated digital computer. In portable scintillation cameras, the detector head and console are joined together in one unit so that it can be moved from one location to another without too much difficulty.

Operationally, a scintillation camera consists of four basic parts (Fig. 11.2, A–D): collimator, detector, multiple PM tubes and position (x, y coordinates) determining circuit, and display. Here, I describe the workings of a scintillation camera. Its operating characteristics such as spatial resolution, sensitivity, and uniformity and quality control are discussed in Chapter 12.

**Collimators** The purpose of a collimator in a scintillation camera is to allow x- or γ-rays originating from a selected area of an organ to reach a selected area of the detector. Thus, a collimator establishes a one-to-one correspondence between different locations on the detector and those within the organ. Another feature of a scintillation camera collimator is that its field of view is large enough to encompass completely the total organ or the desired part of the body to be imaged. Four types of collimators have been used with scintillation cameras (Fig. 11.3).

**Parallel Hole** A parallel-hole collimator is made of a large number (many thousands) of small holes in a lead disc. The diameter of the lead disc is the same as that of the scintillation crystal used. Thickness of the lead disc and the diameter of the holes depend on the desired

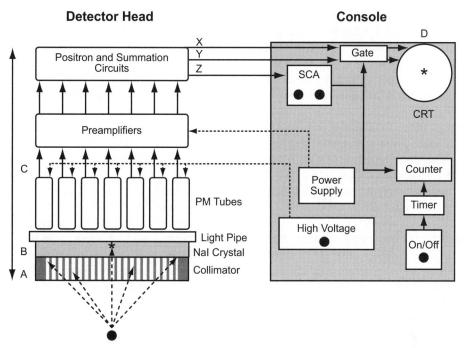

**Fig. 11.2.** Schematics of a typical scintillation camera. Four operational components are identified: A (collimator), B (NaI crystal), C (light pipe, PM tubes, and preamplifiers), and D (CRT for display). Detector head incorporates in it A, B, and C, and the console contains D and power supplies and associated electronics.

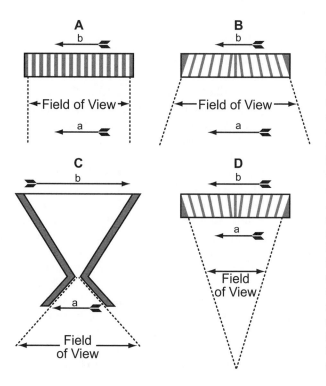

**Fig. 11.3.** Collimators used in a scintillation camera. (A) Parallel-hole collimator: The object a projects the same size image b on the crystal face. The field of view of such a collimator does not vary significantly with distance from the collimator. (B) Diverging collimator: The size of the image b is smaller than the size of the object a, and the field of view increases as we move away from the collimator. (C) Pinhole collimator: A magnified or minified image b of an object a, is produced, depending on its distance from the pinhole. The field of view of a pinhole increases rapidly as we move away from the pinhole. (D) Converging collimator: This collimator produces a magnified image b of an object a. The field of view decreases as we move away from the detector. A converging collimator provides the optimum sensitivity and spatial resolution for an object that is smaller than the crystal size used in the scintillation camera.

spatial resolution and sensitivity of these collimators (discussed in Chapter 12). Lead walls between the holes, called septa, for a well-designed collimator, absorb most, if not all, radiation incident on them. Holes are axial, parallel to each other and circular or hexagonal in shape.

**Pinhole**  A pinhole collimator consists of a single hole, about 5 mm in diameter, at the top of a hollow lead cone. The diameter at the base of the lead cone is the size of the NaI(Tl) crystal. The top of the cone faces the patient. The height of the cone can range from 12 to 20 inches.

**Converging**  A converging collimator is similar to a parallel-hole collimator except that the holes, as we move away from the center of the collimator toward the edge of the collimator, start tilting toward the center, as shown in Figure 11.3. Outermost holes have the most tilt. All holes focus at an axial point, outside the collimator (typically 10–20 inches) and toward the radioactive source or the patient.

**Diverging**  In a diverging collimator, the tilt of the holes is away from the center. As a result, these holes converge toward the detector. In fact, if one flips over a converging collimator, it becomes a diverging collimator and vice versa.

As can be seen, in all these collimators, $\gamma$-rays originating from one area of the arrow reach only a selected area on the crystal. Thus, $\gamma$-rays originating from the front of the arrow reach a different location on the crystal than $\gamma$-rays originating from the middle or back of the arrow. The size of the image formed on the crystal depends on the type of collimator and distance of the object (arrow) from the collimator. In the case of a pinhole collimator, the image is also inverted. The choice of a particular type of collimator is basically dictated by the size of the organ to be imaged. For imaging organs that are similar in size to the size of the detector [NaI(Tl)] crystal, parallel-hole collimators provide the best sensitivity and spatial resolution. For organs larger than the size of the crystal, diverging collimators are preferred. For organs smaller than the size of the crystal, converging collimators have shown great merit. When the size of the organ is small, such as the thyroid, a pinhole collimator is the collimator of choice. One problem that makes the use of pinhole, converging, or diverging collimators less satisfactory than parallel-hole collimators is the fact that for three-dimensional objects (which all organs are), the different planes of the object (front, back, or middle of the organ) are magnified or minified to different degrees by these collimators. This produces distortions in the image that under most clinical circumstances are unacceptable.

Commercially, the collimators, besides being characterized by the above four types, are also classified according to their spatial resolution or sensitivity as high-sensitivity (for dynamic studies), all purpose (for most clinical applications), or high-spatial-resolution (for fine details) collimators and according to the energies of $\gamma$-rays for which they have been optimized as low-energy (0–200 keV), medium-energy (200–400 keV), and high-energy (400–600 keV) collimators. High-energy collimators are used sometimes with positron-emitting radionuclides, as discussed in Chapter 14. The main difference between collimators designed for different energies is the thickness of septum that increases with energy.

## Detector, NaI(Tl) Crystal

**Size and Thickness**  As has already been pointed out, the basic detector element in a scintillation camera is a large disc-shaped [NaI(Tl)] crystal that is viewed from one side by a large number of PM tubes. The diameter of the crystal varies from 11 to 20 inches. Eleven-inch-diameter crystals are used in the standard scintillation camera, whereas 16- to 20-inch-diameter crystals are used in so-called large field of view (LFOV) scintillation cameras. The main advantage of a large crystal is the increased sensitivity for large organs such as lungs or the whole body. For a more effective use of the crystal area, rectangular crystals are also available in some scintillation cameras. The thickness of the crystal is generally 1/2 inch, but scintillation cameras with 3/8- or 1/4-inch-thick crystals are also in vogue, particularly for nuclear cardiology work. Reduced thickness of the crystal improves the intrinsic spatial resolution (to be defined in the next section). The trade-off for improved intrinsic spatial resolution is the reduction in intrinsic sensitivity, particularly for higher energy (>150 keV) $\gamma$-rays.

**Energy Selection** The detection and measurement of energy of the $\gamma$-rays passing through the collimator is performed as in any NaI(Tl) detector system, except that in scintillation cameras a large number of PM tubes are used instead of a single PM tube. To determine the energy of a $\gamma$-ray, one has to determine the total amount of light produced in the crystal (Chapter 8, p. 84). In a scintillation camera, the total light produced is distributed among many or all PM tubes. Therefore, to determine the total amount of light produced, the outputs of all PM tubes have to be summed to produce a pulse equivalent to that produced in a simple NaI(Tl) detector (with only one PM tube). The summated pulse is known as the Z pulse (a misnomer as this should be called E pulse). Pulse-height analysis on Z pulses allows us to select the pulses of the desired energy.

Two important attributes of the Z pulse are linearity with $\gamma$-ray energy and its spatial independence (Z pulse-height should not depend on the location of the point of light production in the crystal). On both scores, newer scintillation cameras have improved significantly. The remainder of the nonlinearity and spatial dependence is reduced further by using online correction methods, as discussed in Chapter 12. Summation of pulses from many PM tubes to obtain a Z pulse in a scintillation camera makes its energy resolution slightly worse than a simple NaI(Tl) detector.

Like any other NaI(Tl) detector, in a scintillation camera there are four controls related to the detection of $\gamma$-rays and their energies: high voltage, gain of the amplifier, peak energy E, and window width $\Delta$E or %$\Delta$E. Energy selection is usually automated; to choose a $\gamma$-ray of a particular energy, one presses a designated button and appropriate pulses are automatically selected. Another useful feature is a provision for simultaneous selection of two or even three $\gamma$-rays of different energies. This feature requires two or three pulse-height analyzers (PHAs) and is useful for imaging the distribution of radionuclides that emit more than one $\gamma$-ray (e.g., $^{67}$Ga, $^{111}$In, or even $^{201}$Tl) or for rejecting the scattered radiation as was pointed out previously (p. 104).

**Automatic Peak Tracking** Scintillation detectors are prone to slow drifts in their outputs, mainly due to the changes in the gain of a PM tube. Changes in the PM gain are caused by small ambient temperature and high-voltage fluctuations. In newer cameras, electronic circuits have been provided that monitor these drifts and readjust the high voltage or amplifier gain to its original value. The automatic peak tracking circuits track the PM gains either on demand or continuously, depending on the manufacturer of a scintillation camera. In either case, the output of PM tubes, and therefore the stability of the scintillation camera itself, has improved tremendously.

**Counting** Pulses selected by the PHA, besides being sent to a logic circuit for generation of X and Y pulses as discussed in the next section, are fed into a counter-timer module. The scintillation camera can count either for a fixed-time interval (preselected time) or for an assigned number of counts (preselected counts). There is also a provision for imaging to stop at preselected time intervals or a preselected number of counts, depending on which happens first. A manual control allows one to start or stop counting at any time. Another feature found only in some scintillation cameras is preselection of the information density in a given area of the image. The scintillation camera will stop when a preselected number of counts have been acquired in the desired area of the image. Scintillation cameras interfaced or integrated with digital computers have these functions—start, stop, time, or number of counts—under computer control.

### Position Determining Circuit (x, y Coordinates)

**Pulse-Height Distribution Among PM Tubes** A collimator in a scintillation camera allows $\gamma$ or x rays originating from one small part of an organ to reach a small part of the crystal in a one-to-one correspondence. To keep this correspondence intact electronically, we should

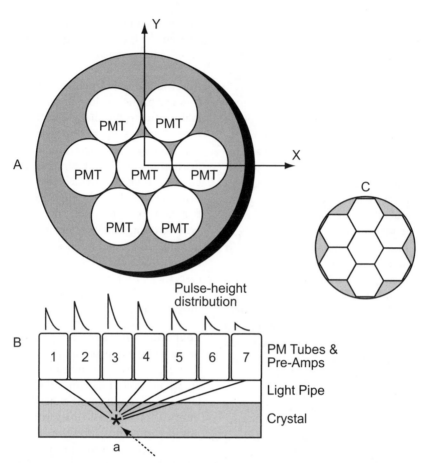

**Fig. 11.4.** Geometric arrangement of PM tubes to localize the point of light-production in a scintillation camera (A). When a γ-ray interacts at point a in the crystal (B), PM tube 3 receives the maximum amount of light, thus providing the appropriate location of the point at which the light is produced. For a γ-ray interaction at a different point, another PM tube will receive the most light. By knowing the PM tube that receives the maximum amount, one can approximately locate the point of light production. However, for more accurate localization, we have to consider the pulse-height distribution produced among many PM tubes. C The shape of PM tubes does not have to be circular; a hexagonal shape is better because of fuller coverage of the crystal area. The same argument is true for the shape of the holes of a collimator where hexagonal-shaped holes are also preferred over circular-shaped holes.

know where the γ rays are interacting in the crystal. This is accomplished with the help of a large number (commonly 37 or 67) of PM tubes, but in Figure 11.4, it is illustrated by considering a simple array of seven PM tubes. In this case, when light is produced at point a in the crystal, it is distributed among all seven PM tubes. However, PM tube 3, being closest to the point a, receives the maximum amount of light. Similarly, when light is produced at other

points in the crystal, different PM tubes will receive the maximum amount of light. Thus, by knowing which PM tube received the maximum amount of light, it is possible to know the rough location (near the PM tube receiving the maximum amount of light) of the point of light production. To locate the point of light production more accurately, the amount of light received by each PM tube, rather than the one receiving the most light, has to be taken into account (i.e., the distribution of light among different PM tubes and therefore the pulse-height distribution produced by the PM tubes is considered). The distribution of light or the pulse heights produced among different PM tubes are directly proportional to the solid angle subtended by each PM tube at the point of light production. This fact is used in the determination of the exact location of the point of light production. The PM tubes can be either a circular or hexagonal cross section. A hexagonal cross section has the advantage of close packing and therefore less dead space between the PM tubes (Fig. 11.4).

**X and Y Pulses, and Z pulse** The output of a PM tube is analog, and it was as such used by Anger to produce two position-determining analog pulses, X and Y and the energy analog pulse, Z. However, in present-day scintillation cameras, the output of each PM tube is digitized (digitization is explained later in this chapter under interfacing with a computer) and all subsequent processing is done with a microcomputer to produce, in digital form, the two position-localizing pulses, X and Y, and the energy pulse Z.

To determine the position-localizing pulses, in analog or digital version, the outputs of various PM tubes are summed with appropriate "weighting factors" (these depend on the distance of the PM tube from the center of the crystal and are not relevant here) to yield four analog signals, known as $X^+$, $X^-$, $Y^+$, and $Y^-$. In commercial scintillation cameras, the number of PM tubes varies from 19 to 96, and the summation circuits are complex and differ from one manufacturer to another.

The position-defining voltages X and Y and the energy-defining Z pulse discussed earlier are generated from the four voltages $X^+$, $X^-$, $Y^+$, and $Y^-$ as follows:

$$Z = X^+ + X^- + Y^+ + Y^- \tag{1}$$
$$X = K(X^+ - X^-) \div Z \tag{2}$$
$$Y = K(Y^+ - Y^- \div Z \tag{3}$$

where K is a constant.

The most desirable property of the X and Y pulses is their linearity with distance of the point of light production along the $x$ or $y$ axis from the center of the crystal. The farther the distance (x, y coordinate) of the source of light from the center of the crystal, the higher the pulse heights, X and Y. However, because of the geometry of light collection, these pulses are not as linear with distance as one would like them to be. Use of light pipe as shown in Figure 11.4 or nonlinear pulse shaping, are two common methods to improve the linearity of X and Y pulses. These methods do not remove the nonlinearity completely. The residual nonlinearity has to be measured and corrected online, as discussed in Chapter 12.

To display the γ-ray interaction, X and Y pulses (if digital, these have to be converted back into analog form) are used to deflect a light spot on a cathode-ray tube (CRT) or oscilloscope in direct proportion to the amplitude (magnitude) of X and Y. The final image of the distribution is formed from the oscilloscope as discussed under display. If a digital computer is used, this information (X- and Y-pulse amplitudes) is stored in memory for further processing or later display.

**Intrinsic Spatial Resolution** Even after considering the amount of light received by all PM tubes and making all the corrections, there is always a small error involved in the exact localization of the point of light production. This error is a measure of the intrinsic spatial resolution of the scintillation camera. Intrinsic spatial resolution is a complex function of the thickness of the crystal, the number of PM tubes used for position determination, the type and shape of PM tubes, and the thickness of light pipe, if used, to couple the PM tubes with the crystal. The most important of these is the thickness of the crystal. Reducing the thickness of the crystal improves the intrinsic spatial resolution, but it also decreases sensitivity of a scintillation camera as a lesser number of γ-rays interact in the crystal. Therefore, a compromise has to be made between the intrinsic spatial resolution and sensitivity of the scintillation camera. The optimum range of thickness for scintillation cameras is 3/8 to 1/2 inches for 140-keV γ-rays. Another factor that also affects intrinsic spatial resolution of the scintillation camera is the energy of γ-rays. This is due to the fact that a higher energy γ-ray produces more light in the crystal (for photoelectric events that are always selected) than a lower energy γ-ray. More light enables better localization of the point of γ-ray interaction, and better localization means better intrinsic spatial resolution. Its exact relationship is shown in the next chapter.

**Display** Gamma-rays originating in the field of view of a collimator interact in the crystal at different locations. These interactions in general occur in a random fashion. A display device should be able to portray such a randomly generated position information (X, Y) quickly (at least $10^6$ events per minute) and accurately. A CRT or an oscilloscope, of which a CRT is an integral part, is effectively used for this purpose.

**Cathode-Ray Tube** A CRT is an evacuated glass tube consisting of five basic components: an electron gun, a focusing electrode, a set of horizontal deflection plates (x direction), a set of vertical deflection plates (y direction), and a phosphor screen. These are shown schematically in Figure 11.5. The electron gun produces a stream of fast electrons. The number of electrons or the intensity of the electron stream can be varied, if desired, by intensity control I. The focusing electrode allows focusing the electron stream to a narrow circular beam (about 0.1 mm in diameter). When voltage pulses are applied to the horizontal and vertical plates, the electron beam moves in the x and y directions in direct proportion to the magnitude of the voltage pulses applied at the horizontal and vertical plates, respectively. The duration for which the electron beam stays at its new location depends on the duration of the voltage pulses applied to

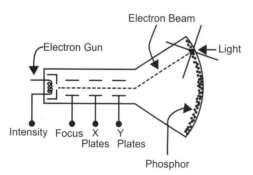

**Fig. 11.5.** Simplified schematic of a cathode-ray tube (CRT).

the horizontal and vertical plates. It is generally less than a microsecond. When there is no voltage pulse applied to the horizontal and vertical plates, the electron beam remains at the center of the phosphor screen. The location of the electron beam on the screen is made visible by the phosphor that emits light at the point where the electron beam strikes it. In this way, when voltage pulses of different magnitudes are applied in succession to the horizontal and vertical plates, the light spot on the CRT screen moves from one place to another but always at a distance that is directly proportional to the magnitude of the applied voltage pulses. The intensity of the light spot is controlled by the intensity control I.

**Display of Individual Interactions** For displaying position information from the scintillation detector, the X and Y voltage pulses are applied to the horizontal and vertical plates of a CRT. The Z signal that carries the energy information exercises a veto on the X and Y signals in such a manner that these are applied to the CRT horizontal and vertical plates only if the Z signal is within the energy range selected by the PHA. If the Z pulses are outside the range selected by PHA, then X and Y are not applied to the CRT horizontal and vertical plates. Thus, only those γ-ray interactions that deposit energy in the crystal in the range selected by PHA are displayed on the CRT screen.

In summary, the display functions as follows. A γ-ray interacts in the detector and the detector produces three signals, giving the location (X and Y pulses) of the γ-ray interaction and the energy transfer (Z pulse) by the γ-ray interaction. The Z pulse is analyzed, and if it is within the selected range, the position signals (X and Y pulses) are applied to the CRT plates, which deflect the light spot from the center of the screen to a distance proportional to the X and Y voltages. When a new γ-ray interacts in the crystal, a new set of X, Y, and Z signals is produced that then deflects the light spot to a new location given by these signals. In this way, as more and more γ-rays interact in the crystal, the light spot on the CRT screen keeps moving from one place to another in correspondence with the location of γ-ray interaction

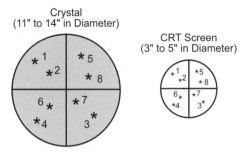

**Fig. 11.6.** Direct correspondence of the location of γ-ray interaction in scintillation detector with the location of light spot on CRT screen.

in the crystal up to 500,000 times or more in a typical image (Fig. 11.6). Because the usual size of CRTs range from 3 to 5 inches in diameter, the image on the CRT screen is displayed in a smaller size than the actual size of the organ or part of the body imaged.

**Integration on a Film** A flying light spot on the screen of a CRT does not constitute an image. This image is formed by point-by-point integration of this information on a photographic film.

*Film Characteristics* On a film, darker areas represent more radioactivity, whereas lighter areas represent less activity. Film darkening is quantitatively measured by a parameter known as optical density or, simply, density. It is defined as the logarithm (base 10) of the ratio of the intensity of incident light on the film to the intensity of light transmitted by the film. According to this

definition, an area of the film with a density of 2 will transmit only 1% light and will therefore appear almost black to the naked eye. A density of 0 represents 100% transmission; therefore, an area with density of zero will appear white. Densities between 0 and 2 will appear as shades of gray. The relationship of density to exposure for a typical x-ray film is shown in Figure 11.7. This curve is known as the H-D curve of the film. The average slope between points A and B determines the contrast of a film, and the relative log exposure between the points A and B (horizontal distance) determines the latitude of a film. A high-contrast film displays smaller exposure variations than a low-contrast film, but a high-contrast film has smaller latitude. Therefore, the range of exposures that can be displayed on a high-contrast film is smaller (Fig. 11.7).

*Film Exposure* It can be seen from the H-D curve that the density is dependent on the exposure or the count rate only in the region that lies between points A and B marked on the curves. The trick in photo display is to correspond this region to the range of the count rates that is of most interest. Normally, count rates in an organ may vary from zero to a maximum $R_{max}$ for effective display, $R_{max}$ (also known as the "hot spot") should correspond to point B and zero count rate to point A on the H-D curve. The $R_{max}$ for individual patients differs because of variations in the administered radiopharmaceutical dose, localization and distribution in the organ, and the size and shape of the organ. Some

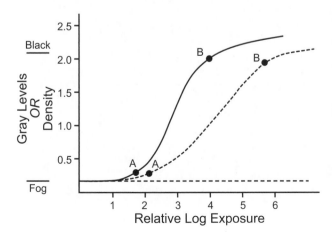

**Fig. 11.7.** Typical H-D curves of x-ray films used to display information. For the proper display of count rate information, the maximum count rate (hot spot) should correspond to point B and the minimum count rate to point A. Two types of films are shown: solid curve, film with high contrast and small latitude; broken curve, film with low contrast and large latitude.

variations are taken care of when one uses fixed number of counts rather than fixed amount of time for exposure. The proper exposure of the film, which is controlled by the intensity I of the CRT, is inversely related to the number of counts. The more counts in an image, the lower setting of I needed and vice versa. Generally, a table is made for the number of counts in an image and I setting needed for proper exposure for those counts.

In fast dynamic studies where the exposure is for a fixed time, I settings are only a guess. This quite often produces bad results. The only solution to this problem is to interface the scintillation camera with a computer, store images, and make exposures after the number of counts in each image has been determined.

*Multiformat Recording* A multiformat recording system is commonly used in nuclear medicine. In this system, multiple images are recorded on a single sheet of x-ray film, usually 8 × 10 or 11 × 14 inches in size. The number of images

and therefore the size of the image that can be recorded on a single sheet can be varied easily with the help of controls provided for such purposes. Thus, a single sheet may contain from one to as many as 64 images. The main advantage of this device is that all views from one patient, including dynamic studies, can be recorded on a single sheet of film, thus consolidating most of the information in one place. A typical study, a bone scan using this format, is shown in Figure 11.8.

# Imaging with a Scintillation Camera

Generally, the following steps are taken to obtain an image with a scintillation camera:

1. Selection of the study to be performed (e.g., brain, liver, etc.);
2. Selection of the radiopharmaceutical and the dose of radiopharmaceutical. A radiopharmaceutical is generally administered

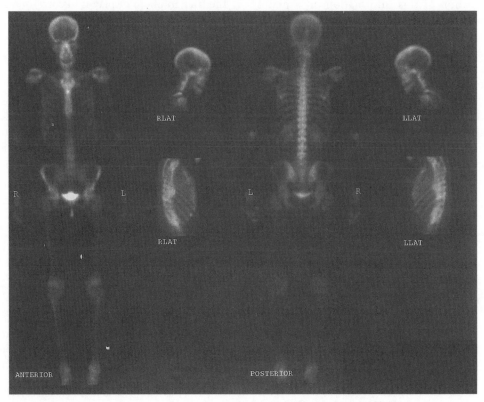

**Fig. 11.8.** Anterior view of a bone scan recorded on a multi-format recording device.

to patients away from the scintillation camera, but sometimes, particularly when fast dynamic studies are to be performed, it may have to be administered with the patient in the appropriate position under the camera (step 7);

3. Selection of the PHA parameters (peak energy and % window corresponding to the γ-ray emitted by the radionuclide to be used);

4. Selection of an appropriate collimator (with respect to energy and spatial resolution);

5. Selection of the mode: accumulation of a certain number of counts or exposure for fixed amount of time;

6. Selection of the appropriate intensity of the CRT for the number of counts expected or to be acquired in the image;

7. Positioning of the patient under the camera and, if the radiopharmaceutical has not been administered, administration of the radiopharmaceutical;

8. Start and finish of the exposure;

9. Development of the film. If more than one view is to be displayed on the same film, then the development of the film takes place at the end of the study.

## Interfacing with a Computer or All-Digital Camera

Digital computers have acquired an important role in nuclear medicine. The main advantage of a computer is the speed and ease with which it can acquire, analyze, store, and display large amounts of complex data. Presently, scintillation cameras either completely integrated with a digital computer (all-digital cameras) or interfaced with a dedicated digital computer are commercially available. Besides SPECT and heart studies, which cannot be performed without a digital computer, many other applications of computers are now an integral part of standard nuclear medicine procedures (e.g., renogram).

**Digitization in General** What does digitization mean? A digital computer handles numbers or digits only and these too in binary (or powers of 2) form only (base 2 instead of base 10).

Therefore, any instrument from which data are to be acquired and analyzed by a digital computer in an automatic fashion has to present the data to the computer in binary (or similar) digital form. Unfortunately, most instruments produce signals or data in an analog form. Analog signals are continuously varying and do not produce data in numbers. For example, the needle of a car speedometer moves in a continuous fashion from one end of the dial to the other as the speed of the car is increased from zero to a certain maximum. The higher the speed of the car, the farther the needle moves. The digital (in numbers) information about the car's speed is derived from a scale printed on the dial. The scale printed on the dial is, in a way, manual digitization of an analog (continuous movement of the needle) signal. Now, if the speedometer has to be coupled to a digital computer to record the speed of the car automatically, some electronic device will have to be used that will digitize the information provided by the speedometer (movement of the needle). Such a device, which automatically changes analog signals into digital (binary) signals, is known as an analog-to-digital converter, or simply an ADC.

Two important parameters of an ADC, accuracy and speed, are relevant for our purpose. Accuracy of ADC tells how close the numeric data is to the analog signal. Let us consider the example of the speedometer again and assume this time for simplicity that the minimum speed of the car is zero and the maximum speed 100 miles/h. Now to read any speed in between these two extremes, the scale on the dial has to be divided into equal divisions. If there are only 10 divisions, then we will be able to measure the speed of a car accurately only in steps of 10 miles/h. When the scale is divided into 100 equal parts, the speed could be read in steps of 1 mile/h. One thousand equal divisions will provide an accuracy of 0.1 mile/h and so on. The more divisions there are on the scale (in a given range), the better the accuracy. Similarly, in an ADC, a given range of signals is broken into divisions; the more divisions, the better its accuracy. The unit of divisions in the case of an ADC is a bit. A one-bit ($2^1$) ADC divides a given range only into two equal parts, a two-bit ($2^2 = 4$) ADC divides it into four equal parts, a three-bit ADC ($2^3 = 8$) into eight equal parts,

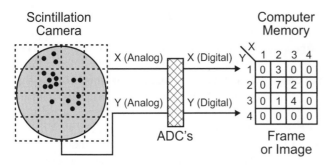

**Fig. 11.9.** Digitization of an image. Analog image produced by a scintillation camera is divided into a number (4000 or 16,000) of square cells or pixels. Counts from each pixel are stored in a separate location in a computer. Here, the X, Y ranges have been divided into four divisions. The resultant 4 × 4 matrix has 16 pixels.

and so on. The more bits an ADC has, the better its accuracy. However, it takes more time to digitize a signal as the number of bits in an ADC increases. This brings us to the second parameter of an ADC, speed. The faster an ADC is, the higher the rate of data it can digitize without any loss of information. Thus, speed and accuracy are inversely related. More accuracy means less speed and more speed means less accuracy.

### Digitization in the Scintillation Camera

In a scintillation camera, unless it is an all-digital scintillation camera, in which case the digitization has already been done at the PM tube, the X, Y, and Z pulses are analog and have to be digitized before being recorded by a digital computer. The ADCs used for digitizing X and Y signals of a scintillation camera are 7 to 9 bits, which means that the X and Y ranges are equally divided into $2^7 = 128$, $2^8 = 256$, or $2^9 = 512$ equal divisions, respectively. In a scintillation camera, the maximum range of X or Y signals will equal the diameter d of the crystal. Therefore, each division of an ADC will correspond to either d/128 or d/256 cm of distance, depending whether the ADC is 7 or 8 bit. For an 11-inch (28 cm) diameter crystal and 7-bit ADC or for an LFOV (20-inch-diameter) crystal and 8-bit ADC, this value equals 0.2 cm. Because the intrinsic spatial resolution of a scintillation camera presently is in this range, greater accuracy is not needed. In terms of the speed of the ADC, it should be able to handle about 100,000 signals per second because higher count rates are seldom encountered in nuclear medicine.

The digitization of X and Y signals into 64, 128, or 256 divisions yields a 64 × 64, 128 × 128, or 256 × 256 matrix. Thus, the analog image (which is a two-dimensional or areal distribution) is divided into 64 × 64 = 4096, 128 × 128 = 16,384, or 256 × 256 = 65,536 equal small areas known as pixels. A specific area on the crystal corresponds to a specific pixel, and each pixel is assigned a specific location in the computer memory. Therefore, when a γ-ray interacts in the crystal, its pixel location is determined by the ADCs and a count is stored in the corresponding location in the computer. As more and more γ-rays interact, they are stored in the appropriate locations, and finally a digitized image is formed. This is graphically illustrated in Figure 11.9 using a 4 × 4 matrix instead of 64 × 64, 128 × 128, or 256 × 256, which are used in practice.

## Some Applications of Computers

The various areas where the computer has helped tremendously in the practice of nuclear medicine are as follows.

**Automatic Acquisition of Images** In the case of static imaging, a digital computer is not as helpful as in the case of fast dynamic studies where images may have to be acquired every 0.5 second for a period of 100 seconds or more. In dynamic studies, a digital ww is the only practical way to acquire such a large amount of data accurately and efficiently. Another type of acquisition, known as multiple-gated acquisition (MUGA), is also made practical by computer acquisition of data. MUGA is desired where the organ to be imaged moves in a periodic fashion (e.g., heart) (Fig. 11.10). To acquire images in various phases of a heart beat (such as systole or diastole), the beat is divided into a number of time segments,

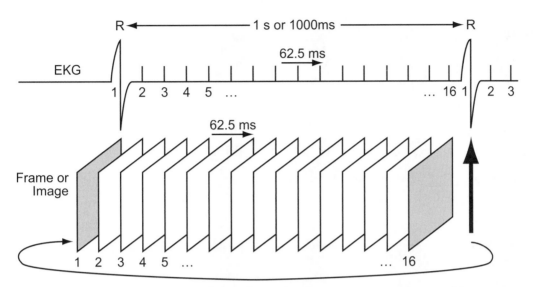

**Fig. 11.10.** Schematic representation of a heart beat and its division into time segments, and the corresponding frames or images of computer memory for heart studies in a multiple-gated acquisition (MUGA).

usually 16. Each time segment corresponds to a particular phase of the heartbeat. Onset of the first-time segment is triggered by the R wave of an electrocardiogram monitor attached to the patient, and data during this segment is collected in a designated area of the computer memory, called frame 1. At the end of this time segment, data acquisition for the second time segment takes place in a different location of the computer memory, called frame 2. Thus, data recorded by the scintillation camera during each time segment (62.5 ms in this example) are stored by computer in different parts of its memory, called frames or images (16 in this case). Each time segment corresponds to a particular frame or image. When the next beat starts, as indicated by the second R wave, the data acquisition reverts back into frame 1 for the first-time segment and frame 2 for the second time segment and so on. This process continues for a large number of beats, quite often up to 1000 or more. The reason for summing the data for each time segment of a heart beat for so many heart beats has to do with the number of counts in the image of each time segment (also called "gate").

Because a heart be at is generally less than 1 second in duration, if one divides it into 16 time segments, each time segment is only 30 to 70 ms

(depending on the actual time of the beat). The number of counts detected by the scintillation camera during a 30- to 70-ms time interval, even for a 20-mCi $^{99m}$Tc dosage to the patient, is quite small. Therefore, by adding counts from a large number of beats for each time segment, images with sufficient numbers of counts (200,000–1,000,000) for each time segment of heart cycle (phase) can be obtained. Images thus obtained from one patient are shown in Figure 11.11.

**Display of Images** In scintillation camera imaging, even with a multi-imager, attaining the proper intensity setting of the oscilloscope light spot in every case is difficult. With computer-acquired digital images, there is no such problem. Images can be stored temporarily or permanently on a disc or magnetic tape and displayed over and over again with any desired intensity level (Fig. 11.12). The dynamic images can be displayed in a movie-like fashion so that the flow of a bolus of radioactivity can be followed. MUGA images of the heart (Fig. 11.11) can be displayed in a cine mode, which shows the motion of the heart during a heart beat. Obviously, this cannot be illustrated here.

**Analysis of the Images** The digitized images can be manipulated individually or added,

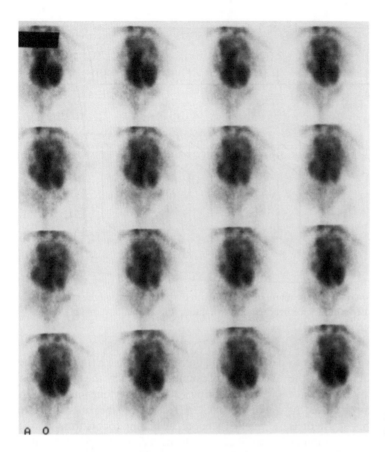

**Fig. 11.11.** Sixteen images in different phases of heartbeat acquired with MUGA.

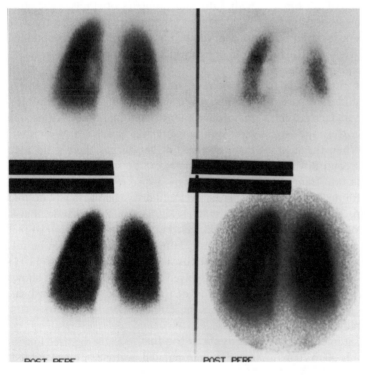

**Fig. 11.12.** Same lung study shown with four different display intensities. Optimum intensity setting is important for accurate diagnosis.

subtracted, multiplied, or divided by one another by the computer to generate another image, which may provide better appreciation of certain clinically important parameters. Also, counts can be determined and compared from areas of interest in the same images or in images taken at different times. An example is the heart study of Figure 11.11. By drawing regions of interest for the left ventricle in each of the 16 frames, one obtains the left ventricle volume in each phase of the heart, and it can be represented as a function of time. From the two phases at diastole and systole, one computes the ejection fraction of the heart. This is shown in Figure 11.13. Another example of the use of the digital computer in a dynamic study in the brain is depicted in Figure 11.14.

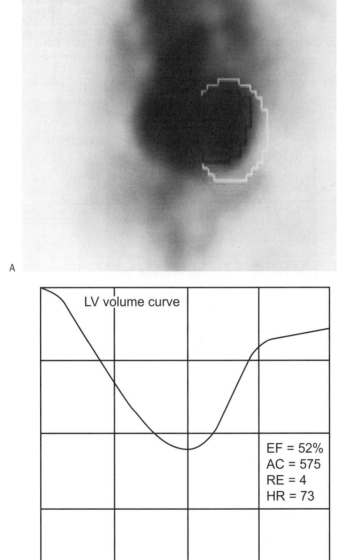

A

LV volume curve

EF = 52%
AC = 575
RE = 4
HR = 73

B

**Fig. 11.13.** (A) Regions of interest (ROI) in systole and distole and (B) left ventricle volume as a function of time during one heart beat.

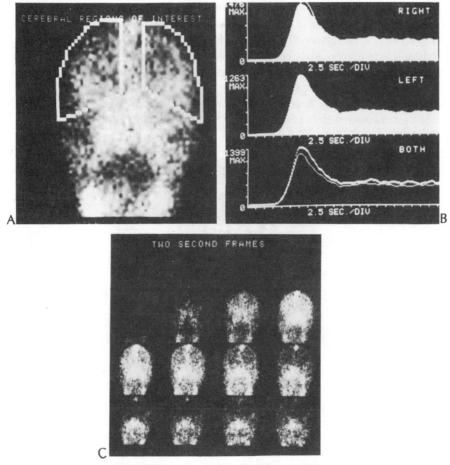

**Fig. 11.14.** Use of a computer to acquire, analyze, and display nuclear medicine images. Sequential brain images of 1-second duration were acquired for 50 seconds. From these data, a composite image consisting of all fifty 1-second images was formed (A). The areas of interest (left and right hemisphere) were chosen. The computer then formed dynamic curves showing time changes in the two regions of interest (B). Also shown (C) are the first sixteen 2-second images formed by adding two 1-second images successively.

## Key Points

1. A scintillation camera can image radionuclidic distributions at a fast rate (20/s). It is available with single, dual, and triple heads and in various crystal sizes.

2. It consists of four operational components, a collimator, a NaI(Tl) crystal, a large number of PM tubes and associated electronics to determine the location of γ-ray interaction in the crystal, and a display system consisting of an oscilloscope and a photographic camera.

3. Four types of collimators—parallel hole, converging, diverging, and pinhole—have been used. A parallel-hole collimator is the optimum collimator for most studies performed in nuclear medicine.

4. The size of the crystal depends on the use of the scintillation camera. For cardiac studies only, small fields of view (10 inch diameter) scintillation cameras are sufficient, but for the whole body studies, LFOV scintillation cameras are needed. The thickness of the

crystal is normally 0.5 inch but slightly less for a dedicated cardiac unit.

5. Thickness of the crystal is inversely related to the intrinsic spatial resolution of the scintillation camera.

6. Output of the PM tubes is combined in a weighted manner to generate three signals: X, Y, and Z. Of these, the two position signals X and Y, are proportional to the x and y distance of the point of $\gamma$-ray interaction in the crystal from the center of the crystal along x and y directions. The Z signal at the photo peak is proportional to the energy of the $\gamma$-ray.

7. The position signals, X and Y, deflect a light spot proportional to the distance from the center of the point of interaction in the crystal on an oscilloscope from where the image is obtained with a camera.

8. Newer scintillation cameras are all digital and have a computer as an integral part. Analog scintillation cameras can be easily interfaced with a computer.

9. A computer allows an automated acquisition, different gray-scale displays, and quantification and processing of images.

## Questions

1. The crystal in a scintillation camera has an optimum thickness. What are the two properties that determine the optimum thickness?

2. How is the geometric efficiency increased in the case of a scintillation camera?

3. If, in the future, a new scintillator material is discovered that produces four times the amount of light produced by the NaI(Tl) crystal for a 140-keV $\gamma$-ray, what factor of the scintillation camera can be affected and how?

4. Name the collimator for which each of the following statements is true. (a) The field of view remains constant. (b) It can only magnify the object. (c) Its field of view increases with distance and it minifies the object. (d) It inverts the object.

5. What is the advantage of multiple PHAs in a scintillation camera?

6. What is the advantage of hexagonal PM tube over circular PM tubes?

7. For optimum exposure of the film, how should the intensity of the light spot of the oscilloscope be changed if the number of counts in the image is increased?

8. An ADC is the most important link between a scintillation camera and a digital computer. If the spatial resolution of the scintillator camera improves by a factor of 10, what effect will it have on the desired accuracy and speed of the ADC?

9. Calculate the area of a pixel if the field of view FOV is 20 cm and the matrix size is 64 × 64.

# Operational Characteristics and Quality Control of a Scintillation Camera

A number of parameters of an imaging device play a major role in the delineation of a radioactive distribution. Of these, two, spatial resolution and sensitivity, are important. For scintillation cameras, two other operational characteristics, uniformity and high count-rate performance, are also considered. These and some routine quality control procedures constitute the subject matter of this chapter.

## Quantitative Parameters for Measuring Spatial Resolution

Spatial resolution is defined as the ability of an imager to reproduce the details of radionuclidic distribution. The finer the details an imaging device reproduces, the better spatial resolution it has. How is spatial resolution measured quantitatively? Two parameters—full-width at half-maximum (*FWHM*) of a point-spread function and modulation transfer function (*MTF*)—are used to measure spatial resolution of an imaging device. Sometimes "bar phantoms" are used as a semiquantitative measure of spatial resolution. These are discussed later in this chapter (p. 139).

**Point-Spread Function and FWHM** If we image a single-point source and plot the intensity profile across its center, a bell-shaped curve similar to that shown in Figure 12.1 results. This curve is known as the point-spread function of an imager. The *FWHM* of this curve can be used to measure spatial resolution quantitatively. The unit of resolution is the same as the unit of length,

centimeter or millimeter, generally. A narrower *FWHM* implies a better spatial resolution of the imaging device. Thus, an imaging device with 2 mm *FWHM* is a better imaging device than one with 5 mm *FWHM*. Measurement of *FWHM* is quite involved and requires a computer interfacing with a scintillation camera.

*FWHM* is a useful parameter for expressing the relationship of spatial resolution to various parameters of an imaging device such as size, shape, and length of the holes of a collimator of a scintillation camera. Its main drawback is that it does not measure spatial resolution under

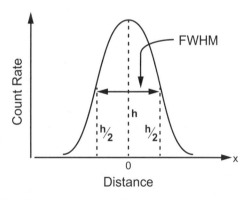

**Fig. 12.1.** Intensity profile through the center of a point-source image taken with a scintillation camera. The width or narrowness of such a profile is a good measure of spatial resolution. The narrower the curve, the better is the spatial resolution of the imager. The full width of this curve at the two points for which the response has decreased to one-half of the maximum *FWHM* is customarily used as a quantitative parameter for measuring the spatial resolution of an imaging device.

varying object contrast conditions. As a result, it is possible to design two imaging devices that have equal spatial resolutions according to this definition, although in practice one performs better than the other.

**Modulation Transfer Function** *MTF* gives the most complete characterization of the spatial resolution of an imaging device, provided that the response of the imaging device is linear. Although the latter condition is not strictly met for imaging devices, the *MTF* is still useful in their evaluation. Its main drawback is the inability to express its relationships with the various parameters of an imaging device in simple and understandable terms.

To understand this parameter fully, knowledge of Fourier analysis is essential. However, to comprehend it conceptually, an analogy with sound is helpful. Any sound—the ding-dong of a bell or the pretty voice of a singer—is made up of a number of sound waves of different frequencies. Once the component frequencies and their strengths (amplitudes) are known for a given sound, it can then be resynthesized (in a laboratory) by proper superimposition of these frequencies. In a similar fashion, any spatial distribution (object) can be broken down into a number of spatial frequencies, and the original distribution (object) can then be resynthesized by the proper superimposition of these spatial frequencies.

How does this breaking up of a spatial distribution into component spatial frequencies aid in evaluating the imaging device? Not per se, but if we measure the degradation produced by an imaging device as a function of various spatial frequencies, the resulting function will provide the information needed to characterize the imaging system completely. The degradation M produced for a spatial frequency $v$ by an imaging device is measured as the ratio of the contrast (amplitude

of the wave) in the image frequency to the contrast in the object frequency (Fig. 12.2).

Measurement of M as a function of $v$, then, produces the *MTF* of the imaging device. When the value of M for a particular spatial frequency is 1, this indicates no degradation of contrast for that frequency. If M equals 0, the imaging device is unable to reproduce this particular spatial frequency; therefore, a value of 0 represents the maximum degradation. Values of M between 1 and 0 represent the extent of degradation for a given frequency. An ideal imager (which produces an exact image of an object) will have a value of M = 1 for all spatial frequencies.

Use of the *MTF* to compare the spatial resolution of two different imaging devices can be appreciated easily by examining Figure 12.3, which depicts the *MTF* for three imaging devices, A, B, and C, respectively. Here, the *MTF* of the imaging device A is higher for all spatial frequencies than the *MTF* of the imaging devices B and C; therefore, the imaging device A possesses the best spatial resolution of the three imaging devices. The choice between B and C is difficult. At low spatial frequencies, B is superior to C, whereas at higher frequencies C is superior to B. The selection of the particular imaging device in this case will depend on the type of objects to be imaged. If an object dominates in high frequencies, device C will be a better choice. If an object contains primarily low frequencies, then device B will be more advantageous to use. The *MTF* of an imaging device is difficult to measure directly. Instead, it is calculated from the line-spread function (LSF) (discussed below) of an imager, which can be easily measured.

**Resolution of an Imaging Chain** Quite often an imaging device can be broken into components, with each component contributing to the final or system resolution of the imaging

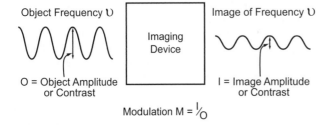

Object Frequency $v$

O = Object Amplitude or Contrast

Imaging Device

Image of Frequency $v$

I = Image Amplitude or Contrast

Modulation M = $I/O$

**Fig. 12.2.** Modulation transfer function. When a spatial frequency v of an object is imaged, its amplitude may change. The ratio of the amplitude in the image of a spatial frequency to that in the object is known as modulation M. Measurement of M as a function of $v$ yields the *MTF* of an imaging device.

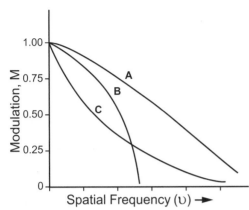

**Fig. 12.3.** *MTF* of three imaging devices. Modulation M for imaging device A is higher than that of B and C at all spatial frequencies. Therefore, it possesses the best spatial resolution of the three. The choice between B and C is difficult because at low spatial frequencies, B is superior to C, whereas at high spatial frequencies, C is superior to B.

device; for example, in the case of a scintillation camera, the final or system resolution is derived from two components, the collimator and the x, y localization mechanism. How does one combine these component resolutions to give the system resolution? If the resolution is expressed using *FWHM* and $R_1$, $R_2$,... are the component resolutions, respectively, then the system resolution $R_S$, is given as follows:

$$R_s = \sqrt{R_1^2 + R_2^2 + \cdots} \quad (1)$$

For *MTF* representation of resolution, the system $MTF_s$ is given by the following expression:

$$MTF_S = MTF_1 \cdot MTF_2 \cdot \ldots \quad (2)$$

## Quantitative Parameters for Measuring Sensitivity

In addition to spatial resolution, the other important parameter of an imaging device is sensitivity. Sensitivity can be defined as the ability of an imaging device to use efficiently all the photons available from an object within a given unit of time. Three parameters—point sensitivity, line sensitivity, and plane sensitivity—have been used to measure the sensitivity of an imaging device. Each has relative advantages and disadvantages.

**Point Sensitivity $S_p$** This parameter is defined as the fraction of $\gamma$-rays detected per unit of time for a point source of radioactivity. In a scintillation camera, $S_p$ is more or less constant in the field of view of the collimator.

**Line Sensitivity $S_L$** This parameter is defined as the fraction of grays detected per unit of time per unit of length of a very long line source of uniform radioactivity. The count profile of a line source, as determined by an imaging device, through a direction perpendicular to the line source is known as the *LSF* (Fig. 12.4). *LSF(x)* is primarily used in the calculation of the MTF of an imager as follows:

$$MTF(\nu) = \frac{\int_{-\infty}^{\infty} LSF(x) \cdot \cos(2\pi\nu x) \cdot dx}{\int_{-\infty}^{\infty} LSF(x) \cdot dx} \quad (3)$$

**Plane Sensitivity $S_A$** Plane sensitivity is defined as the fraction of $\gamma$-rays detected per unit of time per unit of area of a large plane source of uniform radioactivity. This parameter is commonly used to compare the sensitivities of two imaging devices. The principal advantage of $S_A$ is the ease with which it can be measured. Plane sensitivity does not vary with the distance of the plane source from the collimator as long as the area of the plane source is larger than the field of view of the collimator at that distance.

## Factors Affecting Spatial Resolution and Sensitivity of an Imager

The spatial resolution and sensitivity of an imaging device depend on a number of variables described below. Theoretically, the exact relationships of these variables to spatial

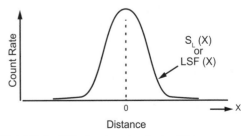

**Fig. 12.4.** *LSF* of an imaging device. Using a gamma camera, *LSF* can be directly obtained from the image of a line source, provided it is interfaced with a computer system.

resolution and sensitivity are difficult to obtain in a generalized case. However, by making certain assumptions, these relationships can be expressed in simplified mathematical form. Using these formulas, an approximation of the dependence of spatial resolution and sensitivity on a given variable can be easily deduced. In the following discussion, we use these simpler formulas. In addition, we use $R(FWHM)$ and $S_A$ as a measure of the spatial resolution and sensitivity, respectively, of an imaging device, assuming that there is no septal penetration by $\gamma$-rays in the collimator of the scanner and there is no scattering of grays in the radionuclide source.

### Scintillation Camera

The spatial resolution, $R_S$, of a scintillation camera comprises $R_1$ and $R_2$, where $R_1$ is the intrinsic spatial resolution of a scintillation camera and $R_2$ is the spatial resolution of the collimator used with the scintillation camera. Spatial resolution $R_S$ is approximately related to $R_1$ and $R_2$ as by equation (1).

The intrinsic spatial resolution $R_1$, which is a measure of the uncertainty in the localization of the point where light is produced in the crystal, is degraded with an increase in the thickness of the NaI(Tl) crystal and is improved with an increase in $\gamma$-ray energy. The improvement in the intrinsic spatial resolution of a camera with the $\gamma$-ray energy is shown in Figure 12.5. Spatial resolution $R_2$ depends on various collimator parameters such as collimator length L and diameter of holes d. We limit our discussion here to a parallel-hole collimator (Fig. 12.6), although similar considerations apply for a converging or diverging collimator. $R_2$ in this case depends on the hole-diameter d, length of the collimator L, thickness of the crystal C, and the distance F of the source from the collimator face. $R_2$ is given by the following expression:

$$R_2 \cong \frac{d(L+F+C)}{L} \qquad (4)$$

When the source is at a distance F from the collimator, to improve $R_2$, we have to either reduce d and/or C or increase L.

The sensitivity $S_A$ depends on d, L, D (crystal diameter), $\in_p$ (intrinsic efficiency), and s (septa thickness), as follows:

$$S_A \cong \frac{\pi d^4}{64L^2} \cdot \frac{3D^2}{4(d+s)^2} \cdot \in_p \qquad (5)$$

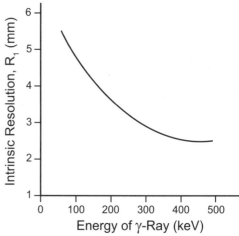

**Fig. 12.5.** Dependence of intrinsic spatial resolution $R_1$ of an Anger camera on $\gamma$-ray energy.

It can be seen from equation (5) that $S_A$ can be increased by either increasing d or decreasing L, the opposite of that required to improve the spatial resolution $R_2$ (for an optimum collimator, $S_A \propto R_2^2$. Therefore, a twofold improvement in $R_2$ (keep in mind that improvement in resolution means that $R_2$ has to decrease in

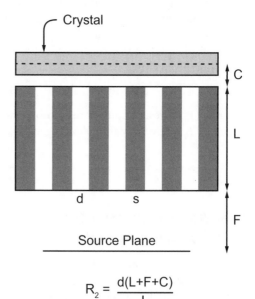

**Fig. 12.6.** Dependence of spatial resolution $R_2$ of a parallel-hole collimator on the length L of the collimator and the diameter d of the holes. Reducing d or increasing L improves $R_2$. Sensitivity of such a collimator also varies as the inverse square of the spatial resolution.

value), either by decreasing d or by increasing L, necessitates a fourfold sacrifice in $S_A$. Sensitivity of a parallel-hole collimator can be increased by enlarging the diameter D of the crystal ($S_A \propto D^2$). Accordingly, a 13-inch-diameter crystal scintillation camera has sensitivity equal to $13^2/11^2$, or 1.4 times that of an 11-inch-diameter crystal scintillation camera. This gain in sensitivity of a large crystal scintillation camera is of value only in cases where the organs to be imaged are of the same size as the crystal. Sensitivity can also be increased by improving $\epsilon_p$ by making the crystal thicker, particularly for higher energy $\gamma$-rays. Of course, that will degrade the intrinsic resolution.

**Loss of Spatial Resolution Resulting from Septal Penetration** In the previous discussion, we assumed that no $\gamma$-ray could reach the radiation detector by penetrating the septa of the collimator. Such an assumption is justifiable only in the case of collimators designed for use with low-energy $\gamma$-rays (<150 keV). In collimators designed for use with high-energy $\gamma$-rays, some septal penetration always occurs because a further reduction of septal penetration, by increasing septal thickness, will produce an unacceptable loss in the sensitivity of the collimator.

The effect of septal penetration on the spatial resolution of a collimator is to degrade it. Septal penetration, in effect, may be construed as an effective increase in the diameter d of the collimator holes. The extent of the degradation of spatial resolution depends on the degree of septal penetration. Higher penetration leads to greater degradation of spatial resolution.

**Variation in Spatial Resolution with Depth** Spatial resolution of a scintillation camera varies with the depth or distance from the face of the collimator. For the scintillation camera, the best spatial resolution is achieved at the face of the collimator. The farther away the source is from the face of the collimator, the poorer the spatial resolution. The dependence of spatial resolution on depth of a typical parallel-hole collimator of a scintillation camera is shown in Figure 12.7, where both R and *MTF* were used as the index of spatial resolution.

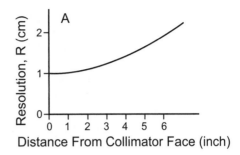

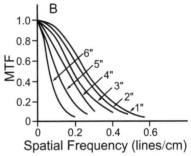

**Fig. 12.7.** Variation of the spatial resolution of a scintillation camera with depth. The best spatial resolution is obtained closest to the collimator. In (A), R has been used as a measure of spatial resolution; in (B), *MTF* has been used for this purpose. Both, however, show similar behavior in variation of spatial resolution with depth. The number on the *MTF* curves in **B** gives the distance from the collimator face.

# Uniformity and High Count-Rate Performance of a Scintillation Camera

Besides spatial resolution and sensitivity, two other characteristics of a scintillation camera, uniformity and high count-rate performance, are also important for the optimal operation of a scintillation camera.

**Uniformity** Uniformity is the ability of a scintillation camera to reproduce a uniform radioactive distribution (mind you, in a uniform source, there are no details or variations of count rate; therefore, spatial resolution has little to do with the uniformity response of a scintillation camera). In practice, all scintillation cameras produce nonuniform or inhomogeneous images of a uniform source to varying extent. These inhomogeneities or the count-rate variations from one area to another in the image of a uniform source may be in amounts up to ±10%.

In the uncorrected image, these areas show as increased ("hot") or decreased ("cold") spots of radioactivity as depicted in Figure 12.8, taken from an old scintillation camera.

Although some inhomogeneity in the image of a uniform source is caused by slight variations in the thickness of the NaI(Tl) crystal and in the transmission of the $\gamma$-rays by the collimator, the dominant cause of nonuniform response is electronic in nature. It is related to differences in response of photomultiplier PM tubes and to the difference in transmission of light produced at different places in the crystal. These differences cause the mis-positioning of some counts. A good demonstration of mis-positioning of counts occurs in scintillation cameras occasionally when a straight-line radioactive source is imaged. The image of a linear radioactive source appears as an arc, which may be curved in or out from the center of the scintillation camera (pin cushion or barrel distortion in optical analogy). Such distortions of linear sources are visible only when the scintillation camera is not properly "tuned." A certain amount of nonlinearity always persists even when it is not discernible on visual inspection of the image and the camera is properly tuned. These small nonlinearities result in a visible nonhomogeneous response of the scintillation camera to a uniform source. To keep the nonhomogeneities to a minimum, scintillation cameras must be properly tuned. Tuning involves the readjustment of individual PM tube gains so as to overcome the individual differences in various PM tube responses. Because the PM tube gain may drift as a result of fluctuations in the line voltage and the ambient conditions, it is essential that the uniformity of response is checked routinely.

Another aspect of the nonuniform response of a scintillation camera is known as edge packing. This is also a manifestation of mis-positioning of the counts. It appears as a bright ring around the edge of an image (Fig. 12.8) and is caused by internal reflection of the light at the edge of the crystal and the fact that the PM tubes are present on one side only. As a result, counts coming from near the edges are bunched together. The region of edge packing is never used in clinical studies; it is always masked by a lead ring around the collimator. Thus, the useful field of view is always smaller than the crystal size.

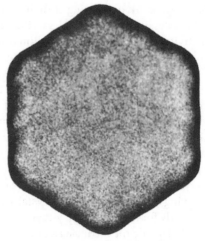

**Fig. 12.8.** Uncorrected "flood" showing the nonuniform response of an old scintillation camera with a hexagonal crystal. The bright outer ring in the image is due to edge packing. In new cameras, this ring is no longer visible.

In modern scintillation cameras, the nonuniformity of response has improved considerably by addressing its causes—local variations in the amount of light transmitted to a PM tube and the nonlinear response of the X, Y pulses due to slightly different PM gains. These nonlinearities are very carefully measured, and from these measurements, a correction matrix formed. This correction matrix then appropriately repositions on line all the subsequent counts detected by the camera using a microprocessor. As a result of these corrections, the uniformity of the scintillation camera has improved tremendously and is 2% or better in the useful field of view (Fig. 12.9). Moreover, the electronic components and the PM tubes used in these cameras are more stable than those used in older cameras. Automatic tuning circuits further enhance the stability. Therefore, the new scintillation cameras generally do not require tuning as often; a monthly or even quarterly interval is adequate for routine maintenance. However, the measurements of the correction matrix are too complicated to be done by in-house personnel; therefore, if a camera detunes significantly from its prescribed limits, a service call is necessary. The nonuniform transmission of $\gamma$-rays by the collimator is tested separately. If it is found unacceptable,

**Fig. 12.9.** Corrected "flood" showing more uniform response of a new scintillation camera with a circular-shaped crystal.

the collimator is replaced. Once a satisfactory collimator is found, occasional physical inspection for the presence of dents or unusual marks ensures the integrity of the collimator.

**High Count-Rate Performance** Because a gamma camera uses a NaI(Tl) crystal to detect γ-rays and to determine the location of γ-ray interaction in the crystal, at high count rates, besides loss of counts due to the finite dead time, mis-positioning of counts also takes place. At high count rates, the probability of two γ-rays simultaneously interacting in the crystal (within the dead time of the detector) increases sharply. If one or both γ-rays interact through the photoelectric effect, the total light produced will be more than the light produced if only one γ-ray interacted that way. Therefore, if the pulse-height analyzer PHA is set on the photo-peak, both of these γ rays, mimicking as one but with higher energy, will be rejected by the PHA. On the other hand, if both γ-rays interact through the Compton scattering and each interaction produces enough light so that the sum of the two is equal to the light produced by the photoelectric interaction of one gray, the two γ-rays, mimicking as one but with correct energy, will be accepted by PHA. However, the location of the interaction will be the mean of the locations of the interactions of the two γ-rays in the displayed image. Thus, a misposition of the count occurs.

The dead time of a scintillation camera is made up of paralyzable and nonparalyzable components. Under ideal conditions, it is between 1 and 2 $\mu$s. However, the dead time of a scintillation camera is a complex function of window width used, scattering material around the source, multiple γ-ray emissions by the radionuclide used, and so on. Therefore, it is essential to determine the dead time of a scintillation camera under conditions typically used in clinical situations. In these circumstances, dead time may be as much as 10 to 15 $\mu$s. Count-rate performance of a typical scintillation camera is shown in Figure 12.10.

# Quality Control of Imaging Devices

Correct interpretation of an image depends on the accuracy of the data in the image. Therefore, it is of utmost importance that nuclear imaging devices operate optimally and reliably. Because these instruments use a variety of electronic components whose response may be affected by changes in line voltage or ambient conditions, the best way to ensure accuracy and reliability of these instruments is through a continuing program of quality control. The quality control procedures are intended to monitor day-to-day variations in some performing characteristics to

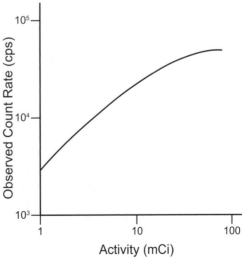

**Fig. 12.10.** Count-rate response of a typical scintillation camera.

be alerted, in time, to the malfunction or unacceptable behavior of these instruments. The gross artifacts, such as one or more PM tube malfunction, cracks in the crystal, dent or other mechanical damage in the collimator or radioactive contamination of the detector head can be easily spotted. However, these are semiquantitative procedures and therefore do not measure the operating characteristics of an imaging device accurately or completely. The procedures given in the following sections are brief and therefore illustrate only the important aspects of such an endeavor.

**Scintillation Camera**  The three most common parameters routinely tested to ensure maximal performance of a scintillation camera are peaking, field uniformity, and spatial resolution.

**Peaking**  This test, which is performed every day, ensures that the window of the PHA is correctly set on the desired photo-peak. The following steps are involved in "peaking" a scintillation camera:

1. Place a small radioactive source under the scintillation camera (if the collimator is removed, 100 to 200 $\mu$Ci of $^{99m}$Tc radioactivity is enough; with the collimator on, 1 to 2 $\mu$Ci of $^{99m}$Tc radioactivity is preferred).
2. Place the camera in Spectrum mode and set the energy and window for the radionuclide being used (for $^{99m}$Tc, 140 keV and 20% window).
3. Observe whether the photo-peak is within the window or not. If not, change the high voltage slowly so as to center the photo-peak in the window.
4. Take a picture of the spectrum and record the high-voltage setting. The high-voltage setting should not change more than 10% from one day to the next. If the change is greater, investigate the cause because this may lead to a malfunction. At this point, also note any fingerprints, dirt, and the like, on the oscilloscope screen.

**Field Uniformity**  This test, which should be performed daily, ensures that the count-rate variations in the image of a uniform source are within

an acceptable range and the scintillation camera is properly tuned. Because the collimator response is not expected to change unless there is evidence of physical damage, sometimes only the intrinsic field uniformity is checked routinely. Occasionally, the system field uniformity can be checked to verify that there are no problems with the collimator. The following steps are involved in the measurement of the intrinsic field uniformity:

1. Remove the collimator and move the detector head at least 5 feet above the floor. This is very important as the radiation from the point source (next step) is not strictly uniform at the face of the scintillation camera. The degree of uniformity of the radiation at the face of the scintillation camera depends strongly on the distance between the point source and the face of the scintillation camera. The farther the point source is from the scintillation camera face, the better is the uniformity of radiation falling on the scintillation camera. Remember that our goal is to measure the nonuniformity produced by the scintillation camera and not to measure the nonuniformity of the radiation source.
2. Place a 100- to 200-$\mu$Ci small volume (0.2 mL) source of $^{99m}$Tc on the floor (use absorbent paper under the source to avoid contamination of the floor).
3. Set the preset count of $10^6$ counts for a small field of view and $2 \times 10^6$ counts for a large field of view on the scintillation camera.
4. Adjust the display oscilloscope intensity to the $10^6$ or $2 \times 10^6$ count level depending on the type of scintillation camera.
5. Turn the scintillation camera on and record the image.

The resultant image is visually evaluated for uniformity, image shape (it should be a nice circle), and other artifacts. Variations greater than $\pm10\%$ are easily detectable in the image and are unacceptable. Present scintillation cameras allow the calculations of the nonuniformity and day-to-day variations of a few percent can be monitored.

For the measurement of the system field uniformity, the collimator remains attached to the scintillation camera and instead of a point source, a uniform planar source of radioactivity ($^{57}$Co, 5–10 mCi activity) is imaged and analyzed for any nonuniformities present.

**Spatial Resolution** Because measurement of the two quantitative indices of spatial resolution, *MTF* and *FWHM*, is time-consuming, a semiquantitative evaluation using a 90-degree quadrant bar phantom is performed. The phantom consists of four sets of parallel lead bars arranged in four quadrants of a Lucite holder as shown in Figure 12.11. The spacing and width of the lead bars vary between each quadrant but are the same within each quadrant. The smallest spacing is chosen to be smaller than the spatial resolution of the scintillation camera. The procedure for evaluation of the intrinsic spatial resolution is identical to that of field uniformity (steps 1–5) except, under step 1, after removing the collimator, the bar phantom is attached in front of the crystal of the scintillation camera. The resultant image is inspected for the separation of the finest bar spacing and linearity of the bars. The recommended frequency for this test is weekly. The system resolution is checked

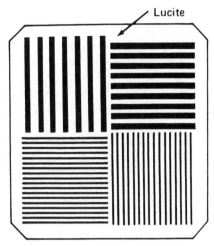

**Fig. 12.11.** A 90-degree quadrant, parallel lead bar, phantom used for quality control of the spatial resolution of a scintillation camera.

with the collimator attached to the scintillation camera. In this case a planar radioactive source ($^{57}$Co, 5–10 mCi activity) is used and the resolution phantom is sandwiched between the source and the scintillation camera. Figure 12.12 is an example of such a measurement.

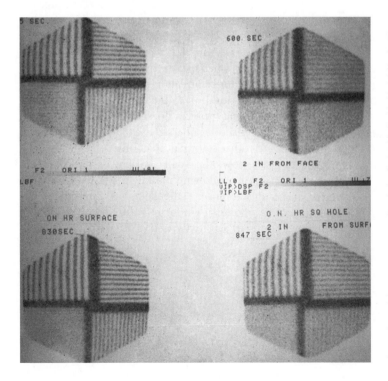

**Fig. 12.12.** Scintillation camera images of a 90-degree quadrant, parallel lead bar, phantom. Image in top left side is with a regular collimator and at the face of the collimator. Image in the top right side is at 2 inch from the face of the collimator. Bottom images (the left at the collimator face and the right at 2 inch away from the face of the collimator) correspond to a high-resolution collimator. For both collimators, resolution shows degradation at 2 inch compared to at the surface. There is slight improvement (barely perceived) in resolution in the case of the high-resolution collimator compared to the regular collimator but the sensitivity is about 30% lower than the regular collimator.

## Key Points

1. Spatial resolution and sensitivity are important in assessing performance of a scintillation camera.
2. Spatial resolution is measured, either as *FWHM* of a point-spread function or in terms of *MTF*.
3. Sensitivity is measured for a point, line, or plane source.
4. Resolution and sensitivity are inversely related.
5. Intrinsic spatial resolution and sensitivity of a scintillation camera depend on the thickness of the crystal and the energy of the γ-ray.
6. Collimator spatial resolution and sensitivity depend on the size of the holes in the collimator and the thickness of the collimator.

7. Collimator resolution degrades with an increase in distance of the source from the collimator.
8. A scintillation camera position-determining circuit produces a nonuniform image of a uniform radionuclidic distribution. To reduce the nonuniformity, on-line correction modules are provided on scintillation cameras. With these modules, typical uniformity is in the range of ±2%.
9. Dead time affects the performance of a scintillation camera at high count rates, typically exceeding 20,000 counts per second.
10. Daily uniformity and weekly spatial resolution tests are recommended for quality control of a scintillation camera.

## Questions

1. The spatial resolution and sensitivity of a scintillation camera are 10 mm and 50,000 cpm/μCi, respectively. What will be the sensitivity of this camera if a new collimator with 5 mm spatial resolution is used instead?
2. Why are there so many indices of spatial resolution? Give the best application for each of them.
3. What is the principal use of a *LSF*?
4. The *MTF* of three scintillation cameras at given spatial frequency are 0.8, 0.5, and 0.7, respectively. Which of these scintillation cameras has the best spatial resolution at this spatial frequency?
5. Determine the overall spatial resolution of a scintillation camera if the spatial resolution of the collimator is 10 mm and the intrinsic spatial resolution is (a) 10 mm, (b) 5 mm, and (c) 1 mm.

6. Which of the two collimators both designed for the same spatial resolution, but one designed for use with low energy γ-rays and the other designed for high-energy γ-rays, will have higher sensitivity?
7. Why is about 1 inch of crystal at the edge not usable for imaging in a scintillation camera?
8. Why must the point source be 5 feet or more away from the face of the scintillation camera when measuring the intrinsic uniformity of the scintillation camera?
9. In addition to the expected loss of counts, what problem does the dead time of a scintillation camera cause that does not occur in other counting situations?
10. How often (daily, weekly, or yearly) should the following parameters of a scintillation camera be checked? (a) Energy resolution, (b) Uniformity, (c) Spatial resolution, (d) Sensitivity, and (e) Energy calibration.

# Detectability or Final Contrast in an Image

The primary goal in imaging is to detect the smallest possible localized or focal abnormalities (lesions) that may be present in an organ. Because of practical limitations, however, it is not possible to attain this goal. There is a lower limit of detectability below which a lesion cannot be visualized. This limit is determined by a number of parameters discussed below.

## Parameters That Affect Detectability of a Lesion

**Object Contrast** The main purpose of any imaging device is to record the details of an object faithfully in its image. What do we mean by the details of an object? These are the spatial variations of a given parameter, such as light intensity in photography, transmitted x-ray intensity in diagnostic radiology, and the concentration of radioactivity in scanning. Such a parameter, in the language of the physicist, is known as object contrast and is most important in the detectability of a lesion. In nuclear medicine, the object contrast is created in the organ of interest by the use of a radiopharmaceutical that either selectively localizes in the abnormal tissue as compared with the normal tissue or vice versa. In either case, the higher the variation between the concentration of radioactivity in the normal and abnormal tissue, the easier it is to detect an abnormality. Therefore, radiopharmaceuticals that produce greater contrast in the lesion have better detectability than those that produce smaller contrast.

For quantitative purposes, we may define the object contrast $C_0$ as follows:

$$C_0 = \frac{\text{(Concentration in abnormal tissue } - \text{ Concentration in normal tissue})}{\text{Concentration in normal tissue}}$$

When there is no differential (variation) between the concentration of radioactivity in the abnormal and normal tissue, $C_0 = 0$ (i.e., there is no contrast). Such a radiopharmaceutical producing zero object contrast will be of no use in the detection of abnormal lesions. When the concentration of the radioactivity is higher in the abnormal area than that of the normal area, then $C_0$ greater than 0, and the radiopharmaceutical produces a positive contrast. For example, radiopharmaceuticals currently used for brain scanning produce positive contrast, with values of $C_0$ generally ranging from 15 to 25. In cases where there is less radioactivity in a lesion than in normal tissue, radiopharmaceuticals produce a negative contrast ($C_0$ less than 0). The value of $C_0$ for negative contrast cannot be increased more than $-1$, a value indicating almost no radioactivity in the lesion. For example, radiocolloids used for liver scanning are preferentially localized in normal tissue with almost no radioactivity in the abnormal lesions. Because radiopharmaceuticals producing positive contrast can achieve higher contrast values ($C_0$ greater than or equal to 1) than those producing negative contrast, the former potentially have far better detectability than the latter.

**Spatial Resolution and Sensitivity of an Imaging Device** An imaging device, such as a scintillation camera, registers the details of the distribution of a radionuclide as a photographic camera records the details of an object or scene. In both cases, a physical device is used to form an image of an object. This is true, in fact, of any imaging process using such diverse instruments as an electron microscope, telescope, or x-ray tube. In all cases, the aim is to reproduce exactly the object contrast in the image.

Unfortunately, no imaging device is capable of reproducing all the details of an object in an image, and a certain loss of detail (object contrast) is inevitable. The parameter of an imaging device that characterizes the extent of the loss of object contrast or measures the faithfulness or the fidelity for reproduction of object contrast is called spatial resolution. An imaging device that possesses better spatial resolution is capable of reproducing finer details of an object (smaller object contrasts) and is able to detect smaller lesions than an imaging device with a poorer spatial resolution. Therefore, the spatial resolution of an imager is an important parameter that strongly influences the detectability of a lesion.

What limits the spatial resolution of an imaging device in nuclear medicine? Theoretically, there are no limitations in designing an imager with fine spatial resolution capabilities. The limitations arise from the two practical constraints: the radiation dose to the patient must be kept low and the time of scanning should be reasonably short.

The effect of these two restrictions is to limit the number of γ-rays that can be detected and displayed in an image. As we see in the following section, the total number of γ-rays (photons) in an image is also an important parameter affecting the detectability of a lesion. To obtain a given number of photons in an image within a limited time, therefore, the imaging device should possess high sensitivity. The sensitivity of an imaging device is a measure of its ability to detect γ-rays efficiently. A more sensitive device will require a shorter interval of time to detect the same number of γ-rays than a less sensitive device.

Unfortunately, the sensitivity of an imaging device is related as the inverse square to its spatial resolution (see Chapter 12). Therefore, an imaging device with a spatial resolution better by a factor of 2 than a given imaging device will have a fourfold loss of sensitivity. This loss of sensitivity theoretically necessitates either a fourfold increase in the scanning or imaging time or a fourfold increase in the radiation dose to the patient. In actuality, the cost to improve the spatial resolution by a factor of 2 will be more than fourfold, as will be seen in the following section.

**Statistical (Quantum) Noise** For reproducing the details of an object, even with high contrast, an imaging device with good spatial resolution is not, in itself, enough. The human eye is capable of seeing minute details of a well-lit object but fails to perceive even large objects in a dark room. Hence, the amount of available light (number of photons) is another important parameter affecting the visualization of the details or contrast of an object.

This point is strikingly demonstrated in Figure 13.1, showing six photographs of a girl taken in succession with increasing numbers of total photons. With a smaller number of photons, only large details with high contrast are visible. As the number of photons increases, finer details of the object become visible in the image. In other words, the number of photons needed to visualize a given detail in an object is related to its contrast in the object. This relationship between the number of photons and the object contrast is not limited only to photography but is a generalized phenomenon of any imaging process.

Consequently, the net contrast in an image (it is the contrast in the image that allows us to determine the presence of a lesion) is derived from two components: the finite spatial resolution of the imaging device and the number of photons that make up the image. The latter component determines statistical noise in the image. In a well-lit object (a large number of photons), the limiting factor for reproducing the object contrast is essentially the spatial resolution of the imaging device, whereas in a dark room (hardly any photons), the limiting factor is the statistical noise in the image. In a moderately lit room (a limited number of photons), the final contrast in the image is determined by both.

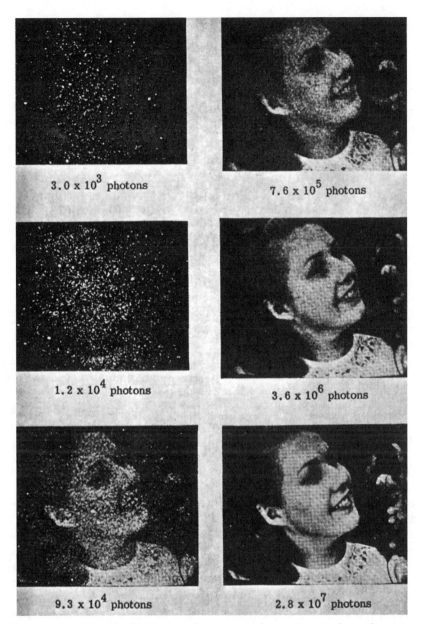

**Fig. 13.1.** Photographs taken under identical conditions except for variations in the total amount of light (number of photons). As the number of photons increases, greater detail is visible. A photographic camera possesses fine spatial resolution, yet without an adequate number of photons, that resolution is useless in providing the finer details in an object. (Reprinted by permission from Rose A. Quantum and noise limitations of the visual process. *J Optic Soc Am* 1953;43:715.)

In nuclear medicine, the statistical noise of an image is related to information density, which is defined as the number of $\gamma$-rays detected per cm$^2$ of an object. If we multiply the information density by the area of the object, we obtain the average number of photons in an image. When performing a scan with a rectilinear scanner, it is convenient to set the information density; in the scintillation camera, it is easier to set the total number of

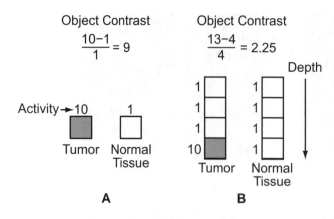

**Fig. 13.2.** Loss of object contrast as a result of the weighted sum in relation to depth of the radioactivity in routine area scanning. In this example, as a result of summation, a tumor with a contrast of 9 appears to have a contrast of 2.25 only. Here, equal weight is given to each box; in actual scanning, their exact contribution to summation will depend on the variation of the sensitivity with depth.

photons. In both cases, the statistical noise can be reduced by increasing either the information density or the total number of photons in the image. The statistical noise or error of N counts in an image equals $\sqrt{N}$ (p. 28). Because the total number of photons or information density needed to visualize a lesion depends on its contrast in the object, an information density of approximately 1000 counts/cm$^2$ of the organ (or approximately 300,000 counts in routine brain scans) is generally accepted as an optimum value for currently available imagers. Use of information densities much lower than this value may cause borderline lesions (with low contrast) to be overlooked. On the other hand, increasing the information density higher than this value will not significantly affect the detectability because, at this level, the limiting factor for detectability is the resolution of the imaging device.

In the future, if imaging devices with improved spatial resolution but without any loss of sensitivity become available, higher information density will have to be used. For example, an improvement in spatial resolution by a factor of 2 will necessitate an increase in information density approximately by a factor of 4. For the present-day imaging devices, however, when we couple this with the fact that improving the spatial resolution will reduce the sensitivity by a factor of 4, we are talking about a factor of roughly 16; that is, an improvement in the lower limit of detectability by a factor

of 2 using present-day imaging devices and radiopharmaceuticals will lengthen the time of the study approximately 16 times.

**Projection of Volume Distribution into Areal Distribution** An imaging device, such as a gamma camera, in essence integrates the radioactivity present in the third dimension (depth) of an organ. The result of such integration (i.e., the weighted sum of radioactivity with depth) is to degrade the detectability of a lesion by lowering the object contrast (see Figure 13.2 for a hypothetical situation).

**Compton scattering of γ-Rays** As explained in Chapter 10, a γ-ray originating outside the field of view of a collimator can still reach the radiation detector as a result of Compton scattering. The effect of such scattering is to reduce the object contrast and therefore to degrade the detectability of a lesion. Pulse-height selection used to discriminate against scattered γ-rays has proven quite effective in restoring some of the object contrast lost as a result of Compton scattering. However, because the energy resolution of a NaI(Tl) detector is not very high, a certain amount of object contrast is still lost. Also, as one narrows the window to reject the unwanted (scattered) counts, some good counts are also rejected. Therefore, too narrow a window may improve the image contrast somewhat, but it will be at the cost of sensitivity. This will not be the case for detectors with better energy resolution, such as Ge(Li) detectors. However, it has other shortcomings, as pointed out in Chapter 8.

**Attenuation** Because attenuation of γ-rays by the tissue of distribution and by the overlying tissue reduces the number of γ-rays reaching a scanner, such a reduction adversely affects the detectability of a lesion. As a result, lesions that are on the surface of an organ are easier to detect than those lying deep within the organ.

**Object Motion** Motion of the patient or the organ (particularly the liver, lung, and heart, which can move as much as 2 cm) also affects the detectability of a lesion in scanning. The effect of motion in an object is to reduce the object contrast, which then results in a diminished contrast in the image. By using a computer with a scintillation camera, it is feasible to eliminate some loss of object contrast due to motion. Because the clinical usefulness of such a procedure, compared with the time and effort involved, has not been convincingly established, we do not go into the details of this method.

**Display Parameters** The ability to visualize an abnormality is also affected by the display parameters, such as exposure settings, the type of film used, Hurter–Driffield (H-D) curve of the film, and so on. For the proper display, the count-rate variations of interest should match the H-D curve's useful latitude (between points A and B of Figure 10.7).

## Contrast-Detail Curve

As detectability of a lesion is affected by so many parameters, can we combine these in a single formula to obtain quantitatively the limit of detectability for a given set of parameters? Unfortunately, it is not feasible to express the dependence of detectability on various parameters in a single equation. However, the performance of an imaging device can be quantified by measuring the contrast-detail curve. To measure the contrast-detail curve, generally a phantom (Fig. 13.3) consisting of several rows

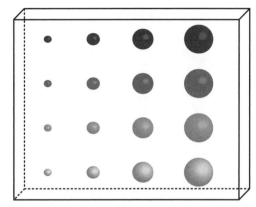

**Fig. 13.3.** A phantom for measuring contrast-detail response of an imaging device. It consists of rows of spheres with varying diameters. The columns provide varying contrasts (different amounts of radioactivity between in each column).

of spheres of different diameters and different amount of activities (contrast) is imaged. From the image, a contrast-detail curve (Fig. 13.4) is obtained by plotting the diameter of the just detectable sphere against the just detectable contrast. As can be seen, the minimum detectable size of a sphere requires high contrast and is dependent on the resolution of the imaging device, and the minimum detectable contrast depends on the noise irrespective of the diameter of the sphere.

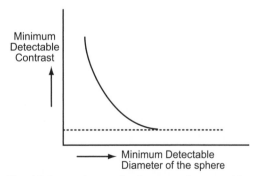

**Fig. 13.4.** By plotting the diameter of a just visible sphere against its contrast from the image of the phantom of Figure 13.3, one obtains contrast-detail curve (solid line) for an imaging device. Also shown is the noise (dotted line) for this imager. Arrows show the direction of increase.

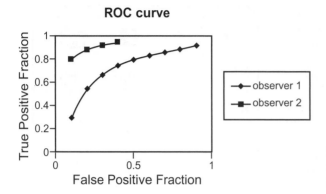

**Fig. 13.5.** Receiver operator characteristic curve for two different observers. Observer 2 has a better performance than observer 1.

# Receiver Operator Characteristic (ROC) Curve

In noise-limited images, the detectability of a lesion is also dependent on the observer (reader, in this case, the nuclear medicine physician). Because in noise-limited images, a decision has to be made whether a given lesion is a manifestation of noise or not (false or true), such a decision may vary from observer to observer. Observer variation can be studied using what is known as receiver operated characteristic ROC curves. A ROC curve can be used to compare not only different observers but also different imaging devices or diagnostic procedures. ROC is a plot of true positive fraction (number of true positives/total number of patients) as a function of false positive fraction (number of false positive/number of patients) for a population of patients for a given test and a given observer. For each patient, there are only four possibilities: patient is normal but the image is read as abnormal (false positive), patient is normal and the image is read as normal (true negative), patient is abnormal and the film is read abnormal (true positive) and the patient is abnormal and the image is read as normal (false negative). Each observer classifies a given set of images in the four possibilities and from these one calculates the true positive fraction and the false positive fraction and then plots the ROC curve for each observer. One such plot is shown in Figure 13.5 for two different observers. Observer 2 performs significantly better than observer 1 because his true positive fraction is consistently higher than observer 1. In general, it is the area under the curves that determines which observer is better. Larger is the area better is the observer.

## Key Points

1. Detectability of a lesion is a complex function of several parameters, which may depend on the patient, the scintillation camera, or the imaging technique.
2. Object contrast depends on the patient (radiopharmaceutical distribution, scatter, and attenuation).
3. Spatial resolution and sensitivity depend on the scintillation camera.
4. The number of counts detected and therefore the statistical noise in the image depends on the technique. Display parameters used also depend on the technique.
5. Contrast-detail curve measures detailed performance of an imaging device and can be used to compare different imaging devices under clinically relevant conditions.
6. The ROC curve is used to compare the performance of observers (readers).

## Questions

1. Concentration of a radiopharmaceutical at 3 hours postadministration is determined to be 5500 counts/mL/min in a brain tumor. It measured 2200 counts/mL/min in the normal brain. Calculate the contrast between the tumor and the normal brain.

2. The same radiopharmaceutical gave the tumor and normal brain concentrations at 24 hours postadministration of 2700 and 1100 counts/mL/min, respectively. Calculate the contrast at 24 hours. Did the contrast improve, degrade, or remain the same at 24 hours compared to that at 3 hours?

3. What should be the minimum contrast between a normal liver and a metastatic lesion (4 cm in diameter) for it to be visualized (at 99% confidence level) when the information density of a liver scintigram is 1000 counts/cm$^2$?

4. Do the radiopharmaceuticals designed to study blood flow in the brain have more or less contrast than the radiopharmaceuticals designed for tumor detection? Which of the two has better detectability?

5. Disregarding the consideration of cost, suggest a way to increase the sensitivity and therefore the detectability of a scintillation camera.

6. Why is the detectability for tumor detection in the brain similar in nuclear medicine and computed tomography when the resolution for computed tomography is an order of magnitude higher than that in nuclear medicine?

7. In contrast-detail curve, what determines the minimum detectable diameter and the minimum detectable contrast?

8. What criterion is used to compare two ROC curves?

# Emission Computed Tomography

Two-dimensional imaging, even with multiple views, does not provide accurate three-dimensional information concerning radionuclide distribution. Because two-dimensional imaging more or less integrates the information from the third dimension (depth), it results in lower contrast of lesions (see Chapter 13). With the advent and success of computed tomography (CT) in diagnostic radiology in the early 1970s, similar concepts and techniques have been applied in nuclear medicine as emission computed tomography (ECT). Tomography, in general, is divided into two categories, transverse and longitudinal. It is the transverse tomography that has found success in routine clinical and research use. Transverse tomography can be performed with radionuclides emitting single photons (x- or $\gamma$-rays) or with radionuclides emitting positrons. Transverse tomography with single photon emitters is commonly known as single-photon emission computed tomography (SPECT), whereas with positron emitters it is known as PET.

This chapter describes the principle of transverse tomography, instruments commonly used for SPECT and PET, and the relative merits of the two types. The mathematical techniques used in reconstruction of a tomogram are highly sophisticated and are beyond the scope of this book. Therefore, I limit myself to a phenomenological description only. Also discussed briefly are the combined instruments, PET and CT, and SPECT and CT.

## Principles of Transverse Tomography

In its simplest form, a detector acquires data from a thin axial section containing radioactivity by linear scanning from multiple directions around the cross section, as shown in Figure 14.1. In its complex form, mainly to reduce the data acquisition time, data are acquired from multiple thin cross sections and multiple directions simultaneously by using a large number of detectors as in PET or a scintillation camera as in SPECT.

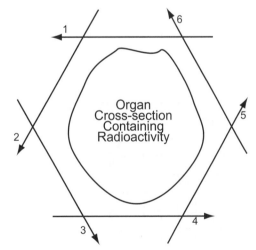

**Fig. 14.1.** Principle of axial tomography. A thin cross section of an organ is scanned from several tangential directions (in this example, six). From these scans, the cross-sectional radioactive distribution is reconstructed, using a variety of superimpositional techniques.

In either case, the principle of transverse tomography is the same and consists of two steps: acquisition of linear projection data of a thin cross section from multiple directions and reconstruction of the cross section or cross sections from these data. In PET, the data, as explained later, are acquired in a coincidence mode that is different than SPECT, but the same following considerations apply.

### Considerations in Data Acquisition
#### Pixel Width, Matrix, and Number of Projections
Let us consider a simple case where a single detector scans a cross section linearly from many directions. Let us also assume that as the detector moves from one position to the next along a line, it receives counts from N columns that are perpendicular to the direction of a scan and chosen to be equally spaced. This is shown in Figure 14.2 for the two positions of the detector in two different linear scans. Two columns perpendicular to each other have only a small area in common. This area is called a pixel, and the entire cross section can be imagined to consist of these small pixels distributed in a square matrix of size N × N. When scans are performed from different directions, different combinations of pixels, but always perpendicular to the direction of scan, contribute to the counts of the detector at different positions along a scan line.

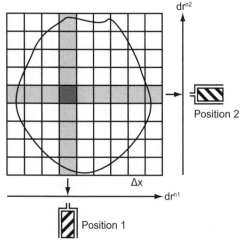

**Fig. 14.2.** Data acquisitions in transverse tomography. $dr^{n1}$, $dr^{n2}$ stand for scan directions 1, 2, and so on.

These are called projections of a plane on a line, and the number M of these projections is a critical parameter in the reconstruction of the cross section. For accurate and artifact-free reconstruction, M should be nearly equal to N. From the projection data, the radioactivity of each pixel is computed using the method described in the next section.

Data acquisition with a single detector is very time-consuming. A variety of methods has been developed to reduce the acquisition time or to increase the overall sensitivity. For example, to avoid the linear motion, a linear array of detectors N can be used simultaneously to gather data from a projection. This increases sensitivity N-fold compared with a single detector. Further gains can be achieved by using multiple linear arrays gathering data simultaneously from multiple directions as well as from many cross sections. Of course, such an increase in sensitivity is accompanied by an increased complexity and cost of such a device. Sensitivity is the main reason why data acquisition with a scintillation camera for SPECT is routinely used in clinical nuclear medicine. In cardiac applications, recently other novel methods of data collection, as described later in this chapter, have been quite successful.

The number of pixels in a cross section is determined by the number of columns, N, in a scan direction and is simply N × N. In the case of Figure 14.2, this number is 9 × 9 = 81. In a given cross section, the number of pixels and the size of the pixel $\Delta x$ are inversely related. The smaller the pixel size is, the larger the number of pixels or matrix size is. In routine clinical nuclear medicine, the matrix size is either 64 × 64 or 128 × 128, resulting in 4096 or 16,384 pixels, respectively. What determines the pixel size is discussed next.

#### Pixel Width, Resolution, and Sensitivity
Pixel width, $\Delta x$ (and therefore the matrix size N × N and number of linear projections M) is an important consideration in data acquisition because it pertains to the amount of time required to complete a scan. Pixel width depends on the resolution obtainable in the tomogram, which in turn depends on the resolution of the collimator used in SPECT or the size of the detector used in PET. A rule of

thumb is that the pixel width $\Delta x$ should be less than or equal to the resolution of the collimator employed in the SPECT or the size of the detector employed in the PET. In general, improving the resolution necessitates reducing the pixel width $\Delta x$ and vice versa. Thus, to improve resolution, one has to reduce the size of the hole in the collimator of the detector (SPECT) or use smaller size detectors (PET), which reduces the sensitivity of the detector. As a result, to achieve the same statistical reliability, one has to spend more time at each location. In addition, the reduction in $\Delta x$ as a result of higher resolution increases the number of pixels N along the scan line that necessitates more linear projections M from different angles for optimum sampling. This again requires more time. Thus, we face a similar (actually worse) dilemma in transverse tomography as we face in areal scanning; that is, improvement in resolution costs dearly in terms of sensitivity and a compromise has to be made between the two.

In CT, where, because of the large number of photons available from an x-ray tube, the typical resolution or pixel size is about 1 mm, the number of linear scans performed is 180 or more. In nuclear medicine, where the available number of photons in a typical cross section is relatively small, typical resolution for SPECT is in the range of 1 cm and the number of linear scans needed is in the vicinity of 64 (128 for higher resolution). For PET, typical resolution is about 6 mm. Newer cardiac specific SPECT systems also have resolution of about 6 mm.

**Other Requirements**  Besides the width $\Delta x$ of the columns, the other important requirements of collimation are

1. An individual detector at a given location picks up counts from only one column (perpendicular to the scan direction);
2. There are no variations in counts detected from a uniform cross section at different locations along scans from multiple directions;
3. The same activity in any pixel in a column contributes equally to the counts at a given location (i.e., the detector response should be uniform with depth);

4. All counts come from only the cross section under consideration and not from adjacent cross sections.

These requirements are not easily achieved in nuclear medicine because of the nature of collimation and attenuation and scatter in the patient, particularly for SPECT (Fig. 10.1 and p. 106).

A major difference between CT and ECT in data acquisition is that in CT, data are acquired within a 180 degree rotation of linear scans, whereas in SPECT (except for heart studies where 180 degree is preferable), a complete rotation (360 degree) of linear scans around the cross section is used.

### Reconstruction of the Cross Section
Reconstruction of a cross section from its multiple linear projections around the cross section is a general problem that is encountered in diverse fields. First analytic solution of this problem was provided by Radon as far back as 1917. However, because of the complexity involved in the computations, practical realization of the solution was achieved only in recent years with the advent and easy access to large digital computers. There are basically two classes of algorithms, analytic and iterative. Of the analytic methods, the most successful method is known as filtered back projection, which is a modified form (therefore more accurate) of back projection. This is widely used in CT, SPECT, and PET. Recently iterative methods have also been successful, particularly in cardiac nuclear medicine.

### Reconstruction with Back Projection (a Simple Explanation)
Let us consider a simple cross section containing two radionuclide sources as depicted in Figure 14.3A. When data are acquired from this cross section with an appropriate detector and by linear scanning from multiple directions, the responses of the detector are shown as scan 1, scan 2, scan 3, scan 4, and so on. Notice that in this case, the detector receives counts only at one or two discrete locations in each scan, and these locations are determined by the intersection of the scan directions and the perpendicular lines from each source to the scan direction, respectively. In the back projection method of reconstruction, as the name implies,

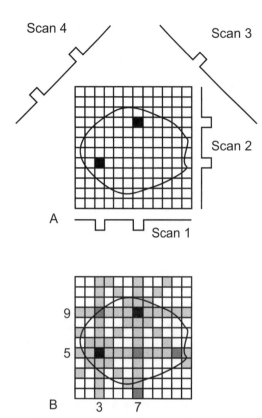

**Fig. 14.3.** Reconstruction of a cross section using simple back projection method.

data received at one location of a linear scan is back projected in the column right above that location and so on. Because no prior knowledge exists about which or how many pixels in that column contain radioactivity (actually, that is what we would like to know), one assumes that counts received at that location came in equal amounts from each pixel in that column. This is done in Figure 14.3B. Counts received by the detector in scan 1 at the two locations are distributed equally in the 12 pixels of columns 3 and 7, respectively. When a similar procedure is repeated for other scans (2, 3, 4, etc.), the reconstruction of the cross section is complete. As can be seen, two radioactive sources have been reproduced at the correct locations, although not as point sources but as star patterns. As a result, a number of pixels (shown as shaded) that contained no radioactivity in the original cross section are reconstructed inaccurately as containing small amounts of radioactivity (starlike artifact).

**Filtered Back Projection (a Better Reconstruction Method): Actual Steps** In a more refined approach, known as filtered back projection, the star artifacts are reduced by adding and subtracting fixed fractions of the counts from the column under consideration to several adjacent columns on both sides. When this is done, a quite accurate and almost artifact-free reconstruction is obtained. Because data acquired are large and the mathematical operations needed for reconstruction are huge, a large digital computer is essential to store and process the data quickly. In practice, the filtered back reconstruction is performed in frequency or Fourier space (similar to modulation transfer function MTF discussed in Chapter 12) where the filter function takes a much simpler form and therefore computations become easier and faster. The following steps are taken:

1. Compute Fourier transform of individual projection data;
2. Multiply it by the filter function;
3. Compute inverse Fourier transform;
4. Back projection to get the cross section.

Filter function is an important parameter in ECT because it affects the noise and resolution characteristics of the reconstruction. A number of filters—ramp, Hanning, Butterworth, and Metz—have been used. Choice of filter depends on the acceptable noise and resolution in the image. Of these, Hanning and Butterworth are most common in clinical nuclear medicine. Figure 14.4 shows a ramp filter and two Butterworth filters,

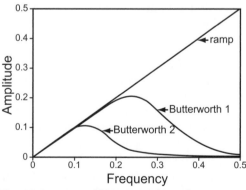

**Fig. 14.4.** A typical filter routinely used in reconstruction of tomographic images in nuclear medicine.

each with a different amount of smoothing. A ramp filter produces an image with the best resolution but with the most noise. Butterworth filter 2 produces the least noisy image but the resolution is worst. Butterworth 1 is a good compromise between loss of resolution and reduction in noise.

**Attenuation Correction in Filtered Back Projection** The requirements for accurate reconstruction of a cross section—the sensitivity for each pixel in a column is the same and the counts at each location originate only from that column—are not met in SPECT because the γ-rays originating from different pixels pass through different thickness of tissues and therefore are attenuated to different degrees. As a result, when reconstruction is done from the data obtained from a cross section of uniform radioactive distribution, it is highly nonuniform. Several methods have been used to solve these problems. These can be classified as analytical or empirical. Analytical methods make some simplifying assumptions about attenuation (e.g., uniformity of attenuating medium) and are incorporated prereconstruction (Sorenson method), simultaneous with reconstruction (Gulberg method), or postreconstruction (Chang method). Of these, the Sorenson and Chang methods are widely available commercially. These methods fail utterly when the attenuating medium is highly inhomogeneous, such as the thorax. With empirical methods, the actual attenuation map is obtained by taking multiple transmission scans from multiple projections (similar to a CT). These methods in theory produce the best results but require additional setup and scan time, and exposure to the patient.

**Scatter Correction in Filtered Back Projection** Compton scattering of γ-rays originating outside the column of interest into the detector and the diverging field of view of a collimator make it hard to collect data at a given location from one column (and one cross section) only (see Figure 10.2). As was suggested in Figure 10.2, the best method to reject scattered events is by using either a narrow window or multiple (two or three, routinely) windows and subtracting the scattered events.

**Iterative Methods** Besides the filtered back projection, a number of iterative methods have been used to reconstruct cross sections from the projection data. Their principal drawback is the computer time needed for reconstruction. However, with the vast improvements in computer data processing speed per unit cost, it is no longer a problem, and these methods have replaced filtered back projection method, particularly in specific applications. The main advantage of these methods is that all the problems encountered in the data acquisition, attenuation and scatter in the patient, collimator response (resolution and its depth variation, septal penetration etc.), and detection characteristics of the detector can be exactly modeled in the algorithm. As resolution recovery is modeled in the algorithm, it allows the use of coarser-resolution collimators. Coarser-resolution collimators have higher sensitivity. The resulting images have better resolution and less noise. There are no streaking artifacts as encountered in filtered back projection. The net result is that images are more quantitative than those produced by filtered back projection. The improvement in noise and resolution comes at the cost of the need of high computer processing power.

In iterative reconstruction, one starts with a gross estimate of the distribution of the radionuclide in the cross section. Projections calculated from the estimated distribution (back projection) are arithmetically compared with measured data. The result is used to update the next estimate (forward projection). This process continues till the errors in the measured projection data and the estimated projection data are minimized. Corrections for attenuation, scatter, and spatial resolution are made by mathematically modeling these factors into the forward and back projection calculations.

Among the iterative methods, maximum likelihood expectation maximization and its relative ordered-subset expectation maximization, and maximum a posteriori expectation maximization algorithms are widely used. There is ongoing work to make these algorithms even more efficient.

## Single-Photon Emission Computed Tomography

Current SPECT techniques employ two methods for data acquisition, with scintillation camera or with multiple detectors arranged in a variety of geometric pattern. The latter are dedicated SPECT systems and do not generate longitudinal projecion images and are mainly used in cardiac applicaions.

**Data Acquisition with a Scintillation Camera**  Of the two current approaches for performing SPECT, using multidetectors or a scintillation camera, the latter is more popular because most of the equipment needed (e.g., a scintillaion camera and a computer) is already available in nuclear medicine departments. Additionally, a rotating gantry on which a scintillation camera head can be mounted and a software program to acquire data and reconstruct the cross sections are needed. To reduce the acquisition time further, SPECT systems with two or three scintillation camera heads are preferred. A commercial dual headed scintillation camera is shown in Figure 14.5.

In this setup (Fig. 14.6), a scintillation camera head (or heads) rotates in a circle around a patient, making a number of stops for a given time to acquire data from multiple directions (64 or 128 in routine procedures). This is a step-and-shoot data acquisition. No data are gathered during its movement from one position to the next. To avoid this dead time and increase sensitivity further, acquisition protocols have been developed where data are either gathered continuously (without a stop) or in a combination of the two (continuous + step-and-shoot). The orbit of detector heads does not have to be circular. Elliptical or body contour orbits, because of their improved sensitivity and resolution characteristics, are now standard features.

Because a scintillation camera acquires data simultaneously from a large area of an organ as opposed to a thin section, data acquired are planar projections of a volume rather than line projections of a cross section. Therefore, it can be easily formatted to produce different cross sections (axial, coronal, sagittal, or oblique) of an organ from just a single acquisition. This is another advantage of scintillation camera–based

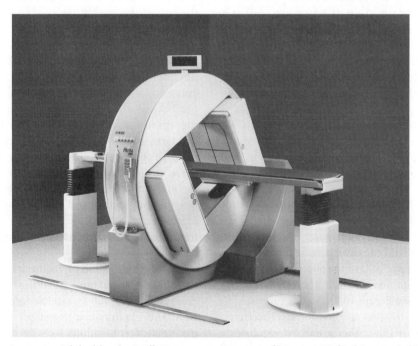

**Fig. 14.5.**  A commercial dual-head scintillation camera (courtesy of Marconi Medical Systems). (From Bushberg JT, Siebert JA, Leidholdt EM Jr, et al. *The Essential Physics of Medical Imaging.* 2nd ed. Philadelphia: Lippincott Williams & Wilkins, 2002, with permission.)

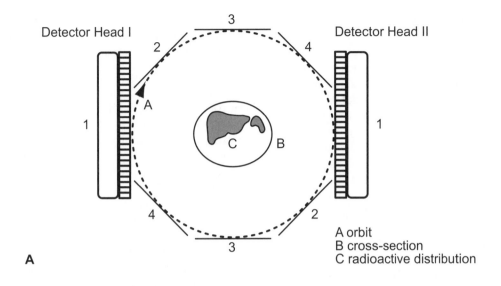

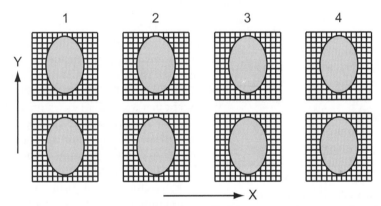

**Fig. 14.6.** (A) Data acquisition with a dual-head scintillation camera making a circular orbit around a patient containing radioactivity. In this example, four pairs of areal projections are acquired. In actual case 32 or 64, such pairs are obtained. (B) Corresponding rows in the four pairs of images (first row in each image, etc.) represent linear projections for an axial cross section at the level represented by that row. These data are then used in reconstruction of that cross section. The thickness of the cross section can be increased by combining adjacent rows.

SPECT over multidetector-based SPECT system that presently reproduce only axial slices.

**Collimators** For optimal performance of SPECT with a scintillation camera, choice of a collimator is very important. For routine use, a general purpose parallel-hole collimator is preferred. A high-resolution parallel-hole collimator may be used in special situations. Special collimators designed for SPECT are also increasingly becoming available. As stated earlier, iterative reconstruction algorithms allow

for the use of coarser (wider radius and shorter length holes) resolution collimators.

**Other Requirements or Sources of Error** For accurate reproduction of a radioactive cross section, the following sources of error are unique for a scintillation camera–based SPECT:

1. Center of rotation: Proper alignment of the center of electronic position- (x, y) determining circuit with the center of rotation. In areal imaging, a shift by one

or two pixels in the x or y direction is hardly noticeable, but in SPECT, such a misalignment produces recognizable artifacts (e.g., a point source is reconstructed as a ring). Proper alignment can be achieved by placing a point source at the center of rotation, imaging it from two opposite directions, and determining the pixel location of the source in the two images. If these are identical, then there is no need for adjustment and the electronic center is properly aligned with the center of rotation. However, if the pixel location of the source is not identical, these are made identical by electronically off setting X or Y voltage, as the case may be.

2. Uniformity: Uniformity of response of a scintillation camera. This requirement is much more stringent in SPECT than routine imaging because errors propagate rapidly in reconstruction of the image. Although in areal imaging uniformity in the range of ±5% is acceptable, in SPECT it should be under ±2%. As explained earlier (p. 134), newer scintillation cameras are capable of such a performance.

3. Invariance of uniformity at different angles: Because images are acquired at a large number of angles, the uniformity of a scintillation camera should be maintained at each angle. The main reason for changes in the uniformity response at different angles is the change in the photomultiplier PM tube gain that occurs when it is oriented at different angles in the earth's magnetic field. In newer cameras where PM tubes are shielded by $\mu$-metal, these effects are reduced considerably.

4. Detector head alignment with the axis of rotation.

Thus, clinical success of SPECT depends on a stringent quality control program; acquisition of a sufficient number of counts in each image; use of properly designed collimators; and proper correction for attenuation, scatter, and, if possible, for system resolution. With proper attention to these points, good quality reconstructed SPECT images can be realized routinely in a clinical nuclear medicine department

(Fig. 14.7). However, these images, although useful clinically, still fall short where accurate quantitative measurements are required.

**Dedicated SPECT Systems** Dedicated systems using multiple scintillator detectors had been tried for many years without any clinical success. However, recently with the emergence of semiconductor detector, CZT, these have made a come back. Primarily, because of smaller size of these detectors, novel geometric arrangements and collimator designs can be utilized to produce clinical images in shorter time (up to 10 times less than the standard scintillation camera–based systems) and with better resolution than those that are produced with scintillation camera–based SPECT. However, because of technical problems, presently these are limited to cardiac applications only. The two commercially successful systems are D-SPECT and GE-Discovery NM 530c.

The D-SPECT (Fig. 14.8) consists of nine detector columns each mounted in an arc mimicking the shape of human torso around the heart as shown in Figure 14.9. Each detector column works like a small scintillation camera except that it uses CZT detectors and not a NaI detector and are capable of imaging heart size objects only. The detector columns are capable of rotation and translation to image from different directions (different projections). Thus nine detector columns (cameras) can generate a large number of projections of heart (more than enough to reconstruct the tomographic slices of the heart). Each detector column (Fig. 14.10) consists of 1024 CZT detectors (each 2.46 x 2.46 in area and 5 mm in thickness). These are arranged in a matrix 16 x 64 making a rectangle of 4 x 16 cm. Collimator on each detector column is a parallel-hole collimator with one rectangular hole for each detector. The size of the hole is larger than the one used in a conventional scintillation camera parallel-hole collimator and the length of the hole is also smaller than the one used in standard parallel-hole collimator, thus producing a poorer resolution than the standard parallel-hole collimator. It sacrifices resolution for a sensitivity gain of up to 10 times; resolution is recovered during the reconstruction, the net effect being up to a 2x increase in resolution over conventional scintillation camera.

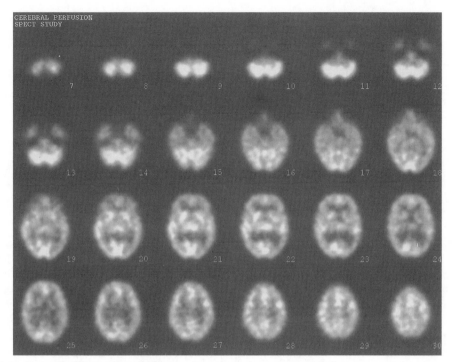

**Fig. 14.7.** Typical SPECT images. Thirty transverse slices showing brain perfusion.

GE-Alcyone NM system employs a large numbers pin holes (at least 27, in a two-dimensional array of 3 x 9) to image the heart from multiple directions, thus gathering enough data for the reconstruction of tomographic slices of the heart without any motion either of the detectors or of the patient. Each pinhole projects heart's image on a 16 x 16 matrix of CZT detectors (each about 2.5 x 2.5 x 5 mm thick)

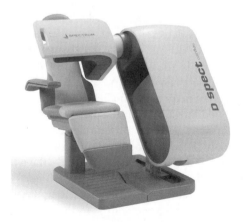

**Fig. 14.8.** A commercial dedicated SPECT system (From D-SPECT with permission).

that acts like a small scintillation camera. The transaxial images of the heart are reconstructed using a three-dimensional algorithm.

## Positron Emission Tomography

**Why PET?** As was discussed in Chapter 5 under radiopharmaceuticals for PET, most radionuclides used in nuclear medicine (e.g., $^{99m}$Tc, $^{67}$Ga, $^{201}$Tl) are not isotopes of physiologically important elements such as hydrogen, carbon, nitrogen, or oxygen. The only $\gamma$-emitting isotopes of these elements are actually positron emitters ($^{11}$C, $^{13}$N, and $^{15}$O) that have short half-lives (in minutes). Fluorine-18, a positron emitter, even though not a physiologically important element, can replace hydrogen in many important biological molecules without changing their function significantly. Therefore, if one is interested in measuring the distribution, physiology, and/or metabolism of a large number of important biomolecules noninvasively, there is no alternative but to use these positron emitters in conjunction with PET. For over the last 25 years, PET has been yielding a wealth of

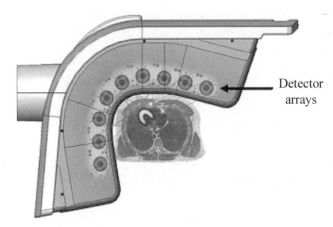

**Fig. 14.9.** Geometric arrangement of the 9 detector heads around the heart of a patient (From D-SPECT with permission).

information as a research tool but now with the easier availability of $^{18}$F-deoxyglucose, PET has finally become an important instrument in a clinical nuclear medicine department.

**Principles of PET** Positron-emitting radionuclides as such do not emit γ-rays, but when an emitted positron has lost its energy by interaction with surrounding medium within a short distance of the site of emission (average range is 0.22 mm in the case of $^{18}$F, see Table 5.2), it annihilates by combining with an electron, and two γ-rays with energies of 511 keV each are produced simultaneously (see Figure 6.2). Such a pair of γ-rays produced by annihilation of a positron always travels in opposite (180 degree apart) directions. In PET or positron scanning, these two γ-rays are used in a coincidence mode where both γ-rays are detected by a pair of detectors (e.g., BGO or

LSO) simultaneously. One or more pairs of small detectors face each other on either side of a radioactive organ as in Figure 14.11 where two such pairs of detectors are shown (detectors 1 and 2 form one pair and detectors 3 and 4 form the second pair). Output of each pair of detectors is relayed to a coincidence circuit to determine whether the output of each detector originated simultaneously or within a short time of each other ($<10^{-9}$ seconds, it is called the resolution time of the coincidence circuit). In this case, output of the detectors 1 and 2 are fed to coincidence circuit 1 and output of the detectors 3 and 4 are fed to coincidence circuit 2, respectively.

**True Coincidences** For the annihilation marked **a**, the two γ rays will interact with the detectors 1 and 2, respectively, and almost simultaneously, and therefore a true coincidence output will result in coincidence circuit 1. As can be seen, this detector pair will produce a true coincidence output only when the annihilation occurs in the area shown by dotted lines between these two detectors. Thus, this detector pair has defined a detection field of view (within the dotted lines) without the presence of a collimator as is required if these detectors were used only in single mode (without coincidence mode). For the annihilation marked **b**, the two γ-rays will interact in the detectors 3 and 4, respectively, and a true coincidence output will result in coincidence circuit 2. In this case, the detection field of view of this pair of detectors is shown by the dotted lines between these two

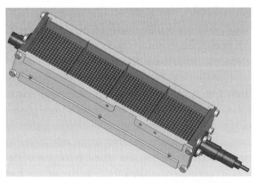

**Fig. 14.10.** The detector head containing the CZT detectors and collimator (D-SPECT with permission).

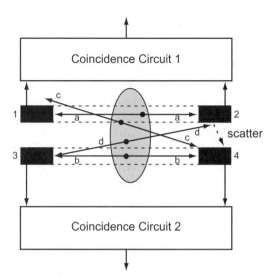

**Fig. 14.11.** Coincidence mode of detection of a positron-emitting radionuclide.

detectors. A similar consideration applies for the annihilation marked **a**, where a true coincidence occurs between detector pair 1 and 2. A coincidence will be detected in coincidence circuit 1 from annihilation occurring only in the area shown by dotted lines between detector 1 and 2. Thus, simultaneous detection of the two annihilation γ-rays by a pair of cylindrical detectors defines uniquely a nice cylindrical (as opposed to a cone for a single detector with a collimator) field of view without the aid of a collimator.

**Sensitivity** Sensitivity of coincidence detection increases with the number of detector pairs employed. To increase the sensitivity of these detector pairs further in the above example, we could connect the output of detectors 1 and 3 in another coincidence circuit 3 and outputs of the detectors 2 and 4 in coincidence circuit 4. This would define two new fields of view, one connecting detectors 1 and 3 and the other connecting detectors 2 and 4 (not shown here but actually done in commercial systems). Thus, two detector pairs with four coincidence circuits produce four distinct areas of detection. The use of multiple coincidence circuits with each detector increases the sensitivity of the coincidence

detection mode greatly when a large number of detectors are used as is the case in commercial PET devices.

**Resolution** The resolution of a coincidence pair is more or less determined by the area of the two detectors. For a square detector, it is the length or the width of the detector. In most commercial systems, it is between 5 to 8 mm. The thickness of the detector determines the intrinsic sensitivity as was discussed in Chapter 8. Also note that in this setup, the sensitivity and resolution in the field of view of such a pair of detectors does not vary significantly with the location of the radioactive source in its field of view. This, as was stated earlier, is an important requirement for ECT that is difficult to achieve in SPECT but is fulfilled easily in PET.

Two other factors that ultimately limit the lowest achievable resolution are the range of positrons and the distance between the detector pair. Range of the positron because the annihilation only occurs at the end of the range. The distance between the detector pair, because the two 511 keV γ rays do not exactly go in opposite direction (the angle is very slightly less than 180 degree. However, in present clinical PET systems, the detector size is the major contributor to the resolution.

**Accidental Coincidences** Annihilations marked **c** and **d** cannot produce a true coincidence output in either of the detector pairs as only one γ-ray strikes a detector in each case. However, if by chance the two annihilations **c** and **d** occur simultaneously, then one γ-ray produced by annihilation **c** can interact with one detector (here detector 4) and one γ-ray produced by annihilation **d** can interact with the other detector (here detector 3) simultaneously and thus producing a coincidence in circuit 2. Such an event is not a true coincidence and is called accidental coincidence. These events are undesirable as they originate outside the field of view of the detector pair. There are two ways to minimize the number of the accidental coincidence: one is to have the coincidence resolution time as short as possible and the other is to keep the radioactivity to be detected small. The second alternative is not a viable option as it will increase the imaging time. However and fortunately, the accidental events can be easily and accurately measured and subtracted. Accidental events are measured by employing another coincidence circuit in parallel to a true coincidence circuit but with a small delay between the outputs of the detector pair. Counts obtained in the accidental coincidence circuit are then subtracted from the counts obtained in the true coincidence circuit.

**Scatter Coincidences** Just as scatter of $\gamma$-rays in SPECT is a serious source of concern, it is also a serious problem in PET. Two types of scatter events occur. One type of scatter is demonstrated by the annihilation marked **d** in Figure 14.11. One of the annihilation $\gamma$-rays interacts with detector 3 and the other with detector 2. As such, there will be no coincidence. However, if the second $\gamma$-ray is scattered by the detector 2 as shown by a dotted arrow in the figure, then a coincidence count will be produced in circuit 2. This is a scatter coincidence and is not a desirable event; it has to be reduced and, if possible, corrected. One way to reduce this kind of scatter is to use shielding between the detectors. The second kind of scattered events occur when the scattering takes place in the patient. Both types of the scattered events are reduced by employing energy discrimination as was discussed in Chapter 10. As LSO detectors have significantly better energy resolution than BGO, LSO detectors are better than BGO in rejecting scattered events.

**Attenuation Correction** The two annihilation $\gamma$-rays taken together pass through the same thickness of tissue irrespective of location of the annihilation in the field of view of the detector pair. Therefore, it is much easier and more accurate to correct for attenuation in PET. First, one measures the attenuation through different locations of the patient by using an external source. This can be done fairly accurately. Then, true coincidences are corrected point by point for the attenuation. Corrected data are then used to reconstruct the image using the filtered back projection method. Again, accurate correction

of the attenuation is one more advantage over SPECT.

**PET Instrumentation** To perform PET, one can acquire data from a thin cross section with a pair of detectors by linearly scanning a cross section from multiple directions. However, the sensitivity of such a device will be low. To increase the sensitivity, multiple pairs of detectors, either in a ring or a hexagonal array, are used in commercially available systems, as shown in Figure 14.12. To increase the sensitivity of these devices, more than one array or ring is sometimes used to acquire data from multiple cross sections simultaneously. A commercial PET instrument is shown in Figure 14.13. The instruments are quite complex as a large number (sometimes exceeding 5000, about 5 mm $\times$ 5 mm $\times$ 30 mm in size) of BGO or LSO crystals

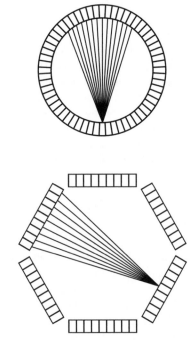

**Fig. 14.12.** Circular or hexagonal arrays of detectors for simultaneous collection of data from various directions in a PET imager. Each detector in the array or ring is in coincidence with a large number of detectors on its opposite side. Here, only one detector is shown in coincidence with several detectors on the opposite side.

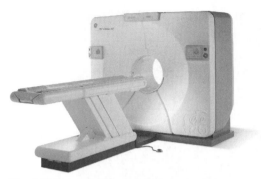

**Fig. 14.13.** A commercial PET system. (From General Electric Medical Systems, Waukesha, WI, with permission.)

are used. It is not practical to use 5000 PM tubes. Instead, to reduce the electronic complexity of the instrument as well as to reduce the cost of the instrument, a large crystal block shown in Figure 14.14, is divided into smaller sections (each serves as one independent detector) by making slits into the crystal block. The block shown is divided into 8 × 8 sections, thus producing 64 detector elements of about 4 to 5 mm width and 3 cm thickness. The large crystal block is coupled to four PM tubes as shown

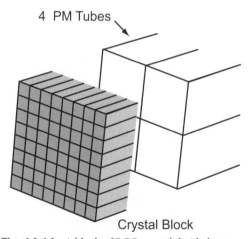

Crystal Block

**Fig. 14.14.** A block of BGO crystal divided into 64 individual detectors but coupled to only four PM tubes. The location of γ-ray interaction among the 64 detectors is determined from the pulse height distribution between the four PM tubes.

in Figure 14.14. Using the Anger logic similar to a scintillation camera, each crystal can be uniquely identified by the pulse height distribution generated in the four PM tubes. Thus, this type of arrangement reduces the number of PM tubes by a factor of 16 compared to if one employed one PM tube for each crystal element. Besides reducing the cost, it increases the electronic stability and performance of the PET instrument. When these crystal blocks are arranged in a circular or hexagonal array, they produce eight or more axial cross sections at the same time.

## PET-CT and SPECT-CT

Recently, the two instruments, PET and CT, have been combined in one unit shown in Figure 14.15. PET produces functional images not obtainable by any other means but with poor resolution and CT produces high-resolution anatomic images. By combining the two, one gets high-resolution functional and anatomic images in one. Of course, the PET image and the CT image of a patient obtained on two independent machines can be fused together using computers, but in practice there are problems related to different formats of images, patient position and motion, time interval between the two studies, and necessity of a separate work station. A combined PET-CT obviates many of these problems. In addition, since, in PET, one needs measurement of attenuation coefficient for the attenuation correction, these can be extrapolated from the CT data and, therefore, there is no need to measure using radioactive sources. This reduces the radiation dose to the patient. Of course, the disadvantage is their cost and the fact that not every patient needs both studies always. Presently, these machines have been shown to be clinically effective in the head and neck tumors. Another area where these have a potential clinical effectiveness is in the abdomen. With the success of the PET-CT combination, there are now SPECT-CT combined units also commercially available. One such unit is shown in Figure 14.16.

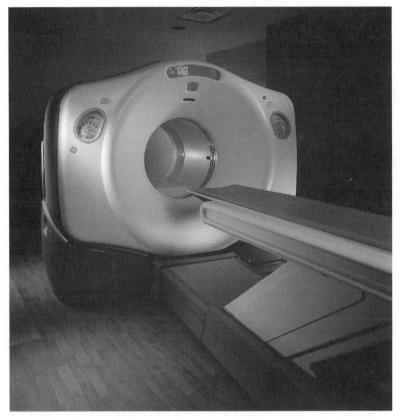

**Fig. 14.15.**  A commercial PET-CT system. (From General Electric Medical Systems, Waukesha, WI, with permission.)

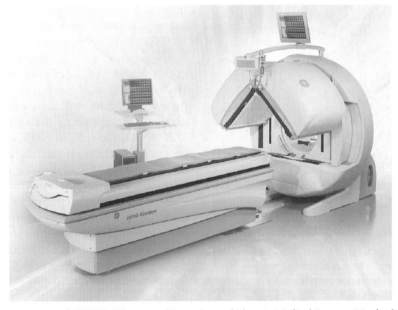

**Fig. 14.16.**  A commercial SPECT-CT system. (From General Electric Medical System, Waukesha, WI, with permission.)

## Key Points

1. ECT determines a radionuclidic distribution in a tissue cross section such as axial, sagittal, or coronal.
2. Linear projection data are collected from multiple directions.
3. The cross section is then reconstructed from these data using mathematical algorithms. Of these, the most common is filtered back projection. However iterative methods are making inroads in clinical SPECT systems.
4. SPECT is easily performed with a scintillation camera attached to a rotating gantry and a digital computer.
5. Dedicated SPECT systems for cardiac studies have many advantages over scintillation camera–based SPECT systems.

6. Two problems that make quantification difficult in SPECT are attenuation and scatter. Recent methods of dealing with these two problems—measurement of attenuation with transmission and scatter correction with triple windows—have reduced the quantification errors significantly.
7. PET uses positron annihilation radiations (two 511-keV $\gamma$-rays traveling in opposite directions) in coincidence mode to collimate (electronic collimation as opposed to mechanical collimators). In coincidence mode, attenuation and scatter can be dealt with easily and reasonably accurately. This leads to accurate quantification of in vivo radioactivity by PET.

## Questions

1. Is it essential to acquire data from all sides (360 degree angle) for accurate reconstruction in SPECT? Can it be less than 180 degree?
2. What is the primary benefit in using a dual- or triple-head scintillation camera in SPECT? What additional problems, if any, do these entail?
3. Why is quality control important in SPECT?
4. What two factors make quantitation with SPECT less accurate than PET?

5. What are the advantages of a CZT detector–based dedicated SPECT system over scintillation camera–based SPECT system?
6. Why is the resolving time of a coincidence circuit an important parameter in a PET scanner?
7. List all the factors that determine the resolution of a PET system.

# Biological Effects of Radiation and Risk Evaluation from Radiation Exposure

Interaction of radiation with biological systems results in a variety of biological changes that can be either deleterious or benign. These changes may become evident immediately or may take years or generations before being manifested. In general, the probability of occurrence and the type and severity of these changes depend on many factors, some related to radiation and its characteristics and others to biological characteristics of the system. Because a detailed account of these changes and the factors affecting them fall under the discipline of radiation biology, the discussion here is limited to only those aspects of radiation biology that are essential for an assessment of the possible dangers in the use of radiation as these relate to nuclear medicine.

## Mechanism of Biological Damage

Manifestation of bioinjury due to radiation is always preceded by a complex series of physiochemical events, as shown in Figure 15.1.

The first step in this series of events is the deposition of energy by radiation in the form of ionization and excitation of some atoms or molecules of the biological system as was explained in Chapter 6. This generally lasts about $10^{-12}$ seconds or less.

The second step, which may last from $10^{-12}$ to $10^{-3}$ seconds, is the transfer of energy either to neighboring molecules (intermolecular) or, quite often, within the molecule itself (intramolecular) to form various short-lived and chemically active species known as free radicals

(atomic or molecular entities with an unpaired electron and shown by a dot to the right side of the chemical symbol). Because water ($H_2O$) constitutes 75% to 85% of the mass of a living

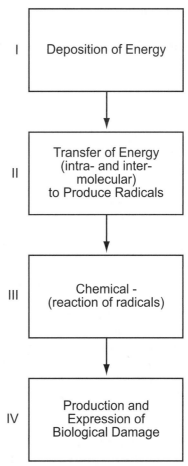

**Fig. 15.1.** Stages in the development of bioinjury by high-energy radiation exposure.

system, most ionization is produced in water, and the two most common radicals formed are H· and OH·.

In the next stage, which may last from milliseconds to several seconds, the free radicals react either among themselves or, more significantly, with other important biomolecules (e.g., DNA, RNA) to produce alterations in them. Reactions of H· and OH· radicals with important biological molecules cause most radiation damage observed in living systems.

The final step (i.e., the expression of the biological alteration produced in the previous stage) is the biological damage that is tied to the fate of these altered biomolecules. Eventual biological damage may be manifested within a short time or may be delayed up to several generations, depending on the type and function of these altered molecules and on the repair capacity of the irradiated biological system.

## Factors Affecting Biological Damage

Biological damage (or effect) to a system caused by radiation depends on the following factors.

**Radiation Dose** Any biological effect of radiation, whether deleterious or benign, strongly depends on the radiation dose. Generally, more effects, and more serious effects, are produced by high than low doses. The exact relationship of the dose to the effect produced, however, depends on the nature of the effect. For example, the dose–effect relationship for the induction of cancer differs from that causing genetic mutation. Depending on the dose–effect relationship, radiation effects are termed as stochastic or deterministic. In stochastic effects, the probability of occurrence, and not the severity of the effect, depends on the radiation dose. Two important examples are induction of cancer and genetic damage, where the probabilities of induction are a function of radiation dose but their severity is not. Stochastic effects do not have a threshold, a dose level below which the probability of occurrence is zero. Therefore, in radiation protection, where stochastic effects are of major concern, a common assumption is made that states that risk from radiation is

directly proportional to dose without a threshold. This assumption forms the basis of the so-called ALARA principle of radiation protection, discussed in Chapter 16.

In deterministic effects, on the other hand, the severity of effect depends on the radiation dose and has a threshold, a dose below which no effect is observed. Two examples of deterministic effects of radiation are production of cataracts and erythema.

**Dose Rate** In the case of low linear energy transfer (*LET*) radiations, if the same dose is delivered to two identical biological systems, one with a short duration (high dose rate) and the other over a longer period (low dose rate), the biological responses of the two systems will differ. High dose rates are more damaging than low dose rates.

**LET or Type of Radiation** Higher *LET* (see p. 57) radiations ($\alpha$ particles and protons) per unit of absorbed dose produce greater damage in a biological system than lower *LET* radiations (electrons and $\gamma$- and x-rays). The relative biological effectiveness (*RBE*) of a radiation for producing a given effect in a biological system under the same conditions is defined as follows:

$$RBE = \frac{\text{Dose of standard (x-ray) radiation needed to produce the same biological effect}}{\text{Dose of a second radiation needed to produce the same biological effect}}$$

For example, the *RBE* of 10-MeV neutrons for killing cells is about 10. In other words, 10-MeV neutrons are 10 times more effective at cell killing than x-rays (generally, 250-kVp x-rays are used as a reference). The "quality factor" Q and radiation weighting factor $W_R$ discussed in the next section are estimated from the *RBE* of a radiation.

**Type of Tissue** Biological response of a system varies widely depending on the type of tissue (e.g., liver, bone marrow, or nerve tissue) involved. Given the same radiation dose and dose rate, bone marrow is much more sensitive than nerve tissue to certain types of radiation damage. The tissue weighting factor $w_T$, discussed later, takes account of this variation when one compares radiation exposures from different sources.

**Amount of Tissue** Injury to a biological system also depends on the amount of tissue irradiated. For example, a mammal can tolerate a much higher dose to a part of the body than irradiation of the total body.

**Rate of Cell Turnover** The rate of cell turnover in tissues is deemed to affect the latent period for the expression of tissue damage. For tissues with a rapid cell turnover (bone marrow), damage appears earlier than for a slow cell turnover (liver).

**Biological Variation** The response of a biological system, even with all other factors constant, may vary enormously even among closely related individuals. One person may survive a total body dose of 400 rad (cGy), whereas a dose of only 200 rad (cGy) in another person may be lethal.

**Chemical Modifiers** The presence of certain chemicals is known to modify the response of a biological system to radiation. Substances that make biological systems more radioresistant are called radioprotectors. A good example of a radioprotector is the protein cysteine. Substances that make biological systems more radiosensitive are called radiosensitizers. An example of a radiosensitizer is molecular oxygen. For a radioprotector or radiosensitizer to have any effect, it must be present in the biological system during irradiation.

## Deleterious Effects in Humans

Deleterious effects in humans may be acute (mainly deterministic) or late (mainly stochastic). Acute effects are manifested within a short period after irradiation and range from transient nausea and vomiting to death. Late effects may take as long as several generations for eventual manifestation. These include stochastic effects, for example, induction of cancer and leukemia, birth defects, and other abnormalities in the offspring of the irradiated person (genetic damage); and nonstochastic effects, for example, cataracts, shortening of the overall life span, and production of temporary or permanent sterility in an individual.

**Acute Effects** These are generally produced when the radiation dose is high and delivered to a large part of the body in a short duration. Five clinically distinct stages can be identified as the radiation dose is progressively increased: no effect, mild damage to bone marrow, severe damage to bone marrow and mild damage to the gastrointestinal tract, severe damage to the gastrointestinal tract, and damage to the central nervous system. Table 15.1 lists the radiation doses and the typical symptoms produced for the four stages.

**Late Effects** Late effects may occur in cases where acute reactions are minimal (i.e., when the radiation dose to the total body is low or only part of the body is involved in the irradiation). In diagnostic uses of radiation, whether in radiology or nuclear medicine, the range of radiation doses generally delivered to a patient falls in this category. Therefore, the dose–effect relationship of late effects is of special interest.

Regrettably, precise information about the risks involving low radiation doses is difficult to obtain for the following reasons. First, the probability of occurrence of any late effect after low doses is small. Therefore, to perform statistically valid studies, large populations have to be considered. In practice, this is difficult to implement. Second, the occurrence of a latent period in the expression of late effects requires a long follow-up (10 years or more). Finally, late effects of radiation also occur naturally and more frequently than those caused by low doses of radiation. Because accurate information is lacking on the natural frequency of these effects, it is difficult to estimate the influence (increase or decrease) of low radiation doses. In addition, the frequency of natural occurrence is influenced by many complex factors such as age, sex, genetic history, geography, and various environmental and socioeconomic factors.

Despite these obstacles, a good estimation has been made of the risks to a person or a

| Table 15.1. | Radiation Doses and Acute Effects | |
| --- | --- | --- |
| **Stage** | **Dose Range (rad)** | **Symptoms** |
| No acute effect | 0–200 (0–2)[a] | Usually unobservable |
| 1 | 150–400 (1.5–4) | Transient nausea and vomiting; some evidence of damage to hematopoietic system, recovering in 1–2 months |
| 2 | 350–600 (5–6) | Severe damage to hematopoietic system; bone marrow transplant essential; survival chances moderate |
| 3 | 550–1000 (5.5–10) | Gastrointestinal damage; severe nausea, vomiting, and diarrhea; very small chance of recovery; death follows in 10–24 days |
| 4 | 1000 and above (10 and higher) | Confusion, shock, burning sensation; death follows within hours |

[a]Values in parentheses are in Gy.

population exposed to low radiation doses. Most information in this regard is derived from two sources: extrapolation from experiments conducted on laboratory animals (e.g., mice) and retrospective studies of the victims of the atomic bomb explosions in Nagasaki and Hiroshima, the inhabitants of Bikini and other Pacific islands who were exposed to radiation as a result of fallout, persons irradiated for medical reasons, and occupational workers such as uranium mine workers and radiation workers (e.g., radiologists). Two scientific committees, the United Nations Scientific Committee on the Effects of Atomic Radiation and the National Academy of Sciences Committee on the Biological Effects of Ionizing Radiations, are actively involved in evaluating these studies and estimating biological risk from radiation.

Of all late effects, the induction of cancer and genetic damage are the most important. The lifetime risk of a fatal cancer (any type) from a single uniform exposure to the total body depends on the age at the time of exposure and the dose and dose rate. The National Council on Radiation Protection (NCRP)

report 116 (1993) takes into account both factors and estimates the fatal cancer risks (probabilities) from 1 Sv radiation exposures as given in Table 15.2.

Information on genetic damage has been deduced mostly from results obtained in experiments with Mediterranean fruit flies (*Drosophila*) and laboratory mice. The present estimate of the doubling dose for genetic effects (the dose needed to double the natural incidence of a genetic or somatic anomaly) is in the range of 60 to 160 rad (0.6–1.6 Gy). This may be an overestimate because recent data indicate that humans are less sensitive to genetic damage than the fruit fly. For radiation protection, NCRP Report 116 estimates a risk value for severe hereditary effects of $0.8 \times 10^{-4}$ rem$^{-1}$ ($0.8 \times 10^{-2}$ Sv$^{-1}$) for workers (18 years or older) and $1.3 \times 10^{-4}$ rem$^{-1}$ ($1.3 \times 10^{-2}$ Sv$^{-1}$) for the general population (all ages). As can be safely inferred from these data, carcinogenic effects of radiation are more significant than genetic effects. Total detriment from radiation for cancer induction and genetic damage is then determined by adding the two risks.

| **Table 15.2.** Radiation Risk of Fatal Cancer to Various Populations | |
| --- | --- |
| **High Dose and High Dose Rate** | **Risk of Fatal Cancer** |
| General population (all ages) | $10 \times 10^{-4}\,\text{rem}^{-1}$ or $10 \times 10^{-2}\,\text{Sv}^{-1}$ |
| Working population (18 years or older) | $8 \times 10^{-4}\,\text{rem}^{-1}$ or $8 \times 10^{-2}\,\text{Sv}^{-1}$ |
| **Low Dose and Low Dose Rate** | |
| General population (all ages) | $5 \times 10^{-4}\,\text{rem}^{-1}$ or $5 \times 10^{-2}\,\text{Sv}^{-1}$ |
| Working population | $4 \times 10^{-4}\,\text{rem}^{-1}$ or $4 \times 10^{-2}\,(\text{Sv}^{-1})$ |

## Radiation Effects in the Fetus

The embryo and fetus are more susceptible to radiation than the adult. Radiation during fetal life may not only cause fetal death and induce cancer, but also produce various gross and behavioral abnormalities and malformations. The most sensitive stage for the production of these abnormalities is between 3 and 15 weeks after conception, and the most common abnormality in humans occurs in the central nervous system (mental retardation). Radiation studies of rodents during this interval suggest that doses as low as 5 rad (cGy) may produce gross congenital malformations. Below 5 rad, the main risk to a fetus is the increased probability of cancer, which at present is estimated to be two to three times that of an adult (i.e., $1 \times 10^{-3}\,\text{rem}^{-1}$ or $1 \times 10^{-1}\,\text{Sv}^{-1}$ for lifetime).

## Different Radiation Exposures and the Concepts of Equivalent Dose (Dose Equivalent) and Effective Dose (Effective Dose Equivalent)

Because biological effects, in addition to being dependent on dose, are modified by many factors, how do we take into account some of these factors when comparing the radiation risk from radiation doses delivered under a variety of conditions? Two advisory groups, the International Council on Radiation Protection (ICRP) and

NCRP, perform this task by considering the most recent scientific data and issuing periodic recommendations on the issues related to radiation protection. These recommendations are subsequently adopted, with minor variations, as rules or regulations by appropriate regulatory agencies. In the United States, the Nuclear Regulatory Commission (NRC) serves this purpose, and its rules and regulations are published in the Code of Federal Regulations under Title 10.

When comparing radiation risks, first factor, type of radiation, has been explicitly incorporated by the NCRP in the definition of a new term, "equivalent dose." The NRC still uses the old term "dose equivalent," which is slightly different as noted below. The second factor is tissue sensitivity. This is taken into account by defining a tissue weighting factor $W_T$. When both radiation weighting factor $W_R$ and tissue weighting are incorporated in risk estimates, NCRP defines a new term, "effective dose." NRC still uses the old term, effective dose equivalent.

### Equivalent Dose (Dose Equivalent)

Because biological effects per unit absorbed dose in a tissue T are dependent on the type of radiation (x- and γ-ray versus proton and a particle), a weighting factor $W_R$ is defined for each type of radiation to account for these differences. The weighted dose is called equivalent dose. To distinguish it from the absorbed dose D it is given in rem in conventional units and sievert Sv in SI units, denoted by the letter H. Thus,

$$H \text{ (rem or Sv)} = W_R \times D \text{ (rad or Gy)} \quad (1)$$

Luckily for radiations used in radiology or nuclear medicine (x- and $\gamma$-rays, electrons, and positrons), the radiation weighting factor, $W_R$ equals 1. Therefore, dose, D and equivalent dose, H are the same in amount but different in units, rem versus rad (Gy versus Sv). Consequently, all doses calculated in Chapter 7 can be easily converted into equivalent doses by simply changing the units from rad to rem (Gy to Sv). For neutrons and $\alpha$ particles, $W_R$ has a much higher value (10–20), but these do not concern us here.

Dose equivalent is used in NRC regulations and defined by an equation similar to equation (1) above except that instead of a radiation weighting factor $W_R$ a radiation quality factor $Q_R$ is used. For radiations used in nuclear medicine, $Q_R$ is also equal to one. Another difference is that, in the above equation, D is an average dose to a tissue, whereas dose equivalent is computed from dose to a point in the tissue. For all practical purposes in nuclear medicine, these two terms are interchangeable.

| **Table 15.3.** | Tissue Weighting Factors, $W_T$, for Different Tissues or Organs According to ICRP and NRC Regulations | |
|---|---|---|
| | **ICRP Report 103** | **NRC** |
| Gonads | 0.08 | 0.25 |
| Red bone marrow | 0.12 | 0.12 |
| Colon | 0.12 | 0.12 |
| Lung | 0.12 | 0.12 |
| Stomach | 0.12 | 0.12 |
| Bladder | 0.04 | 0.05 |
| Breast | 0.12 | 0.05 |
| Liver | 0.04 | 0.05 |
| Esophagus | 0.04 | 0.05 |
| Thyroid | 0.04 | 0.05 |
| Skin | 0.01 | 0.01 |
| Bone surface | 0.01 | 0.01 |
| Remainder | 0.12 | 0.05 |
| Brain | 0.01 | -- |
| Salivary glands | 0.01 | -- |

**Effective Dose, Effective Dose Equivalent, and Tissue Weighting Factors**
Because the risk estimates given in Table 15.2 are for a uniform total body irradiation, risks from a partial body or inhomogeneous irradiation have t o be adjusted appropriately. For this purpose, tissue factor $W_T$, which attempts to take into account the variations in radiosensitivity of different tissues (averaged over age and sex in a given population), is used. The currently recommended tissue factors by NCRP are given in Table 15.3. The NRC regulations still use the older weighting factors. These are also given in Table 15.3. By using NCRP tissue weighting factors, one determines an effective dose E for a given irradiation condition (exposure). However, by using the NRC tissue weighting factors, one determines the effective dose equivalent, or *ede*. The effective doses (or *edes*) are then used to compare the risks from exposures under different conditions such as exposure from background radiation versus radiation exposure from medical procedures to

the U.S. population. An exposure with higher effective dose (or *ede*) proportionally carries a higher risk. The effective dose (or *ede*, in which case NRC tissue weighting factors are used) is defined as follows:

$$E = \Sigma W_T H_T \quad (2)$$

where $\Sigma$ is summation over all irradiated tissues and organs T.

The NCRP recommended limits on exposures to the general public and workers are based on the effective dose that combines doses from both external and internal sources. These have been adopted by the NRC, again with a few modifications, and are given in the next chapter.

**Methodology for Comparison of Different Exposures** How does one compare radiation risks from a variety of radiation exposures? It is not a straightforward proposition because many factors (such as type of radiation, amount and type of tissue irradiated, age at the time of irradiation, sex, dose, and dose rate) are considered.

Recently, the NCRP considered most of these factors when exposure of the general population or radiation of occupational workers is involved and developed the following methodology.

First, estimate the average dose D (rad or Gy) to a tissue or tissues. Second, determine the equivalent dose $H_T$ by multiplying the average dose D by the appropriate radiation weighting factor $W_R$ as given by equation (1). Third, determine the effective dose by using tissue weighting factors and equation (2).

**Committed Equivalent Dose and Committed Effective Dose**    In the case of internally deposited radionuclides, two other terms, committed equivalent dose and committed effective dose, are used. This is to account for a wide range of the half-lives (from seconds to thousands of years) of radionuclides that exists in nature. Calculations of effective doses from internal sources of radiation due to ingestion or inhalation of radionuclides pose a problem, particularly those with half-lives longer than 100 years. Because radiation exposure beyond the average life span of a human (about 70 years) is meaningless, the dose calculation of Chapter 7 has to be modified for long-lived radionuclides (of course, none of these are used in nuclear medicine but are encountered as background). For such cases, the NRC defined two other terms, committed equivalent dose to a tissue and committed effective dose.

The committed equivalent dose to a tissue from an internal source of a radionuclide $H_T(\tau)$ is the integral of the dose rate [see Chapter 7, equation (2)] for time interval $\tau$ (instead of 0 to infinity). The committed effective dose from a radionuclide $E(\tau)$, then is the tissue weighted sum of $H_T(\tau)$ to all tissues as given by equation (2). $\tau$ denotes a specified period of exposure on which integration of the dose rate has to be performed ($\tau$ will vary with age at the time of intake for an individual). For a member of the general public (all ages), it is taken as 70 years and for a radiation worker (18 years or older), 50 years. In the case of a particular individual such as a radiation worker, his or her age at the time of intake will determine $\tau$.

# Sources of Radiation Exposure to U.S. Population

In the United States, people are exposed to radiation for a variety of reasons. These can be classified broadly under three categories, natural background, medical procedures, and technological and commercial uses. Of these, the first two are the major contributors to the radiation exposure of U.S. population.

The first major source of exposure is natural background radiation. Natural background radiation, possibly with no benefit, is present everywhere and all the time. There is little that can be done to eliminate it. It arises from extraterrestrial and terrestrial sources. Cosmic rays and radionuclides produced by them (e.g., $^{14}C$) are the primary source of extraterrestrial radiation. Its amount is lowest at sea level and it increases with altitude. Terrestrial sources of background radiation are long-lived radionuclides such as $^{226}Ra$ (daughter radionuclide, $^{222}Rn$, contributes the major portion of background radiation) and $^{40}K$ that are present in minute but varying quantities everywhere on earth. The radionuclide $^{40}K$ is incorporated in the food chain and as a result is also present in small amounts in humans.

The other major source of exposure is medical procedures that use high-energy radiation, such as CT, nuclear medicine and other radiological procedures.

Technological exposures results from radiation sources used in industry (e.g., nuclear weapons and nuclear energy, x-ray screening devices at the airports, etc.) or from other commercial activities (e.g., uranium mining, etc.). These contribute only a tiny fraction of total exposure of the U.S. population.

The average total effective dose to an individual from all these sources is currently estimated to be 6.2 mSv. This has increased significantly in recent years mainly due to increase in the number of medical procedures being performed. Of the total average effective dose, natural background is 3.1 mSv (50%), medical procedure 3.0 mSv (49%) and technological uses 0.1mSv (1%).

**Table 15.4.**    Effective Doses from Common Nuclear Medicine and Some Radiological Procedures

| Radiopharmaceutical | Radioactivity Dosage | | Effective Dose | |
| --- | --- | --- | --- | --- |
| | mCi | MBq | rem | mSv |
| $^{99m}$Tc-labeled | | | | |
| Pertechnetate | 10 | 370 | 0.48 | 4.8 |
| Phosphate, etc. | 10 | 370 | 0.21 | 2.1 |
| Sulfur Colloid | 3 | 111 | 0.10 | 1.0 |
| MA albumin | 3 | 111 | 0.12 | 1.2 |
| DMSA | 6 | 222 | 0.20 | 2.0 |
| DTPA | 20 | 740 | 0.16 | 16 |
| Red cells | 20 | 740 | 0.52 | 5.2 |
| HIDA, etc. | 5 | 185 | 0.31 | 3.1 |
| Mertiatide (MAG3) | 10 | 370 | 0.26 | 2.6 |
| Sestamibi (Cardiolite) | 30 | 1110 | 1.0 | 10 |
| Tetrofosmin (Myoview) | 30 | 1110 | 0.84 | 8.4 |
| Exametazime (Ceretec) | 20 | 740 | 0.7 | 7 |
| $^{67}$Ga Citrate | 5 | 185 | 1.8 | 18 |
| $^{111}$In-Pentetreotide (OctreoScan) | 3 | 111 | 0.6 | 6 |
| $^{123}$I-Iodide | 0.1 | 3.7 | 0.08 | 0.8 |
| $^{123}$I-MIBG | 10 | 370 | 0.3 | 3 |
| $^{133}$Xe | 10 | 370 | 0.054 | 0.54 |
| $^{201}$Tl-Thallous Chloride | 3 | 111 | 0.18 | 18 |
| $^{18}$FDG | 10 | 370 | 0.7 | 7 |
| Chest x-ray | - | - | - | 0.04 |
| CT (head) | - | - | | 1.8 |
| CT(abdomen) | - | - | | 7.6 |

## Effective Doses in Nuclear Medicine and Comparison with Other Sources of Exposure

Among all sources of medical exposure, CT contributes the most about 49% (1.5 mSv), nuclear medicine about 26% (0.8 mSv). Considering the health benefits they provide, exposure from nuclear medicine procedures is a minor risk factor for the individual patient but is an important contributing factor to the total effective dose received by the U.S. population.

In nuclear medicine, two types of populations are exposed to radiation: patients who receive radiopharmaceuticals for medical benefit (discussed above) and radiation workers such as technologists, physicists, and physicians. What about radiation exposure to nuclear medicine personnel? It is estimated to be about 100 mrem (1 mSv) per year for diagnostic radiology and nuclear medicine personnel and is the lowest among radiation workers such as uranium mine workers (23 mSv), nuclear power personnel

(5.5 mSv), radiation therapy workers (1.7 mSv), and special radiology procedures (18 mSv).

Effective dose is primarily used to compare radiation risks to the general population or a group of radiation workers. However, as a guideline, these can also be used to compare risks to patients from different medical procedures. For example, to compare risks from two nuclear medicine procedures, one first calculates the radiation dose (rad or Gy) to various organs from the two procedures, as was done in Chapter 7. Radiation doses are then converted into equivalent doses (rem or Sv) by multiplying by the radiation weighting factor (1.0 in this case). Radiation doses to various organs from the two procedures are then multiplied by their tissue weighting factors (Table 15.3) and added together to obtain the effective dose for each procedure. The procedures with higher effective doses carry a proportionally higher risk. For example, the radiopharmaceuticals $^{67}$Ga citrate and $^{99m}$Tc-labeled phosphate compounds give effective doses of 22 and 5 mSv, respectively. It means that gallium imaging carries about four times more risk than bone imaging. This is a different, but more realistic, conclusion than if we compared either the total body or critical organ doses listed in Table 7.5 (Chapter 6) for the two procedures. Table 15.4 gives average effective doses from common nuclear procedures for an adult patient. For comparison, effective doses from a few diagnostic procedures are also listed. Note that with the exception of $^{67}$Ga and $^{201}$Tl, effective doses in nuclear medicine are comparable to radiological procedures (not including fluoroscopic procedures where effective doses can be quite high). Also, effective doses given here will change if the administered dosage is different than that given in this table. As these are average doses, these may deviate considerably in the case of a particular individual and in children in particular.

## Key Points

1. Biological effects of radiation are preceded by a variety of physiochemical processes.

2. Biological effects are dependent on total dose, dose rate, *LET* of radiation, type and amount of tissue irradiated, and presence or absence of chemical modifiers in the irradiated tissue.

3. Two kinds of biological effects, stochastic and nonstochastic, are observed. Nonstochastic effects are observed at high doses and high dose rates and have a threshold, and the severity of the effect, depends on the dose. Stochastic effects are assumed not to have a threshold and the probability of occurrence is related to the dose, not the severity of the effect. At low doses and dose rates (most diagnostic exposures), radiation risk to an exposed individual primarily comes from stochastic effects.

4. For the same dose, biological effect may be different for different radiations and different tissues. The two terms, equivalent dose and effective dose, are designed to account for these two variables of the biological effect.

5. In humans, induction of cancer and genetic damage are the two deleterious effects of radiation that are of major concern.

6. Medical radiation exposure to the U.S. population is almost equal to that received from background radiation. Exposure from nuclear medicine procedures is only 26% of all medical radiation exposure to the U.S. population.

## Questions

1. List the various stages in the development of radiation injury.
2. For the same radiation dose, what are the other factors that can modify the biological effects or their intensity?
3. Generally, below what dose are acute effects not observable?
4. Name the most common late biological effect and give its probability of occurrence after 1 rem of total body irradiation at low dose rate to a general population.
5. What is the most sensitive period during pregnancy for the development of a fetal abnormality?
6. What factor relates absorbed dose to equivalent dose or dose equivalent?
7. What is tissue weighting factor and why is it needed?
8. Effective doses from an internally absorbed radionuclide have to be modified. Why? How?
9. What are the two major sources of radiation exposure to U.S. population?
10. What percentage of total medical radiation exposure to U.S. population is contributed by nuclear medicine procedures?
11. What two nuclear procedures give most effective dose to a patient?

# 16

# Methods of Safe Handling of Radionuclides and Pertaining Rules and Regulations

Any use of radionuclides is fraught with the danger of inadvertently exposing an individual to radiation, and therefore to its attendant hazards. This is especially true in the nuclear medicine laboratory where large amounts of unsealed radioactive sources are routinely handled. Each time a generator is milked, a radiopharmaceutical dose is drawn or injected, or a scan is performed on a patient, there is the possibility of exposure and contamination to the user (technician, physicist, or physician) and to the environment. Keeping this in mind, this chapter has two broad objectives: to describe the principles for minimizing radiation exposure, provide some practical ways in which an individual user can minimize exposure to oneself and fellow workers, and reduce contamination of the environment, and to give an overview of the extent and the scope of the pertinent rules and regulations that govern the use of radionuclides in nuclear medicine. For detailed descriptions, reading of the actual and most recent documents (the rules and regulations in this area are subject to periodic changes) is recommended.

## Principles of Reducing Exposure from External Sources

Exposure: Hazard from external radiation sources is measured in terms of exposure. Exposure is a measure of the ability of radiation to produce ionization in air. The unit of exposure is the roentgen R, that level of radiation which produces ionization in air in the amount of $2.58 \times 10^{-4}$ coulomb/kg of air. A milliroentgen mR is one-thousandth of a roentgen. The SI units of exposure are simply coulomb/kg. Therefore, 1 coulomb/kg = 3876 R.

If the exposure is known at a given point, one can calculate the absorbed dose to a person at that point by multiplying the exposure by a term known as f factor. For muscle and soft tissue, f factor is close to unity. Therefore, for purposes in nuclear medicine, we may assume that exposure is more or less equivalent to the absorbed dose, which is equal to dose equivalent, that is, 1 R (1/3876 coulomb/kg) ≡ 1 rad (0.01 Gy) ≡ 1 rem (0.01 Sv).

The principle of reducing exposure to radiation from sources outside the body (x- and γ-ray-emitting radionuclides only) can be summed up in three equally important words: time, distance, and shielding.

**Time** Because the total radiation dose, whether to the total body or part of the body, is directly proportional to the time of exposure, it is extremely important to spend as little time as possible near x- or γ-ray-emitting radionuclide sources. This requires forethought and precaution by the user. For example, when eluting a $^{99}$Mo generator, one should not stand near it while the elution is in progress. When injecting a dose to a patient, one should locate the vein first and then take the syringe containing the radionuclide dose out of the leaded syringe carrier. However, rushing through a procedure is definitely not suggested here; if one has to repeat a procedure because of haste, total exposure time will be doubled.

**Distance** Radiation dose to the body from a small external source varies inversely with the square of the distance of the source from the body (i.e., if we increase the distance from a source of radiation by a factor of 2, the radiation dose will drop by a factor of 4). Therefore, one should use a cart with a long handle when carrying very hot (>50 mCi) radionuclide sources emitting high-energy γ-rays (>300 keV) from one place to another, even though these sources are shielded. When radionuclide sources that are moderate in activity (≈10 mCi) are hand-carried, the source should be held away from the body.

In drawing a dose for injection, use a syringe large enough so that it is no more than half full when the desired volume is added and handle it from the unfilled area. If it is necessary to work with hot sources for long periods, then one should seriously consider the use of various remote-control tools available for picking up a radioactive vial or pipetting a radioactive solution.

**Shielding** γ- and x-rays can be effectively shielded using thick containers, bricks, or partitions made of lead. Mirrors should be used for viewing behind lead partitions. The amount of actual shielding needed to reduce exposure to a minimal level depends on the amount of radioactivity to be shielded and the energy of the γ-rays. Use of a syringe lead shield to reduce exposure during radiopharmaceutical injection is essential in view of the ALARA ("as low as reasonably acceptable") principle. However, lead aprons worn in diagnostic radiology are not very effective in reducing exposure in nuclear medicine and therefore are not recommended.

**Calculation of Exposure from External Sources**
The three variables, time, distance, and shielding, can be combined in a single formula that gives the exposure from a small radioactive source:

$$E = \frac{n\Gamma}{d^2} \cdot e^{-\mu(\text{linear}) \cdot x} \cdot t \qquad (1)$$

Here E is the exposure R, n is the number of millicuries in the source, d is the distance (cm) of the point (at which exposure is desired) from the source, t is the time of exposure (hour), $\mu$(linear) is the linear attenuation coefficient of the shielding material (cm$^{-1}$), and x is the thickness of the

shielding material (cm). Γ* is the exposure rate constant of the radionuclide and its units are R · cm$^2$/mCi · h. The higher the value of Γ of a radionuclide, the more radiation risk it produces. For $^{99m}$Tc, its value is 0.60 and for $^{18}$F, its value is 5.1 R · cm$^2$/mCi · h. As a result, for unshielded sources, $^{18}$F exposes a person 8.5 times more than $^{99m}$Tc for the same amount of radioactivity.

With the increasing use of $^{18}$F and other PET radiopharmaceuticals, this is a potentially serious source of radiation exposure to nuclear medicine personnel. It is more so because the γ-ray energy is 511 keV, which is quite high for shielding to be effective (half value layer of lead for $^{99m}$Tc is 0.3 mm and for $^{18}$F is 3.0 mm. Thus, 3-mm-thick lead will reduce $^{99m}$Tc exposure by a factor of 1000, but it will reduce $^{18}$F only by a factor of 2.), particularly during the administration of injection and when it is in the patient. Short half-life of $^{18}$F does help in this regard. For other radionuclides of interest to nuclear medicine, values of Γ are given in Appendix A.

**Examples**

(1) Calculate the exposure in 1 minute to the tips of the fingers from a syringe held by the tips of the fingers and containing 15 mCi of $^{99m}$Tc radioactivity (assume the distance of the radioactivity from the tips of the fingers is 3 cm).

In this case,

n = 15 mCi    Γ = 0.60 R · cm$^2$/mCi · h

$t = 1 \text{ minute} = \frac{1}{60} \text{ hour}$

x = 0 (no shielding, neglect absorption in the source)

d = 3 cm

Substituting these values in equation (1),

$$E = \frac{15 \times 0.6}{3^2} \cdot e^{-\mu(\text{linear}) \cdot 0} \cdot \frac{1}{60} R$$

$$= 0.017 \text{ R} = 17 \text{ mR}$$

(2) Calculate the same exposure as in example 1 except this time the syringe is shielded by 1-mm-thick lead [$\mu$(linear) = 25 cm$^{-1}$]. In this case, x = 1 mm = 0.1 cm and $\mu$(linear) = 25 cm$^{-1}$.

---

* For radiation protection work, γ- or x-rays with energies less than 20 keV are not included in λ

All other factors are the same.
Therefore, using equation (1), we get

$$E = \frac{15 \times 0.6}{3^2} \cdot e^{-25 \times 0.1} \cdot \frac{1}{60} R$$

$$= 0.017 \, e^{-2.5}$$

$$= 0.017 \times 0.08 = 0.00136 \, R$$

$$= 1.36 \, mR$$

(3)   A patient has been injected with 15 mCi of $^{99m}$Tc radioactivity. Calculate the exposure to a technician who, on average, takes 30 minutes to perform the scan and stays at about 1 m away from the patient during this time. (Assume the radioactivity is localized in a small volume in the patient and that there is no attenuation in the patient.) In this case,

n = 15 mCi, $\Gamma$ = 0.60 R · cm²/mCi · h

d = 1 m = 100 cm

t = 30 minutes = 0.5 hours

x = 0 and $\mu$(linear) = 0

Using equation (1),

$$E = \frac{15 \times 0.6}{100^2} \cdot e^{-0} \cdot 0.5R$$

$$= \frac{15 \times 0.6 \times 0.5}{10,000} = 0.00045R$$

$$= 0.45 \, mR$$

If the attenuation in the patient is also taken into account, the exposure will be further reduced, probably by a factor of 4.

(4)   Same as example 3 but for 15 mCi of $^{18}$FDG.

$$E = \frac{15 \times 5.1}{100^2} \cdot e^{-0} \cdot 0.5R$$

$$= \frac{15 \times 5.1 \times 0.5}{10,000}$$

$$= 0.00382 \, R = 3.8 \, mR$$

These illustrative examples show the extent of the possible exposure in nuclear medicine. The other and very important source of exposure is the radionuclide generator.

## Avoiding Internal Contamination

Internal contamination by a radionuclide is possible by three routes: penetration through skin, ingestion, and inhalation. To avoid ingestion or penetration through the skin, the following steps should be taken.

1.  Wear coveralls or a laboratory coat and disposable gloves each time you handle a radioactive material. Remember that the gloves, once you handle a radioactive material, become contaminated. Because they are the easiest source of spread of contamination in the laboratory, discard them immediately after handling radioactive material. When handling highly radioactive material, it is wise to wear two pairs of gloves.

2.  Do not eat, drink, or smoke in the radionuclide laboratory or pipette radioactive solutions by mouth. Before eating, when you have been handling radioactive compounds, wash your hands thoroughly.

3.  Keep the area neat in which radionuclides are handled. Use a tray with absorbent liners on the bench to limit the spread of radioactive material in case of an accident while working with unsealed radioactive sources.

4.  Because the bed sheets, pillows, and stretchers used when scanning patients may be contaminated as a result of a patient's saliva, blood, or urine, beware of this route of personal contamination.

Contamination by inhalation does not pose a great problem in nuclear medicine except in a few cases where radioactive gases are used or large amounts of radioiodine are handled. To avoid the contamination of the room by radioactive gases, such items should be stored under a fume hood and, while using proper care should be taken to prevent these gases from escaping into the room. In the case of large amounts of radioiodine, all work should be performed under a fume hood if possible. When opening a vial containing high amounts of radioiodine-labeled compounds, the vial should be extended away from you. In the administration of therapeutic doses of $^{131}$I, allow patients to open the vial and drink the dose by themselves.

## The Radioactive Patient

A radioactive patient is an important source of radiation in nuclear medicine. Through penetrating radiations (x- or $\gamma$-rays), the patient can irradiate persons at a distance. Through physical contact or excretion and exhalation into the environment, the patient becomes a source of internal contamination. Presently, a patient has to be isolated in a private room if he or she has received more than 30 mCi (111 MBq) of radioactivity of a radionuclide or the measured dose equivalent at 1 m is less than 5 mrem/h (0.5 Sv/h). There are no such restrictions for radioactivity under this amount. However, because of ALARA, proper health physics principles, some of which have been described earlier, should be followed to keep the radiation exposure to a minimum level. Patients containing radioactivities of $^{131}$I in amounts of 37 to 111 MBq (10-mCi) have a potential of exposing close relatives to more than 100 mrem (1 mSv) of effective equivalent dose (exposure limit for the general public). Therefore, appropriate instructions for limited contact with close family members and contamination containment should be provided to the patient.

With the increasing use of PET radiopharmaceuticals, $^{18}$FDG containing patients are another potential source of exposure to the nuclear medicine personnel as well as to the general population. Since in this case, the $\gamma$-ray energy is 511 keV, shielding is not a viable option; distance and time are the only realistic choices.

**Special Case of a Nursing Mother** A nursing mother is a special case of a radioactive patient that needs to be discussed separately. Because many radionuclides are excreted in milk, an infant dependent on his or her mother's milk may be exposed to undue risk. In such cases, all alternatives should be carefully weighed. For tests performed with technetium-labeled compounds, a simple rule of 2 days' cessation of breast feeding works well. For all of these compounds, the mother's radioactivity will decay by a factor of 1000 or more during this interval and, therefore, little if any will be ingested by the infant. However, for tests using radionuclides such as $^{67}$Ga, $^{111}$In, $^{131}$I, and $^{201}$Tl, the situation is quite complex. Careful assessment and monitoring, coupled with several weeks of cessation, may be required to ensure that the infant is not exposed to undue risk.

# Rules and Regulations

**U.S. Regulatory Agencies** To ensure proper and safe use of radionuclides, a number of federal and state (called agreement states) agencies set standards for protection against radiation and issue regulations for production, transportation, possession, use, and disposal of radionuclides. The standards and regulations are primarily, but not entirely, based on the recommendation of the International Council on Radiation Protection and the National Council on Radiation Protection (NCRP). The U.S. Nuclear Regulatory Commission (NRC) is the federal agency most responsible for these regulations. These are published in the code of Federal Regulations under Title 10. The reader is urged to read this document, particularly parts 20 and 35, which are of direct relevance to nuclear medicine. NRC rules and regulations apply strictly only to the radionuclide produced by a nuclear reactor and not to radionuclides produced by a particle accelerator or cyclotron. The U.S. Food and Drug Administration is responsible for the regulations of the production of radiopharmaceuticals and their clinical or research use in humans. Two other federal agencies with shared responsibility with NRC are the Department of Transportation, which sets regulations for transport of radionuclides, and the Environmental Protection Agency, which sets regulations for the release of radionuclides in the atmosphere.

**Exposure or Dose Limits: Annual Limit on Intake and Derived Air Concentration** Table 16.1 lists the exposure limits to various categories of persons. Both external and internal exposures are included, but exposure from natural sources is excluded from these limits. External doses are for tissues deeper than 1 cm (the deep dose equivalent) and the internal doses are committed effective doses. The dose limits are given as total effective dose equivalent and are based on the current NRC regulations. These are slightly different from those in NCRP Report 116. One major difference between the two is due to the use of different tissue weighting factors, as discussed in Chapter 15.

**Table 16.1.** Current NRC Maximum Permissible Annual Dose Limits

|  | Dose Limit (mSv) |
| --- | --- |
| **Radiation (occupational) workers** | |
| Total effective dose equivalent limits | 50 |
| Dose equivalent limits to tissues and organs | |
| Lens of eye | 150 |
| Skin, hands, and feet | 500 |
| Any other organ or tissue | 500 |
| **General public** | |
| Total effective dose equivalent | 1 |
| **Embryo–fetus (entire pregnancy, 9 months)** | |
| Total effective dose equivalent | 5 |

Normal annual exposures of workers in a clinical nuclear medicine department seldom exceed these limits and generally are about one-tenth of these limits.

Although these limits include internal exposure from radionuclides, calculations of committed effective dose and committed equivalent dose from different radionuclides are complicated (see Chapters 7 and 15). Therefore, to reduce the need of these calculations by the individual user, two new entities that put limits on the intake of radionuclides based on the effective dose equivalent to a "reference man" (similar to the "standard man" of Chapter 7) are defined: the annual limit on intake *ALI* and the derived air concentration *DAC*. These limits are published by the NRC for a large number of radionuclides and should not be exceeded.

*ALI* is defined as the amount of radioactivity of a radionuclide that if taken into the body would give a person (reference man) an effective dose equivalent of 50 mSv in 1 year. The ALI for $^{99m}$Tc compounds is in millicuries and for $^{131}$I in microcuries. These are relatively large limits and are never reached under normal and proper use of radiopharmaceuticals.

For airborne radioactivity, *DAC* is defined as *ALI* divided by the volume of air inhaled by a reference man in a working year ($2.4 \times 10^3$ m$^3$).

**ALARA Principle** The limits in Table 16.1 are legal and are not to be exceeded at any time. However, these limits do not imply that radiation below this level is harmless or safe. The guiding principle in radiation protection or health physics is that radiation doses should be "as low as reasonably achievable" (ALARA). This philosophy is mandated by law and therefore puts the onus on the user to reduce radiation levels in work places to as low a level as is economically and technologically feasible, even if these levels are well below the legal limits.

**Types of Licenses** To practice nuclear medicine, a license issued by the NRC or an agreement state (New York City is one exception where a state has given its authority to a city) is required. The license can be for limited or broad use. A limited-use license is primarily designed for physicians in private practice or hospitals desiring to use radionuclides for specific purposes such as routine and well-established procedures. The broad-use license is issued to large medical centers and it allows, in addition to the use for routine procedures, a wider scope for research and development of new procedures. There are strict educational and training requirements to qualify for the license and a licensee takes upon him or herself to abide by all the conditions of a license.

**Radiation Safety Committee and Radiation Safety Officer** One important requirement of the NRC is the establishment of a radiation safety committee (RSC) consisting of representatives from medical departments using radionuclides and administration. The RSC has the overall responsibility for the radiation safety under the license. It (or a licensee when an RSC is not mandated) designates a radiation safety officer (RSO), who is responsible for the actual implementation and monitoring of the safety program.

**Personnel Monitoring** For the safety of nuclear medicine personnel, monitoring of radiation levels is required. This includes both external and internal monitoring.

**External Monitoring** External monitoring is performed with small inexpensive dosimeters that can be worn on some part of the body externally. Three types of personnel monitors—film dosimeters, thermoluminescent dosimeters (TLDs), and pocket dosimeters—are used for external monitoring of radiation exposure.

Of these, the film dosimeter is the most common and economical, although not the most accurate. It consists of a small film enclosed in a plastic container with four windows covered with different radiation filters (e.g., no filter, aluminum, lead and aluminum, and cadmium and aluminum) to identify the nature and energy of the exposing radiation. The darkening on the film (film density; see Chapter 11) is related to the exposure level. It can measure radiation doses from 0.1 mGy to as high as 15 Gy. Film in the dosimeter is normally changed each month. The old film is developed, exposure measured, and kept as a permanent record.

The TLD, as described in Chapter 8, is made of substances, such as LiF, that store in them the energy deposited by a radiation exposure for a long period and release it as light when they are subjected to heat. The amount of light produced is directly related to the radiation exposure. TLDs are accurate but expensive and, unlike a film dosimeter, do not provide a permanent record.

Pocket dosimeters are small ionization chambers, Geiger–Mueller (GM) tubes, or semiconductor detectors that can measure and instantaneously display the radiation exposure. These are available for different ranges of exposures and used primarily for monitoring high-level exposures of short duration. These do not provide a permanent record.

**Internal Monitoring** Exposure from internal uptake of radionuclides as a result of occupational exposure is monitored through bioassays such as measurement of organ or total body uptake and urine or blood analysis for presence of radioactivity. Bioassay is required whenever $^{131}$I is used for therapeutic purposes.

**Receipt, Use, and Disposal of Radionuclides** A licensee is required to keep detailed records of the radioactivity received, the amount in storage, the amount used, and the amount disposed, if any, for all radionuclides he or she is authorized to possess. In no case should the total activity in possession exceed that allowed by the license.

Disposal of radionuclides for short-lived radionuclides such as $^{99m}$Tc, $^{123}$I, $^{67}$Ga, $^{201}$Tl, and $^{111}$In is through decay in storage for a time period in which the radiation levels are reduced to less than two times the background. Excreta from radioactive patients can be released directly into the sewerage. Any other radioactive waste has severe restrictions on its release in sewerage or, in cases of gases such as $^{133}$Xe, into the atmosphere. Of course, radioactive waste can always be transferred to an authorized recipient. Disposal of the old radionuclidic generators by returning it to the parent company is through such transfer.

**Control and Labeling of Areas Where Radionuclides Are Stored and/or Used** The NRC mandates classification of areas as restricted and unrestricted. For restricted areas, it requires posting of warning signs, symbols, and labels denoting radiation. These include "Caution, Radiation Area" (>5 mrem/h or 0.05 mSv/h dose equivalent at 30 cm from the source), "Caution, High-Radiation Area" (>100 mrem/h or 1 mSv/h at 30 cm from the source), and "Caution, Radioactive Material" (in areas where radioactive material is stored or used and on containers of radioactive material).

**Contamination Survey and Radiation-Level Monitoring** Depending on the level of radiation and the amount of radioactive material used, a licensee is required to monitor periodically the radiation levels and to wipe test for contamination of the areas where radiopharmaceuticals are handled or stored. A weekly survey of ambient radiation levels is performed with a calibrated GM counter. Calibration of the GM counter should be checked annually. Wipe tests are done by swabbing multiple areas with an absorbing material such as paper and counting them with a radiation detector [NaI(Tl) well-type counter if available]. If contamination exceeds the regulatory limits, decontamination of the area is required. These limits are 0.01 $\mu$Ci (370 Bq)/100 cm$^2$ for $^{99m}$Tc and 0.001 $\mu$Ci (37 Bq)/100 cm$^2$ for $^{131}$I.

**Receiving and Shipping (Transport) of Radioactive Packages** Monitoring of all packages labeled "radioactive material" is required. First, a visual inspection to establish the integrity of the package is performed. Then, radiation levels at the surface and 1 m are measured, and a wipe test for possible surface contamination is performed. When the radiation levels exceed 200 mrem/h (2 mSv/h) at the surface or 10 mrem/h (0.1 mSv/h) at 1 m and/or the wipe test shows a reading of 22,000 decays per minute, prompt notification to appropriate authorities should be made.

To protect and warn of possible dangers to persons who may come in contact with a radioactive package, the Department of Transportation has issued specific rules and regulations for shipping radioactive packages. Three types of labels, depending on the surface level of radiation, are required: white—I, surface exposure less than 0.5 mR/h; yellow—II, surface exposure between 0.5 and 50 mR/h and exposure at 1 m less than 1 mR/h; and yellow—III, surface exposure between 50 and 200 mR/h and exposure at 1 m between 1 and 10 mR/h.

**Accidental Radioactive Spills** Despite taking the necessary and appropriate precautions, accidents happen and a spill of radioactive material may occur. A radioactive spill is classified as minor (less than a millicurie) or major (more than a millicurie). For major spills, the RSO has to be notified, who then investigates the incident and recommends corrective action.

In case of a spill, access to the area should be immediately restricted, the spill contained by using liquid absorbers or closing of the room in case of radioactive gases or vapors, and it should be followed by decontamination of the personnel involved and the area of spill.

## Key Points

1. Radiation exposure in the nuclear medicine laboratory can result from both external and internal sources.
2. External exposure can be minimized by keeping one's distance from the radioactive source, spending minimum time necessary near a radioactive source, and shielding radioactive sources appropriately.
3. Internal contamination can be reduced by following proper laboratory procedures.
4. There are regulatory limits (Table 16.1) on exposure to radiation workers and the general public. There are no regulatory limits on radiation exposure to patients except that benefits outweigh the risk of a medical exposure.
5. Monitoring of the external exposure and internal uptake, in certain circumstances, of nuclear medicine personnel is mandatory.
6. There are general rules and regulations for possessing, using, and disposing of radionuclides and some specific rules related to medical use of radionuclides. All persons working in nuclear medicine should be aware of these rules.

## Questions

1. Which radionuclide with the following exposure rate constant $\Gamma$ poses the most danger as an external source of radiation? (a) 2.0 R/mCi/h, (b) 100 mR/mCi/h, (c) 2.0 R/mCi/day, and (d) 1.0 R/mCi/min.

2. A patient who was treated with 100 mCi of radioiodine measured 10 mR/h at 100 cm at the time of administration. By the next day, this measurement dropped to 2 mR/h. How much radioactivity does the patient still have?

3. Why is $^{18}$F more of a concern from the radiation exposure perspective than $^{99m}$Tc?

4. A radioactive syringe produces an exposure rate of 1 R/h at a distance of 20 cm. Calculate the exposures of two persons who were working for 3 hours at 50 and 100 cm, respectively, from the syringe.

5. A nursing mother was given 10 mCi of a radiopharmaceutical. How long should she be asked to stop breast feeding her baby?

6. Which is the larger source of internal contamination: ingestion or inhalation?

7. What does ALARA stands for?

8. What limits are currently imposed on the radiation exposure of a radiation worker, a pregnant radiation worker, member of the general population, and a patient?

9. Does a film-type exposure dosimeter measure total effective dose equivalent?

10. What actions are required when a radioactive package is received?

11. How are major and minor radioactive spills classified?

# Physical Characteristics of Some Radionuclides of Interest in Nuclear Medicine

**Table A.1.** Radiations Emitted in the Decay of $^{123}$I ($\Gamma = 1 \cdot 53$ R $\cdot$ cm$^2$/mCi $\cdot$ h); $T_{\frac{1}{2}} = 13$ h

| Number | Radiation (i) | Frequency of Emission ($n_i$) | Mean Energy (MeV) ($E_i$) |
|--------|---------------|-------------------------------|---------------------------|
| 1 | $\gamma_1$ | 0.84 | 0.159 |
| 2 | K conversion electron | 0.13 | 0.127 |
| 3 | L conversion electron | 0.02 | 0.154 |
| 4 | $\gamma_2$ | 0.01 | 0.529 |
| 5 | X-ray-K ($\alpha$) | 0.71 | 0.027 |
| 6 | X-ray-K ($\beta$) | 0.15 | 0.031 |
| 7 | X-ray-L | 0.13 | 0.003 |
| 8 | LMM Auger electron | 0.92 | 0.003 |
| 9 | MXY Auger electron | 2.19 | 0.001 |

**Table A.2.** Radiations Emitted in the Decay of $^{131}$I ($\Gamma = 2 \cdot 2$ R $\cdot$ cm$^2$/mCi $\cdot$ h); $T_{\frac{1}{2}} = 8.1$ days

| Number | Radiation (i) | Frequency of Emission ($n_i$) | Mean Energy (MeV) ($E_i$) |
|--------|---------------|-------------------------------|---------------------------|
| 1 | $\beta_1$ | 0.02 | 0.069 |
| 2 | $\beta_2$ | 0.07 | 0.096 |
| 3 | $\beta_3$ | 0.90 | 0.192 |
| 4 | $\gamma_1$ | 0.03 | 0.080 |
| 5 | K conversion electron | 0.03 | 0.046 |
| 6 | $\gamma_2$ | 0.06 | 0.284 |
| 7 | $\gamma_3$ | 0.82 | 0.364 |
| 8 | K conversion electron | 0.02 | 0.330 |
| 9 | $\gamma_4$ | 0.07 | 0.637 |
| 10 | $\gamma_5$ | 0.02 | 0.723 |

From *J Nucl Med* 1975; (Suppl 10).

**Table A.3.** Radiations Emitted in the Decay of $^{201}$Tl ($\Gamma = 0.47$ R $\cdot$ cm$^2$/mCi $\cdot$ h); $T_{\frac{1}{2}} = 73$ h

| Number | Radiation (i) | Frequency of Emission ($n_i$) | Mean Energy (MeV) ($E_i$) |
|---|---|---|---|
| 1 | $\gamma_1$ | 0.01 | 0.032 |
| 2 | L conversion electron | 0.21 | 0.018 |
| 3 | M conversion electron | 0.07 | 0.029 |
| 4 | $\gamma_2$ | 0.04 | 0.135 |
| 5 | K conversion electron | 0.10 | 0.052 |
| 6 | L conversion electron | 0.02 | 0.121 |
| 7 | $\gamma_3$ | 0.12 | 0.167 |
| 8 | K conversion electron | 0.18 | 0.084 |
| 9 | L conversion electron | 0.03 | 0.154 |
| 10 | X-ray-K ($\alpha$) | 0.78 | 0.070 |
| 11 | X-ray-K ($\beta$) | 0.22 | 0.081 |
| 12 | X-ray-L | 0.46 | 0.010 |
| 13 | KLL Auger electron | 0.03 | 0.055 |
| 14 | KLX Auger electron | 0.02 | 0.066 |
| 15 | LMM Auger electron | 0.81 | 0.008 |
| 16 | MXY Auger electron | 2.44 | 0.003 |

**Table A.4.** Radiations Emitted in the Decay of $^{133}$Xe ($\Gamma = 0 \cdot 15$ R $\cdot$ cm$^2$/mCi $\cdot$ h); $T_{\frac{1}{2}} = 5.3$ days

| Number | Radiation (i) | Frequency of Emission ($n_i$) | Mean Energy (MeV) ($E_i$) |
|---|---|---|---|
| 1 | $\beta_1$ | 0.02 | 0.075 |
| 2 | $\beta_2$ | 0.98 | 0.101 |
| 3 | $\gamma_1$ | 0.01 | 0.080 |
| 4 | K conversion electron | 0.01 | 0.044 |
| 5 | $\gamma_2$ | 0.36 | 0.081 |
| 6 | K conversion electron | 0.53 | 0.045 |
| 7 | L conversion electron | 0.08 | 0.076 |
| 8 | M conversion electron | 0.03 | 0.080 |
| 9 | X-ray-K ($\alpha$) | 0.39 | 0.030 |
| 10 | X-ray-K ($\beta$) | 0.09 | 0.035 |
| 11 | X-ray-L | 0.08 | 0.004 |
| 12 | Auger electrons | 1.67 | 0.003 |

**Table A.5.**  Radiations Emitted in the Decay of $^{111}$In ($\Gamma = 1 \cdot 9$ R $\cdot$ cm$^2$/mCi $\cdot$ h); T$_{\frac{1}{2}}$ = 67.4 h

| Number | Radiation (i) | Frequency of Emission (n$_i$) | Mean Energy (MeV) (E$_i$) |
|--------|---------------|-------------------------------|---------------------------|
| 1 | $\gamma_1$ | 0.90 | 0.172 |
| 2 | K conversion electron | 0.09 | 0.145 |
| 3 | L conversion electron | 0.01 | 0.168 |
| 4 | $\gamma_2$ | 0.94 | 0.247 |
| 5 | K conversion electron | 0.05 | 0.220 |
| 6 | L conversion electron | 0.007 | 0.243 |
| 7 | K ($\alpha$) X-ray | 0.70 | 0.023 |
| 8 | K ($\beta$) X-ray | 0.14 | 0.026 |
| 9 | L-X-ray | 0.11 | 0.003 |
| 10 | KLL Auger electron | 0.11 | 0.019 |
| 11 | KLX Auger electron | 0.04 | 0.022 |
| 12 | LMM Auger electron | 0.99 | 0.002 |

**Table A.6.**  Radiations Emitted in the Decay of $^{67}$Ga ($\Gamma = 0 \cdot 80$ R $\cdot$ cm$^2$/mCi $\cdot$ h); T$_{\frac{1}{2}}$ = 78.1 h

| Number | Radiation (i) | Frequency of Emission (n$_i$) | Mean Energy (MeV) (E$_i$) |
|--------|---------------|-------------------------------|---------------------------|
| 1 | $\gamma_1$ | 0.033 | 0.091 |
| 2 | $\gamma_2$ | 0.38 | 0.093 |
| 3 | K conversion electron | 0.28 | 0.084 |
| 4 | L conversion electron | 0.038 | 0.092 |
| 5 | M conversion electron | 0.013 | 0.093 |
| 6 | $\gamma_3$ | 0.24 | 0.185 |
| 7 | $\gamma_4$ | 0.025 | 0.209 |
| 8 | $\gamma_5$ | 0.16 | 0.300 |
| 9 | $\gamma_6$ | 0.04 | 0.394 |
| 10 | K-X-ray | 0.46 | 0.009 |
| 11 | Auger electron | 0.66 | 0.008 |

# CGS and SI Units

| Quantity | CGS Units | MKS or SI Units | Conversion Factors[a] (CGS→MKS) |
|---|---|---|---|
| Length | centimeter (cm) | meter (m) | 0.01 |
| Mass | gram (g) | kilogram (kg) | 0.001 |
| Time | second (s) | second (s) | 1 |
| Energy | erg | Joule (J) | $10^{-7}$ |
| Radioactivity | Curie (Ci) | Becquerel (Bq) | $3.7 \times 10^{10}$ |
| Exposure | Roentgen (R) | Coulomb/kilogram (C/kg) | $2.58 \times 10^{-4}$ |
| Absorbed dose | rad | Gray (Gy) | 0.01 |
| Dose equivalent | rem | Sievert (Sv) | 0.01 |
| Equivalent dose | rem | Sievert (Sv) | 0.01 |
| Effective dose | rem | Sievert (Sv) | 0.01 |
| Effective dose equivalent | rem | Sievert (Sv) | 0.01 |

[a]To obtain results in the MKS system, multiply the CGS values by the conversion factor. To obtain results in the CGS system, divide the MKS values by the conversion factor.

# Exponential Table

| x | $e^{-x}$ | x | $e^{-x}$ | x | $e^{-x}$ |
|---|---|---|---|---|---|
| 0.00 | 1.00 | 0.22 | 0.80 | 0.60 | 0.55 |
| 0.01 | 0.99 | 0.24 | 0.79 | 0.65 | 0.52 |
| 0.02 | 0.98 | 0.26 | 0.77 | 0.693 | 0.50[a] |
| 0.03 | 0.97 | 0.28 | 0.76 | 0.75 | 0.47 |
| 0.04 | 0.96 | 0.30 | 0.74 | 0.80 | 0.45 |
| 0.05 | 0.95 | 0.32 | 0.72 | 0.85 | 0.42 |
| 0.06 | 0.94 | 0.34 | 0.71 | 0.90 | 0.41 |
| 0.07 | 0.93 | 0.36 | 0.70 | 1.00 | 0.37 |
| 0.08 | 0.92 | 0.38 | 0.68 | 1.50 | 0.22 |
| 0.09 | 0.91 | 0.40 | 0.67 | 2.00 | 0.13 |
| 0.10 | 0.90 | 0.42 | 0.66 | 2.50 | 0.08 |
| 0.12 | 0.89 | 0.44 | 0.64 | 3.00 | 0.05 |
| 0.14 | 0.87 | 0.46 | 0.63 | 3.50 | 0.03 |
| 0.16 | 0.85 | 0.48 | 0.62 | 4.00 | 0.02 |
| 0.18 | 0.84 | 0.50 | 0.61 | 4.50 | 0.01 |
| 0.20 | 0.82 | 0.55 | 0.58 | 5.00 | 0.007 |

[a]See Chapter 3, p. 24.

# D

## Radionuclides of Interest in Nuclear Medicine

| Radionuclide | Method of Production | Mode of Decay | Principal Photons (keV)$^a$ | Half-Life |
|---|---|---|---|---|
| | *Used clinically, mainly for diagnosis or as a generator* | | | |
| $^{99}$Mo | Fission and reactor | $\beta^-$ | 740(14), 780(5) | 67 h |
| $^{99m}$Tc | Generator | IT | 140(88) | 6 h |
| $^{81}$Rb | Cyclotron | EC, $\beta^+$ | 511(54) | 4.6 h |
| $^{81m}$Kr | Generator | IT | 190(67) | 13 s |
| | *Used clinically, mainly for diagnosis—no generator* | | | |
| $^{51}$Cr | Reactor | EC | 320 (100) | 27.8 days |
| $^{67}$Ga | Cyclotron | EC | 93(40), 184(24), 296(22), 388(7) | 78 h |
| $^{111}$In | Cyclotron | EC | 173(89), 247(94) | 67 h |
| $^{123}$I | Cyclotron | EC | 159(83) | 13 h |
| $^{125}$I | Reactor | EC | 27–31(142) | 60 days |
| $^{133}$Xe | Reactor | $\beta^-$ | 80(37) | 5.3 days |
| $^{201}$TI | Cyclotron | EC | 69–80(94), 167(10) | 73.1 h |
| | *Used clinically, mainly for diagnosis—PET* | | | |
| $^{11}$C | Cyclotron | $\beta^+$ | 511 (200) | 20.4 min |
| $^{13}$N | Cyclotron | $\beta^+$ | 511 (200) | 10 min |
| $^{15}$O | Cyclotron | $\beta^+$ | 511 (200) | 2 min |
| $^{18}$F | Cyclotron | $\beta^+$, EC | 511 (194) | 110 min |
| $^{68}$Ga | Generator | $\beta^+$, EC | 511 (176) | 68 min |
| | *Used clinically mainly for therapy* | | | |
| $^{32}$P | Reactor | $\beta^-$ | None | 14.3 days |
| $^{89}$Sr | Reactor | $\beta^-$ | None | 52 days |
| $^{131}$I | Fission | $\beta^-$ | 364(82) | 8.1 days |
| | *Used as standard source* | | | |
| $^{57}$Co | Cyclotron | **EC** | 122 (86) | 270 days |
| $^{137}$Cs | Fission | $\beta^-$ | 660 (100) | 30 years |

IT = isomeric transition; EC = electron capture.
$^a$Values in parentheses are % emission frequency.

# Organ Masses of a Standard Man

| Organ | Mass (g) |
| --- | --- |
| Total body | 70,000 |
| Bladder | 509 |
| Kidneys (both) | 288 |
| Liver | 1833 |
| Lungs | 999 |
| Ovaries | 8.8 |
| Pancreas | 61 |
| Skeleton with marrow | 10,091 |
| Spleen | 176 |
| Stomach | 402 |
| Testicles | 38 |
| Thyroid | 20 |

## Chapter 1

1. (a) 27.98; (b) 72.14 keV.
2. (a) 2.15, 7.11, and 59.40;
   (b) 1.19, 5.19, and 15.86 keV.
3. H: 0.014, C: 0.07, and I: 5.19 keV.
4. Incoming electron imparts 50 keV to the K-shell electron, of which 33.17 is taken up by the binding energy thus leaving 16.83 keV as kinetic energy for the electron released from the K-shell.
5. For P 17.85 or 19.81 keV, for I 14.81 keV and for Pb 4.14 keV. In P both K or L shell electrons may be emitted. In I and Pb, only L shell electron will be emitted.
6. 0.124, 0.0124, and 0.00124 nm.
7. 10% of 140 keV = 14 keV = 14,000 eV, number of 5 eV light photons emitted = 14,000/5 = 2800.
8. No, not enough energy in a single photon.
9. Energy of Auger electron = x-ray energy − 2 × BE of L shell electron. Therefore, the answers are 19.62, 18.30, and 12.38, respectively.
10. 511 keV and $\gamma$-ray.
11. 2 (exact number is 2.52, one cannot create a fraction of an electron).

## Chapter 2

1. Isotopes: $^{3}_{2}$He, $^{4}_{2}$He and $^{12}_{6}$C, $^{14}_{6}$C; Isobars: $^{3}_{1}$H, $^{3}_{2}$He and $^{12}_{6}$C, $^{12}_{7}$N; Isotones: $^{3}_{1}$H, $^{4}_{2}$He and $^{99}_{43}$Tc, $^{100}_{44}$Ru; and Isomers: $^{99}_{43}$Tc, $^{99m}_{43}$Tc.
2. (a) $\beta$ decay or isobaric transition; (b) positron emission or K capture; (c) electron emission; (d) $\alpha$ decay; and (e) $\gamma$ decay or isomeric transition.
3. 0.0062 and 0.57 MeV, respectively.
4. Excited state and not ionized (electron cancels the charge of one proton in the nucleus, and therefore the atom stays neutral).
5. Yes, there are no laws against it, although it is very rare.
6. Extra amount of energy.
7. (a) 0.021 MeV, (b) 0.172 and 0.247 MeV; (c) $\beta_2$ (0.298 MeV with 0.014 frequency), $\beta_3$ (0.452 MeV with 0.797 frequency), and $\gamma_7 + \gamma_8$ (18.5% combined emission); and (d) x-rays of 70 (78%), 81 (22%), and 10 (46%) keV.
8. $\gamma_1$, 25% and 0%, and $\gamma_2$, 25% and 100% for radionuclide A and C, respectively; 100 keV for both.
9. A, 200 keV (1 hour half-life).
10. 100.
11. 0.75 MeV.
12. 1.77 MeV.

## Chapter 3

1. (a) $2.7 \times 10^{-4}$ mCi; (b) 0.01 MBq.
2. 370 MBq.
3. (a) $10^5$; (b) $3.6 \times 10^8$.
4. (a) 131; (b) 92.5; and (c) 0.370 MBq.
5. 1.32, 1.76, 2.43, and 2.64 mL, respectively.
6. (a) 146; (b) 134; and (c) 156.2 hours.
7. 3 hours.
8. 10,000.
9. 95.
10. $\pm 180$.

11. 20.
12. (a) 5.5% and (b) 9.35%
13. 0.883 (number of 140 keV γ rays emitted per decay of $^{99m}$Tc) $\times 3.7 \times 10^7 = 3.2671 \times 10^7$.
14. $0.9 \times 10^6$.
15. $0.82 \times 10 \times 3.7 \times 10^4 = 3.034 \times 10^5$.
16. SD = 167 and %SD = 0.6%.

## Chapter 4

1. Neutrons, about 0.025 eV.
2. Protons, deuterons, and α particles, above 10 MeV.
3. Capture of neutrons in reactor-produced radionuclides causes an excess of neutrons in the nucleus. Conversion of a neutron into a proton through β decay is the most convenient process for achieving stability in these nuclides. In accelerator-produced radionuclides, protons are in excess and conversion of a proton into a neutron through $\beta^+$ and/or electron capture is favored.
4. The amount of target material, the flux of neutrons or charged particles, the reaction cross section, and the half-life of the radionuclide to be produced.
5. For the same amount of desired radioactivity, carrier-free radionuclides have the least amount of that element or chemical present. Small amount is less toxic and gives high labeling-efficiency.
6. Parent of an almost ideal radionuclide, $^{99m}$Tc, easy availability, inexpensive, little parent breakthrough, and rapid eluting method.
7. No, because of the presence of $^{99}$Tc, which technically is a radionuclide but for all practical purposes is stable (half-life is 200,000 years).
8. Large parent breakthrough increases patient radiation dose without any additional benefit. It may also interfere in imaging.
9. 0.15 μCi (5.6 kBq) of $^{99}$Mo for each mCi (37MBq) of $^{99m}$Tc.
10. 4 GBq.
11. 0.125 GBq.
12. At 12.8-hour intervals (rule is four times daughter's half-life).

## Chapter 5

1. Single γ emission with energy in 100- to 300-keV range, no particulate emission, short half-life.
2. (a) b;   (b) a; and   (c) c.
3. Method of administration, blood flow, protein binding, and extraction efficiency.
4. Hinders.
5. In such a case, the radionuclidic purity of the radionuclide will increase (improve) with time.
6. Pertechnetate and reduced technetium.
7. By reacting with a reducing agent, oxygen decreases the amount of reducing agent needed for pertechnetate reduction.
8. Common examples: $^{99m}$Tc-sulfur colloid, $^{99m}$Tc-phosphate compounds, $^{99m}$Tc-sulfur colloid, $^{201}$Tl-thallous chloride, blood proteins or red cells appropriately labeled, $^{99m}$Tc-DMSA, $^{99m}$Tc-MAA, $^{99m}$Tc-HIDA, $^{123}$Iodide, $^{99m}$Tc-sulfur colloid, $^{67}$Ga-citrate, $^{123}$I-amphetamines.
9. Too short half-lives.
10. Between 20 to 90 minutes after administration.
11. Yes, $^{68}$Ge–$^{68}$Ga is an example. There are many others.
12. Mostly particulate radiations, little if any γ- or x-rays, and a relatively long life.
13. Lack of accurate quantification of localized radioactivity and dosimetry.
14. The FDA approves the human use of radiopharmaceuticals, and the NRC regulates the use of these radiopharmaceuticals from a general radiation safety perspective.
15. 15 days.

## Chapter 6

1. 1-MeV α particle, 1-MeV electron, 50-keV x-ray, 400-keV γ-ray, and 1-MeV x-ray.
2. Mass, energy, and charge of the particle and the density of the interacting medium.
3. (a) Density of the medium; (b) no.
4. Two γ rays of 511 keV and traveling in opposite directions.
5. 5.8, 0.87, and 0.15 cm, respectively.
6. 22% and 55%, respectively.
7. 38%.
8. 0.1% and 71%, respectively.

9. When γ energy is close to the binding energy of electrons in the inner shells of the interacting atoms.
10. 71,167 and 200 keV, respectively.
11. $\mu$(linear) of water = $\mu$(linear) of ice/density of ice = $\mu$(linear) of steam/density of steam.
12. 67% transmitted and 33% interactions.
13. Of the 33% interactions, 26.4% photoelectric and 6.6% Compton.
14. 1.02 MeV.
15. It has a strong effect on the response of a biological system when it interacts with radiation.

## Chapter 7

1. 3.5 Gy, 1.2 mGy, and 50 mGy, respectively.
2. 0.076 Gy.
3. (a) 1.4 Gy and (b) 2 Gy.
4. Radiations emitted and their energies, dosage of radioactivity administered, absorbed fraction in the case of γ-rays, and the effective half-life.
5. Biological data.
6. Same.
7. Different because the absorbed fraction will be different in the three cases.
8. Energy of γ-ray, size and shape of the target organ, and distance between the source and the target organ.
9. $\tilde{A} = 1.44 \times f \times A_0 \times T_{\frac{1}{2}}$ (eff).
10. S factor contains in it all the required physical data of a radionulide. To calculate the radiation dose, one only needs the biodistribution data (cumulative radioactivity). S factors are calculated for a standard man; therefore, these cannot be used for a specific patient who may be quite different from a standard man, as in the case of children.
11. 6 mGy.
12. (a) Yes; (b) brain, being the farthest, will receive the least amount of radiation dose.
13. Gallium citrate.

## Chapter 8

1. Linear attenuation coefficient and thickness of the sensitive material of the detector. It allows reduction of either radiation dose or imaging time.
2. Inversely. The shorter the dead time, the higher the count rate for which a detector can be used.
3. Proportional counters; however, these are not used in nuclear medicine.
4. Because the current produced by the interaction of a single radiation is too small to be detected by an ionization chamber.
5. About 60,000 counts/min.
6. (1) GM counter; (2) NaI(Tl) scintillator detector; (3) dose calibrator; and (4) Ge(Li) detector.
7. High linear attenuation coefficient for γ-ray energies used in nuclear medicine, high light output, short dead time, inexpensive, and easy availability in large sizes.
8. Better intrinsic efficiency for 511 keV γ-rays.
9. Even though the intrinsic efficiencies for 511 keV γ-rays are similar, LSO has better energy resolution and shorter dead time.
10. To select pulses in a given range.
11. Narrowing the window will decrease the observed count rate.
12. 13%, 14%, and 16%, respectively. The detector with 13% energy resolution is the best.
13. It has better sensitivity and energy resolution. In addition it does not require a bulky PM tube.

## Chapter 9

1. Either by using a large-area detector or by decreasing the distance between the source and the detector. No, it does not depend on the type of the detector. This gives the maximum geometric efficiency.
2. Decay rate and the observed count rate differ because of the overall detection efficiency. Decay rate of a sample is generally higher than the observed count rate.
3. Assuming one γ-ray emission per decay, 0.225%.
4. 2775 counts/s.
5. 0.675.
6. 1240.
7. 2400 (overall efficiency drops to 80%).
8. Yes, unless this is taken into account by some other means.
9. Because of short range of β particles.
10. 4π.

## Chapter 10

1. Unknown shape and size of radionuclidic distribution in the body makes it difficult to correct for the attenuation and scattering of γ-rays.
2. By allowing the rejection of scattered γ-rays.
3. Detector with very good energy resolution, for example, Ge (Li) detector. CZT detector is next best thing.
4. Narrowing window will decrease the scattered counts as well as the true counts. Therefore, the sensitivity will also decrease.
5. Heart, because of very heterogeneous attenuations (soft tissue, bone, and lungs). For brain and kidneys, the attenuation is more or less homogeneous.
6. Multiplying the two images pixel by pixel and then taking the square root.
7. To select a well-defined field of view. Lead is a high atomic number and high-density material and is inexpensive. Other high atomic number and high-density materials (e.g., gold) are comparatively expensive.
8. Compromise between efficiency and the uniformity of response in the thyroid gland.
9. To detect the radioactive uptake in surgical procedures called intraoperative lymphatic mapping (ILM) or sentinel lymph node biopsy.
10. These had no capability for fast dynamic studies.

## Chapter 11

1. Intrinsic spatial resolution and intrinsic efficiency.
2. Use of multiple detector-heads, size of the crystal at least as large as the organ to be imaged.
3. More light will improve the energy resolution of the scintillation camera. This will improve the intrinsic spatial resolution and the rejection of more scattered γ-rays.
4. (a) Parallel-hole; (b) Converging; (c) Diverging; and (d) Pinhole.
5. Increases the sensitivity for radionuclides that emit γ-rays with different energies. Also, it can be used to image simultaneously two radionuclides emitting γ-rays with different energies.

6. Improves the uniformity.
7. The intensity should be decreased.
8. More bits will be needed and higher speed will be desirable.
9. $9.76 \text{ mm}^2$.

## Chapter 12

1. An improvement by a factor of 2 in resolution will decrease the sensitivity by a factor of 4. Therefore, sensitivity of the new collimator will be 12,500 cpm.
2. FWHM is best suited to study the relationships with various parameters of an imaging device. Point-spread function or modulation transfer function gives most general and complete descriptions of the spatial resolution of an imaging device. Good for comparison of diverse imaging devices. Resolution phantoms, such as parallel bars, are good to monitor gross changes in spatial resolution of an imaging device and are therefore used in quality control.
3. Mainly to measure MTF of a scintillation camera.
4. Scintillation camera with MTF of 0.8.
5. 14.14, 11.18, and 10.05 mm, respectively.
6. One designed for low energy γ-rays because it will have thinner septa.
7. Because of edge packing, localization of interaction of a γ-ray in this area of the crystal is not very accurate.
8. For lesser distance, the radiation incident on the crystal will not be uniform.
9. Mis-localization.
10. (a) yearly, (b) daily, (c) weekly, (d) yearly, and (e) daily.

## Chapter 13

1. 1.5.
2. 1.45, almost no change from problem 13-1. Better to image at 3-hour postadministration than at 24 hours.
3. 10%. This is a simple calculation. It assumes that the resolution of the imaging device very good and the detectability is determined by the noise only.
4. Radiopharmaceuticals for tumor detection have higher contrast than those used for

blood flow in the brain. Higher contrast means higher detectability.

5. Large-area and multiple-head scintillation cameras have higher sensitivity that can be used to increase the detectability or to reduce the study time.

6. The contrast in nuclear medicine is much higher than that in computed tomography, but the spatial resolution in computed tomography is much better than that in nuclear medicine.

7. Resolution of the imaging device and noise.

8. Area under ROC curve.

## Chapter 14

1. In general, a 360 degree angle improves the result in SPECT, but when an organ is located near the surface (e.g., heart), a 180 degree angle is preferable. No.

2. Increase in the sensitivity. It requires more rigorous quality control.

3. Because small errors in scintillation camera response are magnified during the reconstruction process.

4. Field (volume) of view in SPECT is not cylindrical and attenuation cannot be easily corrected. However, the newer algorithms are capable to correct for these to some extent.

5. Better sensitivity and rejection of scattered radiation in the patient.

6. The shorter the resolving time, the lesser the accidental counts in the detector pair.

7. The size of the detector pair, range of positron, and the distance between the detector pair.

## Chapter 15

1. Energy deposition, energy transfer to other molecules, chemical reactions, and production and expression of the damage.

2. Dose rate, type of radiation, type and amount of irradiated tissue, presence of chemical modifiers, and biological variation.

3. Under 200 rads (2 Gy).

4. Cancer, 0.0005 excess mortality.

5. Between 3 and 15 weeks after conception.

6. Radiation weighting factor (quality factor).

7. Biological risk from the same dose to total body and individual organs is different. Tissue weighting factors make risk comparison for different types of exposure (total body versus an organ) possible.

8. The normal life span of humans is about 70 years, but many radionuclides have half-lives in thousands of years.

9. Natural background and medical procedures.

10. 26%.

11. $^{67}$Ga and $^{201}$Tl.

## Chapter 16

1. d.

2. 20 mCi.

3. Because the same amount of radioactivity of $^{18}$F gives 8.5 times the exposure given by $^{99m}$Tc.

4. 0.48 and 0.12 R, respectively.

5. 3 days minimum.

6. Ingestion.

7. As low as reasonably achievable.

8. 5 rem (50 mSv) and 0.1 rem (1 mSv).

9. No, it basically measures dose at a specific point.

10. Physical inspection, monitoring of radiation levels at 1 meter and the surface, and contamination check with a wipe test.

11. minor spill <1 mCi and major spill >1 mCi.

1. Cherry SR, Sorenson JA, Phelps ME. *Physics in Nuclear Medicine*, 3rd ed. Philadelphia: W. B. Saunders; 2003.

2. Shapiro J. *Radiation Protection—A Guide for Scientists and Physicians*. Cambridge, MA: Harvard University Press; 2002.

3. Hall, EJ, Giaccia, AJ. *Radiobiology for the Radiologist*, 6th ed. Philadelphia: Lippincott Williams and Williams; 2006.

# Index